P9-CSA-116

Health Information Management Case Studies

Dianna M. Foley, RHIA, CCS, CHPS

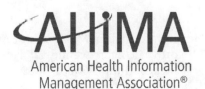

AHIMA
American Health Information
Management Association®

Copyright ©2016 by the American Health Information Management Association. All rights reserved. Except as permitted under the Copyright Act of 1976, no part of this publication may be reproduced, stored in a retrieval system, or transmitted, in any form or by any means, electronic, photocopying, recording, or otherwise, without the prior written permission of the AHIMA, 233 North Michigan Avenue, 21st Floor, Chicago, Illinois, 60601-5809 (https://secure.ahima.org/publications/reprint/index.aspx).

ISBN: 978-1-58426-458-3
AHIMA Product No.: AB125115

AHIMA Staff:
Chelsea Brotherton, MA, Assistant Editor
Katherine M. Greenock, MS, Production Development Editor
Pamela Woolf, Director of Publications

Limit of Liability/Disclaimer of Warranty: This book is sold, as is, without warranty of any kind, either express or implied. While every precaution has been taken in the preparation of this book, the publisher and author assume no responsibility for errors or omissions. Neither is any liability assumed for damages resulting from the use of the information or instructions contained herein. It is further stated that the publisher and author are not responsible for any damage or loss to your data or your equipment that results directly or indirectly from your use of this book.

The websites listed in this book were current and valid as of the date of publication. However, webpage addresses and the information on them may change at any time. The user is encouraged to perform his or her own general web searches to locate any site addresses listed here that are no longer valid.

CPT® is a registered trademark of the American Medical Association. All other copyrights and trademarks mentioned in this book are the possession of their respective owners. AHIMA makes no claim of ownership by mentioning products that contain such marks.

For more information, including updates, about AHIMA Press publications, visit http://www.ahima.org/publications/updates.aspx

American Health Information Management Association
233 North Michigan Avenue, 21st Floor
Chicago, Illinois 60601-5809
ahima.org

TABLE OF CONTENTS

ABOUT THE AUTHOR

Dianna Foley, RHIA, CHPS, CCS, has been an HIM professional for 20 years, holding jobs as coder, department supervisor, department director, and now as a coding consultant. She earned her bachelor's degree from the University of Cincinnati subsequently achieving her RHIA, CHPS, and CCS certifications. Ms. Foley recently served as the program director for medical coding and HIT at Eastern Gateway Community College. She is an AHIMA-approved ICD-10-CM/PCS trainer and has been part of OHIMA's coding roundtable committee, facilitating roundtables held at the OHIMA annual meeting. She has been a presenter at several regional Ohio meetings, the OHIMA annual meeting, and an OHIMA-sponsored webinar. She is a second-year OHIMA board member working as a project leader under the academics endeavors and leadership strategy. Ms. Foley mentors new AHIMA members and also provides monthly educational lectures to coders and clinical documentation specialists. Ms. Foley has also served on AHIMA's item writing committee and the RHIT exam development committee.

ACKNOWLEDGMENTS

AHIMA Press would like to thank LisaRae Roper MS, MHA, CCS-P, CPC-I for her technical review of this textbook.

ONLINE RESOURCES

For Instructors

AHIMA provides supplementary materials for educators who use this book in their classes. Materials include an answer key, curriculum maps, and discussion questions. Visit **http://www.ahimapress.org/Foley4583** and click the link to download the files. Please do not enter the scratch-off code from the interior front cover, as this will invalidate your access to the instructor materials. If you have any questions regarding the instructor materials, contact AHIMA Customer Relations at (800) 335-5535 or submit a customer support request at https://secure.ahima.org/contact/contact.aspx.

ICON KEY

These icons appear throughout the book to indicate the Bloom's Taxonomy level of each case and the tasks within. This key can also be found on the chapter opener.

 Bloom's Taxonomy Level 1: Remember

 Bloom's Taxonomy Level 2: Understand

 Bloom's Taxonomy Level 3: Apply

 Bloom's Taxonomy Level 4: Analyze

 Bloom's Taxonomy Level 5: Evaluate

 Bloom's Taxonomy Level 6: Create

The subdomains from the associate level curriculum will be presented in gray text in the print book and red text in the online instructor key. The subdomains from the baccalaureate level curriculum will be presented in blue text in both the print book and the online instructor key.

CHAPTER 1

Domain I: Data Content, Structure, and Standards

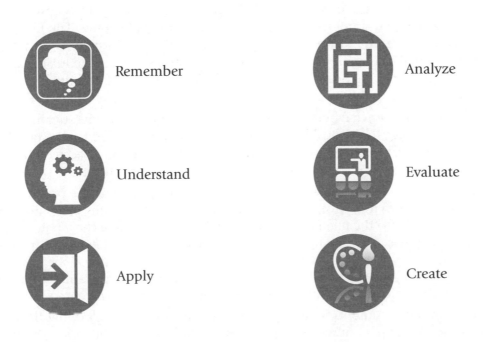

Remember

Analyze

Understand

Evaluate

Apply

Create

Classification Systems

1.0

Taxonomies, nomenclatures, and terminologies

Subdomain I.A.1
Apply diagnosis or procedure codes according to current guidelines

Subdomain I.A.2
Identify the functions and relationships between healthcare classification systems.

Select the appropriate healthcare data set that should be used in each scenario.

- A 42-year-old male comes to the emergency room with chest pain which has been occurring more frequently after meals in the last week. Today, the chest pressure was intense and did not ease so the patient came to the hospital. The ER doctor runs cardiac enzymes, troponin level, and has an EKG performed, all of which return normal. The patient is diagnosed with gastroesophageal reflux disease, given a prescription for medication, and told to follow up with his family doctor in a week.

- The Human Resource Director of Pinewood Nursing Home is investigating a potential change to the healthcare insurance currently provided to the staff. He is comparing several different health plans to determine an overall accreditation status and their outcomes related to asthma, diabetes, and hypertension.

- Margaret is an admitting clerk at Valley View Hospital. She is in the process of collecting information from Mrs. Williams, an emergency room (ER) patient, who is being admitted to the telemetry floor after arriving with severe chest pain. Elevated cardiac enzymes and a slightly abnormal electrocardiogram (EKG) prompted the ER physician to have her admitted for further study to determine if she has had a myocardial infarction (MI). Margaret gets Mrs. William's demographic information, along with her insurance information, and enters the admission date.

- Nurse Barnes documents in the patient's electronic medical record that the expected outcome for the patient was to improve their condition and that upon discharge the patient's condition was resolved.

- Tammy is transferring to the home health division of Metzger Health Care. It is her responsibility to enter the data elements collected such as medications, ADLs, and care management into HAVEN. This information is then used for purposes of reimbursement, monitoring outcomes, and assessing quality.

Examine the following scenarios and answer the questions.

- You've been contacted by the lab department because they are reviewing lead testing data. They have the following lead tests that are performed:

Lead screening assessment	5673-9
Lead in the hair (mass/mass)	8202-4
Lead in the nail (mass/mass)	17052-2
Presence of lead in the blood	39193-8

They ran a report to determine how many screenings they had performed last quarter and feel the results were incorrect. Analyze the tests and determine the following:

1. What terminology is being used?
2. What error(s) was(were) found?
3. What corrective action should be taken?

- The classification system for cancer is based on morphology and topography.

1. What is it called?
2. Examine the following codes and provide the type of cancer and behavior signified.

   - M9821/3
   - M8042/3
   - M8081/2
   - M8140/0
   - M8010/6
   - M8140/1

- You work for a podiatrist who is working on incorporating meaningful use measures in his practice. This month you are focusing on two diabetic measures: foot exam and Hemoglobin A1c-poor control. For each of the following data elements, indicate the vocabulary(s) that will be used for reporting purposes.

  - HbA1c Laboratory Test
  - Visual exam of foot
  - Diabetes
  - Preventive Care Services, Established Office Visit, 18 and up
  - Annual Wellness Exam

- Nomenclatures undergo periodic evaluation and update. Discover some of the major changes evidenced in DSM-IV to DSM-5. Include discussion of the multi-axial change, terminology change related to mental retardation, reclassification of Asperger's syndrome, and use of codes that reflect factors that influence health status.

- The DSM has a built-in crosswalk to what other classification system(s)?
- Discover the components of a national drug code and outline below.
- Given the following NDC codes, map to the specific drug it represents and breakdown the information contained in the code for further detail.
  - 0056-0174-01

    54868-5322-1
- Supply the NDC code for the following medications.
  - Xarelto 20 mg oral 90 film-coated tablets in 1 bottle Janssen Pharmaceuticals, Inc.
  - Caduet 10 mg oral 30 film-coated tablets in 1 bottle Pfizer Laboratories

References

American Psychological Association. 2016. http://www.dsm5.org/Documents/changes%20from%20dsm-iv-tr%20to%20dsm-5.pdf

Brinda, D. 2016. Data Management. Chapter 6 in *Health Information Management Technology: An Applied Approach*, 5th ed. Sayles, N.B. and L. Gordon, eds. Chicago: AHIMA.

Giannangelo, K. 2016. Clinical Terminologies, Classifications, and Code Systems. Chapter 5 in *Health Information Management Technology: An Applied Approach*, 5th ed. Sayles, N.B. and L. Gordon, eds. Chicago: AHIMA.

LOINC. 2016. www.loinc.org

US Food and Drug Administration. 2016. http://www.fda.gov/Drugs/InformationOnDrugs/ucm142438.htm

US Food and Drug Administration. 2016. http://www.accessdata.fda.gov/scripts/cder/ndc/default.cfm

US National Library of Medicine Data Element Catalog. May 2015. http://www.nlm.nih.gov/healthit/dec/

1.1

Ambulatory surgery data collection

Subdomain I.B.2
Verify the documentation in the health record is timely, complete, and accurate

Subdomain I.D.2
Apply graphical tools for data presentations

Ambulatory surgery data collection

Northwest Ambulatory Surgery Center provides urology, endoscopy, orthopedic, otolaryngology, and ophthalmology procedures. Physicians for each service are listed below. The Center has a documentation requirement that every patient's health record must have an H&P prior to surgery. A data collection is being done to verify compliance with that requirement.

1. Determine which data elements should be included in the data collection.
2. Create a data collection checklist to be used in the chart review.

Urology – Dr. Westerly, Dr. Columbia
Endoscopy – Dr. Southcliffe, Dr. Harvard, Dr. Cornell, Dr. Penn
Ophthalmology – Dr. Easton, Dr. Northrop
Orthopedic – Dr. Yale, Dr. Princeton
Otolaryngology – Dr. Princeton

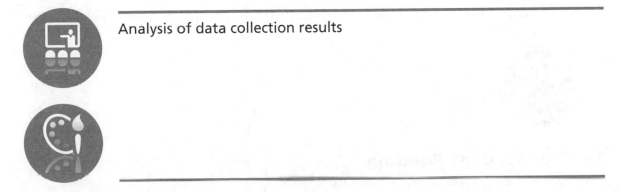

Analysis of data collection results

In June, Northwest Ambulatory Surgery Center conducted a chart audit to determine compliance with the H&P on the chart prior to surgery requirement. The results are as follows:

A total of 1220 surgeries were performed in May:
    640 endoscopies
    160 urological procedures
    240 ophthalmologic procedures
    120 otolaryngology procedures
    60 orthopedic procedures

100 total charts were reviewed:

Dr. Northrop	7 charts	6 with H&P	1 w/o H&P
Dr. Easton	22	22 with H&P	
Dr. Westerly	33	30 with H&P	3 w/o H&P
Dr. Southcliffe	28	20 with H&P	8 w/o H&P
Dr. Penn	10	10 with H&P	

Examine the results of the data collection and answer the following questions.

1. What deductions can be made about the data collection itself?

2. Propose a more meaningful data collection.

3. What deductions can be made regarding the results of the data collection?

Create a graph to depict the data collection results

1. Based only on the data collection above, create a graphic design which illustrates the missing H&Ps by service.

Further Student Reading

Shaw P.L. and Carter, D. 2015. *Quality and Performance Improvement in Healthcare: A Tool for Programmed Learning,* 6th ed. Chicago: AHIMA.

1.2

Evaluate CAC systems

Subdomain I.A.1
Evaluate, implement, and manage electronic applications/systems for clinical classification and coding

Your organization is in the final stages of selecting a vendor for computer assisted coding. You have narrowed the choices to two vendors and will be conducting conference calls with a current client for each vendor. Formulate a list of questions that will help you assess which product to choose.

References

Reynolds, R. 2016. Health Record Content and Documentation. Chapter 4 in *Health Information Management: Concepts, Principles, and Practice*, 5th ed. Oachs, P. and A. Watters, eds. Chicago: AHIMA.

1.3

ICD mapping exercise

Subdomain I.A.3
Map terminologies, vocabularies, and classification systems

Distinguish the ICD codes below, identifying them as ICD-9-CM or ICD-10-CM or ICD-10-PCS and then perform a mapping to its counterpart in the other classification. Provide an explanation for the mapped code assignment.

Example: Chronic kidney disease in ICD-9 585.9 maps to N18.3 ICD-10 code—this is a one-to-one match

Example: Closed fractured shaft of clavicle in ICD-9 810.02 maps to S42.021(A, D, G, K, P, or S)—this is a one-to-many match

1. T50.0x6A
2. 86.59
3. E11.311
4. 91.44
5. 789.63

References

Centers for Medicare and Medicaid Services. 2015. General Equivalence Mappings Frequently Asked Questions. https://www.cms.gov/medicare/coding/icd10/downloads/gems-crosswalksbasicfaq.pdf

1.4

Coding audit

Subdomain I.A.2
Evaluate the accuracy of diagnostic and procedure coding

Subdomain I.A.4
Evaluate the accuracy of diagnostic and procedural coding

As coding supervisor you are auditing the coding accuracy of two outpatient coders on the following orthopedic charts. You are auditing ICD-10-CM diagnoses and CPT procedures.

1. First, create an audit checklist. Decide what data elements are relevant to collect and include them in the checklist.
2. Perform the audit of the following 10 scenarios.
3. Create three different meaningful data display of the results.
4. Formulate an educational plan to address any inaccuracies found.

Coders will need to focus on four main areas:

Op Report 1. Coder DEF
Acct. # 0632175   DOS: 2/05/16
Pt. Name: Mr. John Jones   Physician: Dr. M. Patrick
PREOPERATIVE DIAGNOSIS:
Left knee medial meniscal tear

POSTOPERATIVE DIAGNOSIS:
Posterior horn tear around medial meniscus

NAME OF OPERATION:
Left knee arthroscopy with partial medial meniscectomy.

ANESTHESIA: General

PROCEDURE: Patient arrived in OR and was prepped and draped in the normal method for knee surgery. Tourniquet applied and a stab incision made for the anterolateral portal. The arthroscope was then introduced via the trocar.

Examination of the suprapatellar pouch was performed first with slight chondromalacia found and debrided. I moved to the medial compartment where I found a posterior horn medial meniscus tear which I debrided back to a stable rim. Lateral compartment was examined and found to be in good shape with no abnormalities.

I removed the scope and repaired the incision sites with 4-0 nylon suture. Marcaine 0.5 percent injected into the knee for pain relief and then the patient was taken to the recovery room in stable condition.

Op report 2. Coder DEF
Acct. # 0648461   DOS: 2/15/16
Pt. Name: Mrs. Martha Mason   Physician: Dr. J. Harris
PREOPERATIVE DIAGNOSIS:
Meniscal tears (medial and lateral)

POSTOPERATIVE DIAGNOSIS:
Complex lateral and complex medial meniscus tears.
Patellar chondromalacia

SURGERY TO BE PERFORMED:
Lateral and medial meniscectomy.
Chondroplasty.

PROCEDURE:
General anesthesia was administered once the patient was brought to the operating room.
Appropriate draping of the right knee was done and then a timeout to verify the correct
patient and procedure was performed.

Tourniquet was applied and an arthroscope introduced into the suprapatellar pouch
where a chondroplasty of the patella for the chondromalacia that was identified was
performed. I moved to the medial compartment where it was immediately evident there
was a complex medial meniscus tear. I did a meniscectomy of the complex tear and then
shifted focus to the lateral compartment. There another complex tear, this time of the lateral
meniscus, was found. I performed a lateral meniscectomy and then withdrew the scope.
Local anesthetic injection of 0.5 percent Marcaine was given to assist with pain control.
Tourniquet was removed and the patient was taken to recovery in excellent condition.

Follow up in 2 weeks or earlier if any problems arise.

Op report 3. Coder DEF
Acct. # 0634899   DOS: 2/13/16
Pt. Name: Mr. Jason Johnson   **Physician: Dr. M. Patrick**

PREOP DX:
Left knee tear medial meniscus

POSTOP DX:

1. Peripheral medial meniscal tear, left
2. Bucket-handle tear lateral meniscus, left
3. Degenerative joint disease, primary, left
4. Patellar chondromalacia, left

PROCEDURE PERFORMED:

1. Diagnostic arthroscopy, left knee.
2. Medial and lateral meniscectomy, left knee.
3. Patellar chondroplasty.

ANESTHESIA:
General.

PROCEDURE: Patient brought to the OR where general anesthesia was given. After
appropriate sterile prepping, portals were created medially and laterally and the arthroscope
introduced into the knee for a diagnostic arthroscopy. Suprapatellar pouch investigated first
where grade II chondromalacial changes were found necessitating a patellar chondroplasty.
No loose bodies were found. I moved to the medial compartment and shaved the tear to
achieve a smooth rim. The same technique was used on the lateral meniscus tear. The knee

was then irrigated and suctioned. I injected Marcaine at 0.25 percent to help control any post-operative pain. The patient went to recovery in stable condition and will be followed in the office in three weeks.

Op report 4. Coder DEF
Acct. # 0627765   DOS: 2/2/16
Pt. Name: Mr. Donald Davison   **Physician: Dr. M. Patrick**
Preoperative diagnosis:
Right knee lateral meniscus tear

Postoperative diagnosis:
Same with medial meniscus tear (both peripheral in nature)

Anesthesia:
General

PROCEDURE:
After arrival in the OR, general anesthesia was given to the patient. Sterile prep and drape was performed and the arthroscope was introduced into the patient's right knee. I examined the patellofemoral joint and found no evidence of disease. Moving to the medial compartment showed a peripheral tear in the medial meniscus which I repaired with two sutures. The same technique was then used on the peripheral tear of the lateral meniscus. Instrumentation was removed following irrigation and suctioning. The small portal sites were closed. Patient was then taken to post-anesthesia care unit (PACU) in good condition.

OP report 5. Coder DEF
Acct. # 0646923   DOS: 2/18/16
Pt. Name: Miss Shirley Shields   **Physician: Dr. J. Harris**

PREOPERATIVE DIAGNOSES:
Right ACL tear

POSTOPERATIVE DIAGNOSES:
ACL tear right knee
Posterior horn lateral meniscus tear, complete, right

PROCEDURES PERFORMED:
Diagnostic arthroscopy
Right ACL reconstruction
Repair of lateral meniscus

ANESTHESIA:
General

PROCEDURE:
The 28-year-old male arrived in the OR and general anesthetic was administered. His right knee was immobilized and a tourniquet applied. Appropriate sterile, prepping, and draping occurred and then the procedure was begun by harvesting the hamstring tendon. I created the portal sites and examined the knee compartments, noting no pathology in the medial compartment but a posterior horn lateral meniscus tear which I repaired with sutures.

After the knee was cleaned of loose debris, a tibial guide was used and tibial and femoral tunnels were drilled. A U-shaped guide was utilized to pull the harvested tendon up and then pinned. Cycling of the knee was then done with no impingement noted. Scope removed from the knee which was then irrigated and suctioned. The tourniquet was removed and immobilizer placed. Patient tolerated the procedure well and went to PACU in good condition. Follow-up instructions provided to spouse along with instruction to make appointment for office visit in two weeks.

Op report 6. Coder LMB
Acct. # 0631167   DOS: 02/04/16
Pt. Name: Mr. Carl Collins   Physician: Dr. J. Harris

PREOP DX:
Medial meniscus tear, right
Right osteochondral defect, distal femur

POSTOP DX:
Right medial and lateral meniscus tears complex in nature
Right osteochondral defect, distal femur
Loose bodies

OPERATIONS PERFORMED:

1. Right knee diagnostic arthroscopy, with complex medial and lateral meniscectomies.
2. Microfracture.
3. Loose body removal.
4. Extensive debridement of knee.

ANESTHESIA:
General

OPERATION: Patient arrived in OR where sterile prep and drape took place. A surgical timeout was taken prior to applying the tourniquet to the right lower extremity. The arthroscope was inserted through the portals and substantial synovitis was noted in the suprapatellar pouch which I debrided. Moving the medial compartment, loose bodies, three small ones, were identified and removed from the region. A complex tear of the medial meniscus was noted as we moved to the medial compartment. I shaved the meniscus and moved to the lateral compartment where an identical procedure was completed on the lateral meniscus. It was also evident that distal femoral area would benefit from a microfracture procedure that I performed. The knee was irrigated then and suctioned clean. Marcaine injected. The tourniquet was removed and sterile dressings applied to the knee. The patient was taken to recovery and given instructions for follow up in two weeks.

Op report 7. Coder LMB
Acct. # 0631832   DOS: 02/11/16
Pt. Name: Mr. Kevin Kendrickson   Physician: Dr. J. Harris

PREOPERATIVE DIAGNOSIS:
ACL tear, left

POSTOPERATIVE DIAGNOSES:
ACL tear, left

OPERATION PERFORMED:
ACL repair with arthroscopy, left

ANESTHESIA:
General

DESCRIPTION OF OPERATION: Patient was transported to the OR. Antibiotics were given pre-operatively. A tourniquet was placed and the patient was then prepped and draped in the normal manner. I began by dissecting hamstring tendons to use in the reconstruction. Once that was accomplished, I created a port site and inserted the arthroscope performing a diagnostic arthroscopy. All three compartments were examined and no pathology found except for the ACL tear. Initially, I debrided the ACL with a shaver, and using a bur created a notchplasty. Then I used the tibial guide to make a tunnel, after which I pulled the graft back through the tunnel. I t was secured with pins and tested for impingement, none found. The graft was secured distally and then the knee was irrigated and suctioned. Post operative pain was mitigated with injection of Marcaine. Instrumentation was removed and the small incision sites were closed by suture. Dressings applied and the patient went to recovery in stable condition.

Op Report 8. Coder LMB

Acct. # 0641919   **DOS: 02/16/16**
Pt. Name: Miss Rita Reynolds   **Physician: Dr. M. Patrick**

PREOP DX:
Lateral meniscus tear, right

POSTOP DX:
Lateral meniscus tear, right

OPERATION:
Arthroscopy right knee, lateral repair

ANESTHESIA:
General

DESCRIPTION OF OPERATION: Patient arrived in the OR, and was then prepped and draped in sterile manner. Preoperative IV antibiotics were administered and general anesthesia given. Surgical timeout taken. Portal established and suprapatellar pouch examined and found to be clean. Medial compartment was examined next with no disease found. The lateral compartment was found to contain a tear which was suture-repaired. Instrumentation was removed; knee irrigated and suctioned. Marcaine injected for postoperative pain management. Portal sites closed and tourniquet removed. Patient taken to PACU in good condition.

OP Report 9. Coder LMB

Acct. # 0627345   **DOS: 02/01/16**
Pt. Name: Mr. Mark Monroe   **Physician: Dr. J. Harris**

PREOPERATIVE DIAGNOSIS:
Left ACL tear

POSTOPERATIVE DIAGNOSES:
Left ACL tear
Left, medial meniscus tear, bucket-handle variety

OPERATIONS:
Left, diagnostic arthroscopy
Left, ACL repair
Left, medial meniscus repair

DESCRIPTION OF OPERATION: After the patient's arrival in the OR, a surgical timeout was taken, followed by prep and drape of knee, and administration of general anesthesia. Hamstring tendons were harvested, port sites opened, and then scope inserted. The suprapatellar pouch had no pathology on examination. Medial compartment had a bucket-handle tear which was repairable with sutures. The lateral compartment exhibited no disease processes, so I began the ACL repair performing a notchplasty. A guide was used and followed by tibial tunnel reaming. Guidewire affixed to the graft and pulled back through the tunnel, pinning it in place. I pinned the graft distally after no impingement was found through cycling. The procedure was terminated. Instruments were removed, and irrigation and suctioning done. Postoperative pain was mitigated with Marcaine injection. Sterile dressings were wrapped around the knee and then we released the tourniquet. I sent the patient to the recovery room in excellent condition.

OP Report 10. Coder LMB
Acct. # 0631864   DOS: 02/11/16
Pt. Name: Mrs. Leona Leonard   Physician: Dr. J. Harris

PREOP DX:
Right knee pain.

POSTOP DX:
Tears medial and lateral meniscus

OPERATIONS PERFORMED:
Meniscectomy, medial and lateral

ANESTHESIA: General.

DESCRIPTION OF OPERATION: Patient arrived in OR and given IV antibiotics pre-operatively. Sterile prepping and draping was done. A tourniquet was applied to the patient's leg and the procedure was begun. Portal sites were created and the scope inserted. The suprapatellar pouch showed no evidence of pathology. The medial compartment exhibited a complex tear of the meniscus which had to be shaved. I discovered a lateral meniscus tear upon moving to examination of that compartment. Again, I shaved the meniscus. With no other pathology found, I irrigated and suctioned the knee, and then removed the instruments. The small portal sites were closed with sutures and Marcaine injected for pain relief. The patient went to recovery in good condition.

Acct. #	Pt. Name	DOS	Physician	ICD-1D DX codes (assigned)	ICD-1D code errors	ICD-1D correction	CFT codes (assigned)	CFT code errors	CFT code correction
0632175	John Jones	2/5/2016	M. Patrick	583.242A			27332-LT	open vs. arthroscopic	29881-LT
0648461	Martha Mason	2/15/2016	J. Harris	538.231A 583.271A M22.41			29880-RT 29877-RT	chondroplasty (29877) not separately coded when performed with other knee px	29880-RT
0634899	Jason Johnson	2/13/2016	M. Patrick	583.222A 583.252A M22.41 M17.12			29870-LT 29880-LT 29877-LT	diagnostic arthroscopy (29870) not coded when any surgical knee px performed; chondroplasty (29877) not coded separately when performed with other knee px	29880-LT
0627765	Donald Davison	2/2/2016	M. Patrick	583.221A 582.261A			29883-RT		
0646823	Shirley Shields	2/18/2016	J. Harris	583.511A 583.281A			29870-RT 29888-RT 29882-RT	diagnostic arthroscopy (29870) not coded when any surgical knee px performed	29888RT 29882-RT
0631167	Carl Collins	2/4/2016	J. Harris	583.271A 583.231A M21.851 M32.41			29870-RT 29880-RT 29879-RT 29874-RT	diagnostic arthroscopy (29870) not coded when any surgical knee px performed; loose body removal (29874) not coded when performed in same compartment as other knee px	29880-RT 29879-RT
0631832	Kevin Kendrickson	2/11/2016	J. Harris	583.511A	583.512A	left vs. right	27407-LT	open vs. arthroscopic	29888-LT
0641919	Rita Reynolds	2/16/2016	M. Patrick	583.281A			27403-RT	open vs. arthroscopic	29882-RT
0627435	Mark Monroe	2/1/2016	J. Harris	583.511A 583.212A	583.512A	left vs. right	29870-LT 29888-LT 29881-LT	diagnostic arthroscopy (29870) not coded when any surgical knee px performed; meniscus repair not meniscectomy	29888-LT 29882-LT
0631864	Leona Leonard	2/11/2016	J. Harris	583.231A 583.281A			27333-RT	open vs. arthroscopic	29880-RT

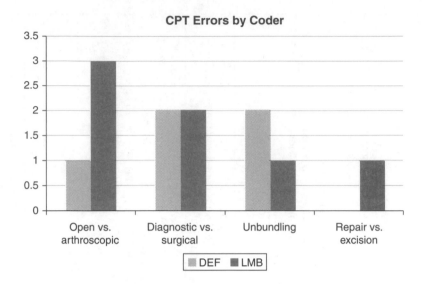

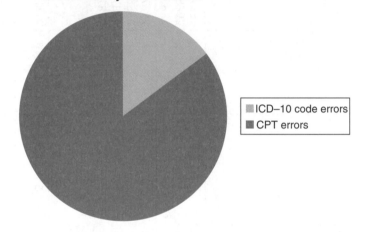

CPT Errors by Type

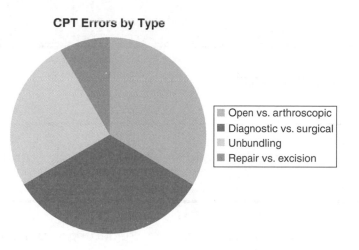

Further Student Reading

Edgerton, C.G. 2016. Healthcare Statistics. Chapter 16 in *Health Information Management: Concepts, Principles, and Practice*, 5th ed. Oachs, P. and A. Watters, eds. Chicago: AHIMA.

Malmgren, C. and C. J. Solberg. 2016. Reimbursement Methodologies. Chapter 8 in *Health Information Management: Concepts, Principles, and Practice*, 5th ed. Oachs, P. and A. Watters, eds. Chicago: AHIMA.

1.5

Trauma registry audit

Subdomain I.E.2
Validate the reliability and accuracy of secondary data sources

As HIM supervisor at Valley View Hospital, you are conducting a trauma registry audit. You are auditing only the following data elements:

- Inclusion criteria
- Sex
- Work related
- Emergency Department discharge disposition
- Protective devices
- Alcohol use indicator

1. One of the records you have chosen to audit is listed below. Use this ER report and the Ohio Trauma Registry data dictionary to compare the results and determine accuracy of the data reported.

CC: Closed head injury

HPI: A 34-year-old male was delivering the mail when he lost control of his car on ice and hit a tree. The man said that he was fully conscious throughout the event; however, the EMTs tell a different story. They indicate that he was unconscious for at least two minutes after their arrival on the scene as they worked to remove him from the three-point restraints. The airbag did not deploy despite the cracked windshield. The young man remained stable during transport, although there were complaints of a severe right-sided temporal headache accompanied by some blurred vision.

PMH: Hypertension.
ROS: All systems reviewed and negative unless otherwise noted in the physical exam. Patient has no known allergies.

MEDICATIONS: Lisinopril.

PHYSICAL EXAMINATION:
VITALS: Blood pressure 142/88, pulse 95, respirations 22, temperature 97.9°.
HEENT: Contusion over right temporal area.
NECK: Tender on the right side.
CHEST: Tender on the right.
LUNGS: Clear.
ABDOMEN: Flat, nontender.
BACK: Tender in the c-spine area.
PELVIS: Normal.
EXTREMITIES: Contusion right thigh.
RECTAL: Not performed.

NEUROLOGIC: Patient intact.
LABORATORY DATA: Hematocrits 42.9, and 41.7. WBC 8.5. Ethanol: None. Urinalysis: normal. PT 13.0, PTT 31. Chemistry normal.

X-rays: C-spine, LS- spine, and pelvis x-rays completed and all returned as normal. X-ray of chest shows 1 broken rib on the right. Right distal clavicle fracture noted.

ASSESSMENT:
1. Concussion.
2. Rib fracture
3. Fracture right clavicle.

PLAN: Admit the patient to the ortho service for treatment of fractures and have trauma follow for the concussion.

Data Element	Reported Value	Audit finding
Inclusion criteria	Yes	
Sex	1	
Work related	2	
ED discharge disposition	1	
Protective devices	2	
Alcohol use indicator	1	

References

Ohio Trauma Registry. 2014. Trauma Acute Care Registry Data Dictionary. http://www.publicsafety.ohio.gov/links/ems_otr_data_dictionary14.pdf

Sharp, M. 2016. Data Management. Chapter 6 in *Health Information Management: Concepts, Principles, and Practice*, 5th ed. Oachs, P. and A. Watters, eds. Chicago: AHIMA.

1.6

Secondary data

Subdomain I.E.1
Identify and use secondary data sources

Specialized data collection systems, like those for cancer or trauma registries, may utilize edits to ensure data validity. Consider that you are training to become a trauma register in Mayfield, Ohio.

1. Determine what validation checks will be available to you as you complete your data collection entries for the mandatory state trauma reporting on-line.
2. Identify the source document for your responses.

References

Ohio Trauma Registry. 2014. Web Entry Training Manual. http://www.publicsafety.ohio.gov/links/EMS-Acute-Care-Training-Manual.pdf

Sharp, M. 2016. Data Management. Chapter 6 in *Health Information Management: Concepts, Principles, and Practice*, 5th ed. Oachs, P. and A. Watters, eds. Chicago: AHIMA.

1.7

Videotaping policy

Subdomain I.B.3
Interpret health information standards

Pine Valley Community Hospital, a critical access hospital, is considering participation in an educational project for medical students. Under the proposal, they will videotape the events of the emergency department 24/7 for one week. In your role as HIM director, you have been asked to identify and interpret any Joint Commission standards that might impact such an agreement and report back to Administration.

1. Assess and interpret any Joint Commission information on the topic of videotaping.
2. Formulate a policy that would ensure compliance with the intent of the standard.

References

LeBlanc, M.M. 2016. Human Resources Management. Chapter 23 in *Health Information Management: Concepts, Principles, and Practice*, 5th ed. Chicago: AHIMA.

The Joint Commission. 2016. Videotaping in a critical access hospital. *Standards Interpretation*.

https://www.jointcommission.org/standards_information/jcfaqdetails.aspx?StandardsFAQId=834&StandardsFAQChapterId=31&ProgramId=0&ChapterId=0&IsFeatured=False&IsNew=False&Keyword=videotaping

https://www.jointcommission.org/standards_information/jcfaqdetails.aspx?StandardsFAQId=833&StandardsFAQChapterId=60&ProgramId=0&ChapterId=0&IsFeatured=False&IsNew=False&Keyword=videotaping

https://www.jointcommission.org/standards_information/jcfaqdetails.aspx?StandardsFAQId=832&StandardsFAQChapterId=31&ProgramId=0&ChapterId=0&IsFeatured=False&IsNew=False&Keyword=videotaping

https://www.jointcommission.org/standards_information/jcfaqdetails.aspx?StandardsFAQId=835&StandardsFAQChapterId=31&ProgramId=0&ChapterId=0&IsFeatured=False&IsNew=False&Keyword=videotaping

1.8

Emergency department documentation

Subdomain 1.B.2
Verify the documentation in the health record is timely, complete, and accurate

Subdomain I.B.1
Verify the documentation in the health record supports the diagnosis and reflects the patient's progress, clinical findings, and discharge status

Subdomain I.B.2
Compile organization-wide health record documentation guidelines

Subdomain 1.D.1
Analyze information needs of customers across the healthcare continuum

The Emergency Department Chair has asked for an audit of ED records in preparation for an upcoming Joint Commission survey. Your staff conducted the audit against the Joint Commission standard that addresses ED documentation. The results were very poor, with no consistency in documenting the required components. You check the medical staff by-laws and realize that there are no specifics related to ED documentation.

1. Determine the Joint Commission documentation requirements for Emergency Department reports. List them here.

2. Audit the five representative ED cases below to determine the major areas in need of documentation improvement. As HIM director, present your results in a short memo to the ED Department Chair, Dr. Wilkerson.

3. Create a new section for the medical staff by-laws that incorporates ED documentation requirements. Include this in the memo to the Chief of the ED for his approval before it continues through the formal process for inclusion into the by-laws.

4. The timing for this coincides with the transition of ED documentation into an electronic format. You propose to utilize the electronic record to facilitate the appropriate data collection. Create a screen design that encompasses the required ED documentation data elements.

<u>ER Report 1:</u>

HPI: Four year old female arrived after fall on trampoline. Patient fell and landed on her right elbow. Complaining of pain. Tearful.

PMH: Child currently on antibiotics for an acute otitis media infection of her left ear. Tympanum still inflamed.

IMMUNIZATIONS: Up-to-date.

ALLERGIES: None known.

PHYSICAL EXAMINATION:

VITAL SIGNS: Temperature 36.8 Celsius, pulse 95, respirations 22, blood pressure 114/77, weight 18 kilograms.
GENERAL: Alert, minimal distress upon palpation of elbow.
SKIN: Negative
HEENT: Head: Normal. Eyes: PERRL. Nose and throat normal. Ears: Left tympanum inflamed.
NECK: Supple, no lymphadenopathy, no masses.
LUNGS: Clear bilaterally.
HEART: Normal S1, S2. Regular rate.
ABDOMEN: Soft, non-tender. Bowel sounds are present.
EXTREMITIES: Warm. Right elbow tender to palpation.

NEUROLOGICAL: Alert.

X-RAY: Right elbow shows supracondylar fracture.

EMERGENCY ROOM COURSE: Patient had an x-ray of the right upper extremity which showed a displaced supracondylar fracture. A long arm splint was applied. No lab work was done.

DX: Displaced, right supracondylar fracture.

DISPOSITION: Home with parents.

<u>ER Report 2:</u>

CHIEF COMPLAINT: Ankle pain.

HISTORY OF PRESENT ILLNESS: A 67-year-old female fell off a curb while crossing the street. Complains of pain in left ankle and right wrist, as she landed on the wrist when she fell. No other injuries are apparent.

PMH: COPD. Hypertension. Diabetes. Smoker.

PAST SURGICAL HISTORY: Appendectomy 10 years ago.

SOCIAL HISTORY: Denies alcohol.

ALLERGIES: NKDA.

MEDICATIONS: Spiriva. Lisinopril. Humulin.

ROS: Ten systems reviewed and negative unless noted above.

PHYSICAL EXAMINATION:
VITAL SIGNS: Temperature 98.7, pulse 81, respirations 19, blood pressure 130/83, and pulse oximetry 93 percent on room air.

GENERAL: No acute distress.

EXTREMITIES: Full range of motion in his right knee. Palpation of the ankle and Achilles tendon elicit no pain. Pulses are intact, with strong capillary refill. Normal sensation. There is pain on the lateral aspect of the right foot. Contusion and swelling noted as well. Dorsal foot pain present too.

X-RAY: Left ankle shows lateral malleolus fracture. Right wrist film shows an intraarticular distal radius fracture.

DX: Fractures of left ankle and right wrist as evidenced on x-rays. Contusion of lower left leg.

DISPOSITION: Splints applied on both extremities (arm and leg) and prescription given for Motrin 800mg. to be taken four times a day. Home to follow with ortho tomorrow.

ER Report 3:

CHIEF COMPLAINT: Shortness of breath brings this 72-year-old Caucasian female to the ER transported by her husband.

HPI: Patient is in ER often due to her COPD exacerbations. Today the patient experienced severe respiratory distress. Her husband states the patient was admitted two weeks ago with bronchial pneumonia and discharged last week. Patient continued to have a chronic cough after discharge and today all her symptoms worsened.

PMH: Hypertension, emphysema, and lupus.

MEDICATIONS: Dyazide, and Atrovent inhaler.

ALLERGIES: NKDA.

SOCIAL HISTORY: The patient is florist, married, with 2 children.

REVIEW OF SYSTEMS: Ten system review normal except as noted above.

PHYSICAL EXAMINATION:
VITAL SIGNS: Temperature 101.3. Pulse 91. Respirations 22. Blood pressure 136/88. Initial oxygen saturations on room air are 84.
GENERAL: Breathing is labored.
HEENT: Head is normal.
NECK: The neck is supple.
LUNGS: Auscultation of the chest reveals faint breath sounds, on the right, no obvious rales.
HEART: Sinus tachycardia.
ABDOMEN: Nontender.
Extremities: Slight pedal edema.

DIAGNOSTIC DATA: White blood count 16.5, hemoglobin 15, hematocrit 41.3, Sodium of 137, chloride 80, CO2 45, BUN 7, creatinine 0.8, glucose 192, albumin 3.4 and globulin 4.0. Urinalysis normal.

X-RAY: Early infiltrates noted on chest x-ray.

EMERGENCY ROOM COURSE: One gram of Rocephin was administered intravenously as there is evidence that pneumonia is persisting. Further medication orders included Atrovent q. 2h. and Levaquin 500 mg IV. Patient appears to have a degree of respiratory failure and possible sepsis.

FINAL DIAGNOSIS: Pneumonia.

DISCHARGE INSTRUCTIONS: Patient admitted to medical floor. Will require close observation and care.

ER Report 4:

CHIEF COMPLAINT: Abdominal pain.

HPI: This 58-year-old Caucasian complains of unrelenting right lower quadrant abdominal pain. Began in the early hours of the morning, actually awakening the patient from his sleep. Has not abated and patient decided to come to ER for evaluation.

PMH: Healthy.

REVIEW OF SYSTEMS: Nausea with one episode of emesis after arrival in ER.

SOCIAL HISTORY: Married, no children.

FAMILY HISTORY: Negative.

MEDICATIONS: None.

ALLERGIES: NKDA.

PHYSICAL EXAMINATION: VITAL SIGNS: Temperature 100.5, heart rate 95, blood pressure 125/76, respiratory rate 21. GENERAL: Patient in acute abdominal distress. HEENT: Unremarkable. NECK: Supple. LUNGS: Clear. CARDIAC: Slight tachycardia. ABDOMEN: Soft, tender at McBurney's point.

ED COURSE: Lab work done which resulted in elevated white count. Abdominal CT scan done which supported diagnosis of appendicitis.

IMPRESSION: Acute appendicitis.

ASSESSMENT AND PLAN: Admit patient and take to surgery for appendectomy. Surgeon on call notified of admission.

<u>**ER Report 5:**</u>

HPI: A 32-year-old black male arrived in the ER. He was incoherent and barely able to stand. Companion states he may have "gotten some bad drugs". Companion indicates patient did heroin 45 minutes ago and had a bad reaction, so he brought him here.

ALLERGIES: NKDA.

MEDICATIONS: Unknown.

PAST SURGICAL HISTORY: Unknown.

FAMILY HISTORY: Unknown.

SOCIAL HISTORY: Smokes, consumes 6 beers a day, uses street drugs.

PHYSICAL EXAMINATION:
VITAL SIGNS: temperature of 99.2 degrees, pulse 66, respiratory rate is 14, and blood pressure is 90/51, recheck blood pressure was 90/50.
GENERAL: Disoriented.
HEENT: Pupils dilated.
NECK: Supple.
CHEST: Clear.
HEART: Regular.
ABDOMEN: Soft.
SKIN: Color is normal.
EXTREMITIES: Laxity in all extremities.
NEUROLOGIC: Decreased reflex responses.

ER COURSE: Labs were drawn and IV fluids started. Narcan was administered and patient had good response. Patient admitted to ICU in critical condition.

IMPRESSION: Heroin overdose.

1.9

HIE data stewardship and integrity

Subdomain I.C.1
Apply policies and procedures to ensure the accuracy and integrity of health data

1. You have just been hired as the HIM director at a 465 bed hospital. In preparation for participation in a regional HIE, your predecessor had just completed a data collection on duplicate entries in the MPI. She found a 1 percent duplication rate on 21,000 registrations last month. She found that rate acceptable. You interpret the findings differently. Explain your interpretation and assess what the next steps should be.

2. The hospital listed above services a large population of immigrants. As a result, you discover that the registration staff often searches for patients in the ADT system by date of birth rather than name, as a language barrier is evident. You observed this process and realized that most of the duplicates are arising from this process as the dates of birth are not always entered correctly. Decide what other criteria the staff should search on if they do not search by name. Create a priority list of the criteria.

References

AHIMA. 2009. Managing the Integrity of Patient Identity in Health Information Exchange. *Journal of AHIMA* 80(7):62–69.

Altendorf, R.L. 2007. Establishment of a Quality Program for the Master Patient Index. Proceedings of AHIMA's 79th National Convention and Exhibit.

1.10

MPI screen design evaluation

Subdomain I.D.1
Collect and maintain health data

Subdomain I.D.1
Analyze information needs of customers across the healthcare continuum

1. Study the MPI screen design on the next page. All those entries are for the same person. Deduce from the screen how the patient could have ended up with multiple MPI entries. Then explain the type of MPI error that has occurred and the importance of correcting these errors.

2. Assume that the registration staff now enters a patient by the name of Ann K. Black and mistakenly assigns her the same medical record number (154360) as Kathryn Ann Black. Which type of MPI error is this and what issues do you perceive as a result of this error?

Search   ○ All Patients ○ Current Patients ○ My Patients ● MPI

Search by Patient Name ⬇

   Birth date
   Social Security Number
   Medical Record Number
   Admit date

Pt. Name	MR Number	Date of Birth	Social Security Number	Admit Date
Gray, Kate Ann	073251	15/12/1968	123–45–5533	07/09/2015
Gray, Karthryn Ann	021485	15/12/1968	123–45–5533	02/07/2015
Black, Kathryn Ann	154360	15/12/1968	123–45–5533	10/15/2015
Black, Kathryn Ann	159667	15/21/1968	123–45–5533	11/16/2015

References

Reynolds, R. 2016. Health Record Content and Documentation. Chapter 4 in *Health Information Management: Concepts, Principles, and Practice*, 5th ed. Oachs, P. and A. Watters, eds. Chicago: AHIMA.

1.11

Screen design evaluation

Subdomain I.D.1
Collect and maintain health data

Study the screen design below. This design was to facilitate data collection for immunizations.

1. Identify the design flaws.
2. Diagram a better layout.

Immunization Record

Patient Name		Date Vaccine given	
Gender		Address	
Vaccine given		Date of Birth	
Lot Number		Phone number	
Age		Height	
Weight		Hair color	
Eye color			

Additional consideration
High risk
First responder
Pregnant
Chronic medical condition
Health care worker

1.12

Providers/roles/documentation

Subdomain I.B.4
Differentiate the roles and responsibilities of various providers and disciplines, to support documentation requirements, throughout the continuum of healthcare.

A 50-year-old woman has been experiencing a chronic cough for the past two months. She is a two pack a day smoker and has been for the past 30 years. She sees her PCP for the cough and is given an order for a chest x-ray at the local hospital. The x-ray report states "nodule in lower lobe of right lung, worrisome for malignancy." The PCP refers her for a biopsy of the nodule at the ambulatory surgery clinic which substantiates the diagnosis of cancer in the pathology report. Two weeks later, the same physician who did the biopsy performs a right lower lobectomy. Prior to discharge after surgery, the patient develops an infection and the infectious disease specialist is asked to evaluate her and recommend the appropriate treatment course. Upon discharge, she receives care in her home for the next two weeks. Four weeks after surgery, radiation therapy is initiated, but her condition continues to deteriorate over the next few months with metastasis to the brain noted, at which point she decides to receive only palliative care.

1. Classify the providers for each stage of the patient's care noted above and outline their responsibilities.

2. Explain the documentation that each provider will be creating as part of the patient's record.

Further Student Reading

Fuller, S. 2016. The US Healthcare Delivery System. Chapter 1 in *Health Information Management: Concepts, Principles, and Practice*, 5th ed. Oachs, P. and A. Watters, eds. Chicago: AHIMA.

1.13

Health record completion

Subdomain I.B.3
Identify a complete health record according to, organizational policies, external regulations, and standards

As an HIM chart analyst, you are reviewing the chart of a patient who was admitted on 2/17 with gallstone pancreatitis. She arrived through the emergency room on Wednesday afternoon in severe abdominal pain. After lab work was performed showing an increased lipase level, she was admitted. Her family physician evaluated her the next morning and ordered an ultrasound, and repeat lab work. The ultrasound showed gallstones and the lab work indicated the lipase was coming down. He consulted a general surgeon who evaluated the patient and agreed to perform a cholecystectomy on Friday if the lipase level returned to near normal levels. Surgery was then performed on Friday morning, and after an uneventful night, the patient was discharged home on Saturday morning. On 2/25, you have the following documentation available in the EHR:

H&P	dictated 2/18	authenticated 2/18
Consultation report	dictated 2/18	authenticated 2/23
Immediate post-op note	written 2/19	authenticated 2/19
Operative report	dictated 2/20	authenticated 2/21
Discharge summary	dictated 2/22	authenticated

Lab work from all dates of stay
Nursing notes from all dates of stay
Anesthesia documentation from surgery
Physician orders from all dates of stay -all signed
Progress notes—all signed
Medication list—signed

You analyze the above information and identify that the record is not complete.

1. List the reason(s) for your determination of an incomplete record.
2. List the steps that must be taken to get the record complete in the required time frame.

1.14

MPI integrity

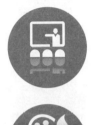

Subdomain I.C.1
Apply policies and procedures to ensure the accuracy and integrity of health data

Analyze the MPI report that follows.

1. What deductions can you arrive at as a result of the analysis?
2. Create a policy that can address one of the issues you discovered.

MRN	SSN	Last Name	First Name	Middle	DOB	Payment
47233	546-23-XXXX	Baker Sr.	Louis	Howard	5/18/1954	Medicaid
158237	315-24-XXXX	Watson	Michelle	Lee	7/22/1942	Medicare
520613	588-32-XXXX	Jones	Lynn	Tara	10/12/1963	Commercial
723341	213-22-XXXX	Harris	Ann	Marie	9/10/1952	Self
894231	588-32-XXXX	Jones	Tara	Lynn	10/21/1963	Commercial
189011	533-44-XXXX	Marshall	Tucker	B.	11/4/1961	Commercial
218220	151-24-XXXX	Leonard	Timothy	Allen	6/17/1943	Medicare
797536	213-22-XXXX	Harris-Smythe	Ann	Marie	9/10/1952	Commercial
36524	315-24-XXXX	Watson	Michelle	Lee	7/22/1924	Medicare
466100	546-23-XXXX	Baker	Louis	Howard	5/18/1945	Medicare
744183	626-26-XXXX	Baker	Louis	Howard	4/18/1965	Commercial
118231	641-58-XXXX	Thomas	Paul	Carlson	1/16/1971	Self
237352	641-58-XXXX	Carlson	Thomas	Paul	1/16/1971	Self
898233	213-22-XXXX	HarrisSmythe	Ann	Marie	9/1/1952	Commercial
789321	151-24-XXXX	Allen	Timothy	Leonard	6/17/1934	Medicare
664455	213-22-XXXX	SmytheHarris	Ann	Marie	9/1/1925	Commercial
98723	315-42-XXXX	Watson	Michelle	Lee	7/22/1924	Medicare
587532	546-23-XXXX	Baker	Howard	Louis	5/18/1954	Medicaid

References

AHIMA. 2009. Managing the Integrity of Patient Identity in Health Information Exchange. *Journal of AHIMA* 80(7):62–69.

Altendorf, R.L. Establishment of a Quality Program for the Master Patient Index. Proceedings of AHIMA's 79th National Convention and Exhibit, October 2007.

Reynolds, R. 2016. Health Record Content and Documentation. Chapter 4 in *Health Information Management: Concepts, Principles, and Practice*, 5th ed. Oachs, P. and A. Watters, eds. Chicago: AHIMA.

1.15

Patient-generated health data

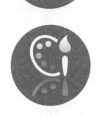

Subdomain I.E.1
Validate data from secondary sources to include in the patient's record, including personal health records

The physician you work for is concerned about incorporating patient generated health data into his EHR. Help him design a policy that not only addresses his concerns but employs sound data stewardship principles as well.

1. For the purpose of this exercise, formulate a list of the topics that should be covered.

2. Create a policy.

References

AHIMA. 2015. Including Patient-Generated Health Data in Electronic Health Records. *Journal of AHIMA* 86(2): 54–57.

LeBlanc, M.M. Human Resources Management. Chapter 23 in *Health Information Management: Concepts, Principles, and Practice*, 5th ed. Oachs, P. and A. Watters, eds. Chicago: AHIMA.

1.16

Assign MS-DRG and APC groupings

 Subdomain I.A.3
Apply diagnostic/procedural groupings

1. Identify the MS-DRG for the following scenario:

A 78-year-old female is discharged home with the following diagnoses:

> Principal Dx – acute systolic, CHF
>
> Additional Dx – Lupus (SLE), Insulin-dependent diabetes uncontrolled

MS-DRG_____

2. If the same patient also had a diagnosis of an acute exacerbation of COPD, what is the MS-DRG?

MS-DRG_____

3. If the patient in the first example also had a diagnosis of gram negative pneumonia, what is the MS-DRG?

MS-DRG_____

4. Now consider that the same patient in the first example had to have a total system, open biventricular pacemaker inserted while admitted, with leads into the right atrium and ventricle inserted percutaneously. What MS-DRG do you get now?

MS-DRG_____

5. A 72-year-old male has an ESWL performed for a right renal calculus. At the same operative session, the same physician removes a malignant lesion from his back resulting in a 3 cm. defect and performs an intermediate repair.

6. Provide the CPT codes that should be assigned for this case along with their corresponding APC.

- When this case is coded using the encoder, an edit is given. Explain the edit.
- Identify if you should bypass the edit and the step(s) that would be required.

Further Student Reading

American Medical Association. 2017. *CPT Professional Edition*. Chicago: AMA.

Centers for Disease Control and Prevention. 2016. ICD-10-CM Official Guidelines for Coding and Reporting. http://www.cdc.gov/nchs/data/icd/10cmguidelines_2016_final.pdf

Centers for Medicare and Medicaid Services. 2016. ICD-10-PCS Official Guidelines for Coding and Reporting. https://www.cms.gov/Medicare/Coding/ICD10/Downloads/2016-Official-ICD-10-PCS-Coding-Guidelines-.pdf

1.17

Evaluate MS-DRG and APC groupings

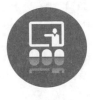

Subdomain I.A.3
Evaluate the accuracy of diagnostic/procedural groupings

Evaluate the following MS-DRG assignments for accuracy. Defend your answers and provide corrections if necessary.

1. A 12-year-old, intellectually disabled male (IQ=19) was admitted from home with high fever (105.2) and chills. He had been experiencing a hacking cough for two days prior to admission and was very lethargic. Lab work, sputum culture, rapid flu test, and chest x-ray were performed. Flu test was negative and chest x-ray indicated acute bronchitis. Due to the patient's severely weakened condition and low O_2 levels, he was admitted. After two days in the hospital where he received IV antibiotics and respiratory treatments for the acute bronchitis, he was much improved and ready for discharge back to his home.

    MS-DRG assigned 203

Admit diagnosis	R50.9
Principal diagnosis	J20.9

2. A 68-year-old female was admitted from skilled nursing with complaints of right flank pain and fever. This developed one day after her last dialysis treatment for CRF. Lab work was drawn, urinalysis performed, and a KUB showed evidence of a renal calculus. The urinalysis indicated a UTI, and the patient was admitted for definitive treatment of the streptococcal B UTI and renal calculus. IV antibiotics were administered and increased fluids flushed the stone. By the third day, the UTI seemed to be clearing so the patient was discharged back to skilled care. Her hypertension was controlled during her admission with Atenolol.

    MS-DRG assigned 694

Admit diagnosis	R10.9
Principal diagnosis	N20.0
Secondary diagnosis	N39.0
	B95.1
	I10
	N18.9

3. A 69-year-old male was admitted after arrival in the ER with extreme shortness of breath. He was found to be experiencing an acute exacerbation of his COPD and therefore admitted for treatment. On the second day of his admission, he began complaining of right knee pain. Examination indicated a pyogenic arthritis and an aspiration of the joint was done and appropriate antibiotics started. Two days later both the patient's respiratory and knee conditions were much improved and the patient was discharged home.

MS-DRG assigned 192

Admit diagnosis	R06.02
Principal diagnosis	J44.1
Secondary diagnosis	M25.561
Procedure performed	0S9C3ZZ

4. A 72-year-old black male was admitted to the hospital with four-vessel CAD. A diagnostic, left heart catheterization was done and it was determined that the patient needed an immediate bypass procedure. An open, aortocoronary bypass was done of the four vessels with heavy disease utilizing a right leg saphenous vein graft that was harvested percutaneously. The patient's pre-existing diabetes and hypertension were monitored and treated with Metformin and Lisinopril respectively. Discharged to home six days after surgery in good condition.

MS-DRG assigned 236

Admit diagnosis	I25.10
Principal diagnosis	I25.10
Secondary diagnosis	E11.9
	I10
Procedure performed	021309W, 06BP3ZZ

Further Student Reading

Centers for Disease Control and Prevention. 2016. ICD-10-CM Official Guidelines for Coding and Reporting. http://www.cdc.gov/nchs/data/icd/10cmguidelines_2016_final.pdf

Centers for Medicare and Medicaid Services. 2016. ICD-10-PCS Official Guidelines for Coding and Reporting. https://www.cms.gov/Medicare/Coding/ICD10/Downloads/2016-Official-ICD-10-PCS-Coding-Guidelines-.pdf

1.18

Special health record documentation requirements

 Subdomain I.B.1
Analyze the documentation in the health record to ensure it supports the diagnosis and reflects the patient's progress, clinical findings, and discharge status.

You have been asked to audit a pediatric group's medical records. In addition to verifying the appropriate E&M code assigned, you are tasked with ensuring that all relevant documentation is present in the record.

1. Develop a checklist of the documentation that should be included in a pediatric record.

2. Use the scenario below and the checklist you have developed to determine if all relevant documentation is present in the record.

3. Verify the E&M code assigned. If the code is incorrect, select the appropriate code. Defend your selection whether you determine it is correct or incorrect.

OFFICE NOTE: 7/15/16

Timothy is a nine-month-old male who presents today with bilateral earaches. Timothy's mother states that the child has been crying and pulling at his ears for the last two days. She has also noticed a mild fever. Otoscopic examination revealed bulging tympanic membranes indicative of fluid buildup. Amoxicillin prescribed for ear infection. Script e-faxed to pharmacy.

CPT code assignment for visit: 99202

BIRTH HISTORY

10/09/15 Timothy had an uneventful, full-term, vaginal birth. Uncomplicated pregnancy, natural childbirth. No forceps used in delivery. APGAR score at birth 8, repeat APGAR 10.

PERSONAL, SOCIAL, AND FAMILY HISTORY

11/10/15/ Second child, one older sister who is four years old. Parents are married. Non-smoking environment. No pets in the home. Will attend daycare after mother's maternity leave ends in three months. Circumsized prior to discharge at birth.

NUTRITIONAL HISTORY

11/10/15 Timothy is breastfed initially.
12/13/15 Breastfeeding continues.
2/16/16 Breastfeeding continues.
4/18/16 Cereal has been introduced into diet, rice.
7/15/16 Infant eats rice and oatmeal cereal, variety of fruits. No reactions noted to new foods.

<u>OFFICE NOTE:</u> 11/10/15

Well-child visit. No problems. Child thriving. Growth appropriate.

<u>OFFICE NOTE:</u> 12/13/15

Well-child visit. No problems. Growth appropriate. First set of vaccines administered.

<u>OFFICE NOTE:</u> 2/16/16

Well-child visit. No problems. Growth appropriate. Developmental milestones met. Second set of vaccines administered.

<u>OFFICE NOTE:</u> 4/18/16

Well-child visit. No problems. Growth appropriate. Developmental milestones met. Third set of vaccines administered.

<u>MEDICATIONS</u>

7/15/16 Amoxicillin BID for 10 days.

References

American Medical Association. 2017. *CPT Professional Edition*. Chicago: AMA.

Bricker, M.R. 2016. Health Record Content and Documentation. Chapter 4 in *Health Information Management Technology: An Applied Approach*, 5th ed. Sayles, N.B. and L. Gordon, eds. Chicago: AHIMA.

1.19

Physician assistant documentation practices

Subdomain I.B.4
Differentiate the roles and responsibilities of various providers and disciplines to support documentation requirements throughout the continuum of healthcare.

Rockville Family Practice in Florida is considering hiring physician assistants (PA). The physicians need some clarification on the scope of work permitted by law and want you, their HIM manager, to find out the answers to several questions. You identify the following website as a resource to find the answers: http://www.bartonassociates.com/nurse-practitioners/physician-assistant-scope-of-practice-laws/

1. Research the questions and provide your conclusions to the physicians in a memo.

- Is there a limit to the number of PAs that can be supervised by a physician?
- Can a PA write prescriptions?
- Are the physicians required to co-sign PA documentation?

2. Do some further research and answer the following questions.

- Compare the results for Florida with those from Texas, Alabama, and Pennsylvania. Outline the differences.
- Offer an opinion for the difference in the number of PAs physicians can supervise among these states.
- Critique Alabama's co-signature requirement. As an HIM manager, what difficulty do you see with that state's co-signature requirement?

References

Barton Associates. 2016. Physician Assistant Scope of Practice Laws. http://www.bartonassociates. com/nurse-practitioners/physician-assistant-scope-of-practice-laws/

Sayles, N.B. 2016. Health Information Management Profession. Chapter 1 in *Health Information Management Technology: An Applied Approach*, 5th ed. Sayles, N.B. and L. Gordon, eds. Chicago: AHIMA.

1.20

Meaningful use and vocabularies

Subdomain I.A.1
Apply diagnosis/procedure codes according to current guidelines

Subdomain I.A.2
Identify the functions and relationships between healthcare classification systems.

Explore the relationship between meaningful use and vocabularies.

- Determine why vocabularies are a necessary part of the meaningful use process.
- Identify the vocabularies that have been selected to support meaningful use.
- Explain why vocabularies are needed for meaningful use rather than classification systems.

References

Amatayakul, M.A. 2016. Health Information Technologies. Chapter 11 in *Health Information Management Technology: An Applied Approach*, 5th ed. Sayles, N.B. and L. Gordon, eds. Chicago: AHIMA.

1.21

Interoperability

Subdomain I.C.1
Format data to satisfy integration needs

Read the Office of the National Coordinator for Healthcare Information Technology's paper "Connecting Health and Care for the Nation: A Ten-Year Vision to Achieve Interoperable Health IT Infrastructure". Within the paper, the ONC presents five building blocks for interoperability. Give your opinion on which one will be the most challenging and provide support for your position.

References

Office of the National Coordinator for Health Information Technology. 2016. Connecting Health and Care for the Nation: A Ten-Year Vision to Achieve Interoperable Health IT Infrastructure. http://www.healthit.gov/sites/default/files/ONC10yearInteroperabilityConceptPaper.pdf

1.22

Information governance advocacy

Subdomain I.C.4
Advocate information operability and information exchange

1. Two months ago, as HIM director, you broach the subject of information governance (IG) with your immediate boss, the chief financial officer, stating that the formation of a new committee dedicated to IG would be advantageous. Appraise the value of an IG committee and plan for your boss.

2. At the time, the CFO gave you little support for the endeavor. However, today, you hear from your counterpart in IT that she was asked last week to serve on a new committee for information governance that is to have their first meeting in two days. You decide to schedule a meeting with the CFO to defend the value that an HIM representative could bring to an IG committee by compiling a comparison of the IG Principles of Healthcare to the responsibilities that HIM already upholds. Justify your position to add HIM to the IG committee with that information.

References

AHIMA. 2016. Information Governance: Principles for Healthcare. http://www.ahima.org/topics/infogovernance/igbasics?tabid=overview

AHIMA. 2016. Information Governance Toolkit. http://www.ahima.org/topics/infogovernance/igbasics?tabid=overview

1.23

Encoder replacement

Subdomain I.A.1
Evaluate, implement, and manage electronic applications/systems for clinical classification and coding

Subdomain III.B.2
Take part in the planning, design, selection, implementation, integration, testing, evaluation, and support of health information technologies

As the coding supervisor for a mid-size acute care hospital, you have been hearing complaints about the current encoder product for the past year. The present contract with the encoder vendor you now have expires in one year. You have received approval to investigate an encoder change.

1. Construct a timeline for the entire process and assume that you will make a definite change to a new vendor.
2. Incorporate the steps of the Systems Development Life Cycle in your plan.

References

Amatayakul, M.A. 2016. Health Information Technologies. Chapter 11 in *Health Information Management Technology: An Applied Approach*, 5th ed. Sayles, N.B. and L. Gordon, eds. Chicago: AHIMA.

1.24

Screen design eMPI

Subdomain I.D.1
Collect and maintain health data

Experiment with building a screen design. Choose the data elements that you would want in an eMPI and then build a layout of those data elements.

References

Reynolds, R. 2016. Health Record Content and Documentation. Chapter 4 in *Health Information Management: Concepts, Principles, and Practice*, 5th ed. Oachs, P. and A. Watters, eds. Chicago: AHIMA.

1.25

Cloud computing pros and cons

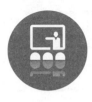

Subdomain I.D.2
Evaluate health information systems and data storage design

The IT Director has asked for a meeting with you to discuss the possibility of utilizing cloud computing.

1. Prepare for the meeting by researching cloud computing in healthcare and creating a list of at least three pros and cons related to the implementation or use of cloud computing. Focus on areas such as cost, access, privacy and security, and performance.

2. Reach a recommendation to share with the IT Director at the meeting justifying your position on whether or not implementing cloud computing is a sound practice.

References

Amatayakul, M.A. 2016. Health Information Technologies. Chapter 11 in *Health Information Management Technology: An Applied Approach*, 5th ed. Sayles, N.B. and L. Gordon, eds. Chicago: AHIMA.

Dinh, A.K. 2011. Cloud Computing 101. *Journal of AHIMA* 82(4):36–37.

1.26

SNOMED CT vs. ICD

 Subdomain I.A.2
Identify the functions and relationships between healthcare
classification systems

A fellow classmate is having difficulty understanding the difference between SNOMED-CT
and ICD-10. Compare the terminologies and distinguish reasons for their usage to assist
your classmate with comprehending these concepts.

References

Bowman, S. 2005. Coordinating SNOMED-CT and ICD-10: Getting the Most out of Electronic Health
Record Systems. *Journal of AHIMA* 76(7):60–61.

Giannangelo, K. 2016. Clinical Terminologies, Classification Systems, and Code Systems. Chapter
5 in *Health Information Management Technology: An Applied Approach*, 5th ed. Sayles, N.B. and L.
Gordon, eds. Chicago: AHIMA.

1.27

Patient registration impact on HIM

Subdomain I.B.4
Differentiate the roles and responsibilities of various providers and disciplines, to support documentation requirements, throughout the continuum of healthcare

On your first day as HIM director at a small community hospital, your coding staff has come to you complaining about the number of errors originating from patient registration. Over the course of the next week, you see how these errors are impacting the entire revenue cycle from duplicate medical record numbers to wrong insurances listed.

1. First, assess the possible reasons for the errors.
2. Decide how to present this information to the patient registration director to reduce the number of errors.

References

Amatayakul, M.A. 2016. Health Information Technologies. Chapter 11 in *Health Information Management Technology: An Applied Approach*, 5th ed. Sayles, N.B. and L. Gordon, eds. Chicago: AHIMA.

Cummins, R. and J. Waddell. 2005. Coding Connections in Revenue Cycle Management. *Journal of AHIMA* 76(7):72–74.

Reynolds, R. 2016. Health Record Content and Documentation. Chapter 4 in *Health Information Management: Concepts, Principles, and Practice*, 5th ed. Oachs, P. and A. Watters, eds. Chicago: AHIMA.

1.28

Privacy and security concerns related to interoperability

Subdomain I.C.1
Format data to satisfy integration needs

One of the biggest concerns about interoperability for health records is safeguarding privacy and security. For instance, consider the impact that various state laws and HIPAA have on information exchange. Propose a solution, supported by research, to solve two conflicts between current laws and HIPAA. Provide justification for your solution.

References

Heubusch, K. 2006. Interoperability: what it means, why it matters. *Journal of AHIMA* 77(1):26–30.

Rinehart-Thompson, L.A. 2016. Data Privacy and Confidentiality. Chapter 9 in *Health Information Management Technology: An Applied Approach*, 5th ed. Sayles, N.B. and L. Gordon, eds. Chicago: AHIMA.

1.29

Data dictionary and The Joint Commission

Subdomain I.C.2
Construct and maintain the standardization of data dictionaries to meet the needs of the enterprise

A new hospital is preparing to open. They want to ensure that, when it is time to report on the national quality measures to The Joint Commission, the data flows properly.

1. Assist in creating the data dictionary for the following data elements to be reported by noting the correct format and allowable values.

2. Identify and use the appropriate source document for this information.

Admission date
Discharge disposition
Sex
Race
Hispanic
Payment source

References

Joint Commission. 2016. Specifications Manual for Joint Commission National Quality Measures. http://www.jointcommission.org/specifications_manual_joint_commission_national_quality_core_measures.aspx

1.30

Data warehouse and modeling

Subdomain I.D.4
Apply knowledge of database architecture and design to meet organizational needs

1. Explain the concept of a data warehouse and differentiate it from a clinical repository.
2. Compare and contrast two data models for data warehouse design: the snowflake schema and the star schema.

References

Sayles, N.B. and L. Gordon. 2016. *Health Information Management Technology: An Applied Approach*, 5th ed. Chicago: AHIMA.

1.31

Data dictionary maintenance

Subdomain I.C.2
Construct and maintain the standardization of data dictionaries to meet the needs of the enterprise

Currently, in your organization, pediatric patients are considered those that are under 13 years of age. Patients that are admitted to the pediatric unit are registered as PEDS. Reports to your state pediatric disease registry are run based on the location of PEDS. Suppose the state's data dictionary for the pediatric disease registry supplies the definition of pediatric patient as one that is 18 years of age or younger.

1. How will you design or modify reports based on the current data dictionary?
2. Elaborate on what changes will need to be made going forward to collect the appropriate information for reporting.

References

AHIMA. 2012. Managing a data dictionary. *Journal of AHIMA* 83(1):48–52.

Brinda, D. 2016. Data Management. Chapter 6 in *Health Information Management Technology: An Applied Approach*, 5th ed. Sayles, N.B. and L. Gordon, eds. Chicago: AHIMA.

1.32

Data dictionary flaw

Subdomain I.C.3
Demonstrate compliance with internal and external data dictionary requirements

Subdomain III.A.6
Create the electronic structure of health data to meet a variety of end user needs

It has been discovered that there are issues with reporting your organization's Joint Commission core measures because several data elements are incorrectly formatted. You must review the following data elements to isolate the problems and provide the appropriate modification which will correct your data submission.

Data element	Current depiction	Revision needed	Correction
Admission date	MM-DD-YY		
Discharge disposition	1-8		
Sex	0, 1, 2		
Race	1-7		
Hispanic	1, 2		
Payment Source	1-12		

References

The Joint Commission. 2016. Specifications Manual for Joint Commission National Quality Measures (v2013A1). https://manual.jointcommission.org/releases/TJC2013A/DataDictionaryIntroductionTJC.html

AHIMA. 2012. Managing a data dictionary. *Journal of AHIMA* 83(1):48–52.

1.33

HEDIS report card

Subdomain I.D.3
Manage clinical indices/databases/registries

Your 73-year-old uncle Henry lives in Pennsylvania and is looking for a Medicare PPO to join. He has several chronic diseases including diabetes, hypertension, and Parkinson's disease. In particular, he wants to join a PPO that is highly rated for helping individuals live with their illnesses. Help him create a report card on the HEDIS website to evaluate the health plans. Which health plan would be the best selection and why?

References

National Committee for Quality Assurance. 2015. Health Plan Report Card.
http://reportcard.ncqa.org/plan/external/plansearch.aspx

1.34

Data dictionary mapping

Subdomain I.C.2
Construct and maintain the standardization of data dictionaries to meet the needs of the enterprise

Subdomain I.C.3
Demonstrate compliance with internal and external data dictionary requirements

Subdomain III.A.6
Create the electronic structure of health data to meet a variety of end user needs

Create a table to map the data element patient race to Joint Commission, MEDPAR, and HL7 data requirements. Your organization lists eight race choices and uses the first two letters of each race as the data value.

Patient Race	Facility Code	HL7	MEDPAR	Joint Commission
White	WH	2106-3	1	1
Black	BL	2054-5	2	2
Asian	AS	2028-9	4	4
Native American	NA	1002-5	6	3
Hispanic	HI		5	
Pacific Islander	PA	2076-8		5
Other	OT	2131-1	3	
Unable to determine	UN		0	7

References

AHIMA. 2011. Data mapping best practices. *Journal of AHIMA* 82(4):46–52.

AHIMA. 2012. Managing a data dictionary. *Journal of AHIMA* 83(1):48–52.

Joint Commission. 2016. Specifications Manual for Joint Commission National Quality Measures (v2013A1). https://manual.jointcommission.org/releases/TJC2013A/DataDictionaryIntroductionTJC.html

HL7. 2016. Appendix A. Data Definition Tables. https://www.hl7.org/special/committees/vocab/V26_Appendix_A.pdf

Research Data Distribution Center Medicare Provider Analysis and Review (MEDPAR) Record. 2016. Dictionary For SAS and CSV Datasets. https://www.cms.gov/Research-Statistics-Data-and-Systems/Files-for-Order/IdentifiableDataFiles/Downloads/sasIDmedpar.pdf

1.35

Cancer reporting

Subdomain I.D.5
Evaluate data from varying sources to create meaningful presentations

As cancer registrar, the cancer committee chairman at your hospital in Napoleon, Ohio, has requested that you create a presentation comparing cancer statistics in the state of Ohio. She wants comparisons among the counties represented by Columbus, Cleveland, Cincinnati, Toledo, and Marietta, along with your own county. You will use the Cancer County Profiles data from Ohio Department of Health website to gather this data.

1. Determine the top three cancer sites by county based on number of cases. Create a table that illustrates this data.

2. Create a bar graph to compare your county's top cancer site incidence rate to the other counties, the state, and the nation for the same site.

3. Create a graph that compares the percentage of early and late diagnosis stage for Henry County's top cancer site with the state and national rates.

References

Geology.com. 2016. Ohio County Map with County Seat Cities. http://geology.com/county-map/ohio.shtml

Ohio Department of Health. 2016. 2015 County Cancer Profiles. http://www.odh.ohio.gov/en/healthstats/ocisshs/profiles.aspx

Further Student Reading

Edgerton, C.G. 2016. Healthcare Statistics. Chapter 16 in *Health Information Management: Concepts, Principles, and Practice*, 5th ed. Oachs, P. and A. Watters, eds. Chicago: AHIMA.

CHAPTER 2

Domain II: Information Protection: Access, Disclosure, Archival, Privacy and Security

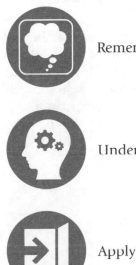 Remember

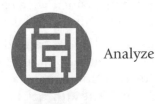 Analyze

 Understand

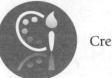 Evaluate

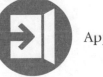 Apply

Create

Health Law

2.0

Legal terminology

Subdomain II.A.1
Apply healthcare legal terminology

Subdomain II.A.1
Identify laws and regulations applicable to healthcare

Identify the appropriate healthcare legal terminology from the following scenario.

Mrs. Jean Harper was admitted to Richmond Medical Center for hip replacement surgery. Pre-operatively she was administered a prophylactic medication to reduce post-operative gastrointestinal complications as part of the surgeon's, Dr. Gilchrist, standing orders. Unfortunately, Mrs. Harper had an allergy to the medication which was listed in her medical record, but went unnoticed by staff. Once the error was recognized, Benadryl was given to counteract the original medication but that caused a steep drop in her blood pressure which led to a stroke. Mrs. Harper suffered dysphasia and hemiplegia which continue to this day.

Mrs. Harper sued Dr. Gilchrist and the nursing staff for damages as a result of the injuries she sustained. Her attorney, Monique LeClair, recognized the need to move quickly to preserve the documentation related to the case.

1. Based on that necessity, the attorney's first step should be to ask the court for what?
2. Demonstrate why that is a necessary step in this proceeding.

Next, knowing that RMC's medical records were hybrid, Ms. LeClair needed access to the electronic documents which were part of her patient's record along with any e-mails that may have been pertinent to the case.

Documents were then exchanged between the various lawyers and members of the hospital staff gave pretrial oral testimony. Upon reviewing documents from the hospital, Ms. LeClair's team found a metadata discrepancy on an e-form used to document the patient's vital signs. The attorney had the court issue an order for nurse responsible for the documentation to appear at the trial. Based on the nurse's statement at trial that the document had been altered to reflect constant vital sign monitoring with no substantial change, the deciders of fact supported Mrs. Ramsey and awarded 4.3 million dollars in damages.

3. Plaintiff
4. Defendant
5. Court issued order requiring the nurse to appear at the trial
6. Deciders of fact
7. Pretrial exchange of documents between lawyers

8. Pretrial oral testimony
9. Electronic documents
10. Statement at trial

References

Brodnik, M. S., L. A. Rinehart-Thompson, and R. B. Reynolds. 2012. *Fundamentals of Law for Health Informatics and Information Management*, 2nd ed., revised reprint. Chicago: AHIMA.

2.1

Healthcare laws and HIM

Subdomain II.A.1
Identify laws, regulations, and events applicable to healthcare

1. Put the following laws/regulations/events related to healthcare in chronological order. Provide a brief synopsis of key features of each.

1. Medicare Modernization Act
2. Founding of the Joint Commission on Accreditation of Hospitals
3. ARRA-HITECH
4. National Academies of Sciences, Engineering, and Medicine-*To Err Is Human*
5. Hill-Burton Act
6. Medicare and Medicaid Patient Protection Act
7. Patient Protection and Affordable Care Act
8. Title XIX of the Social Security Act
9. *Darling v. Charleston Community Memorial Hospital*
10. National Academies of Sciences, Engineering, and Medicine-*Crossing the Quality Chasm-A New Health System for the 21ˢᵗ Century*
11. EMTALA
12. *Tarasoff v. Regents of the University of California*
13. GINA
14. The Flexner Report
15. Stark Law
16. HIPAA
17. Title XVIII of the Social Security Act
18. Tax Relief and Health Care Act
19. Hospital Standardization Program
20. Inpatient Prospective Payment System

1. Identify the year that the following HIM related events occurred. Then explain their individual significance in relation to the healthcare laws, regulations, and events above.
   a. Association of Record Librarians of North America formed
   b. CCS certification established
   c. CHPS certification established
   d. RRL certification established
   e. Association name changed to American Health Information Management Association

References

Brodnik, M. S., L. A. Rinehart-Thompson, and R. B. Reynolds. 2012. *Fundamentals of Law for Health Informatics and Information Management,* 2nd ed., revised reprint. Chicago: AHIMA.

Fuller, S. 2016. The US Healthcare Delivery System. Chapter 1 in *Health Information Management: Concepts, Principles, and Practice,* 5th ed. Oachs, P. and A. Watters, eds. Chicago: AHIMA.

Hazelwood, A. and C. Venable. 2016. Reimbursement Methodologies. Chapter 7 in *Health Information Management: Concepts, Principles, and Practice,* 5th ed. Oachs, P. and A. Watters, eds. Chicago: AHIMA.

O'Dell, R. M. 2016. Clinical Quality Management. Chapter 21 in *Health Information Management: Concepts, Principles, and Practice,* 5th ed. Oachs, P. and A. Watters, eds. Chicago: AHIMA.

Further Student Reading

Klaver, J. C. 2012. Risk management and quality improvement. Chapter 14 in *Fundamentals of Law for Health Informatics and Information Management,* 2nd ed. revised reprint. Brodnik, M. S., L. A. Rinehart-Thompson, and R. B. Reynolds, eds. Chicago: AHIMA.

2.2

Release of information form

Subdomain II.C.1
Apply policies and procedures surrounding issues of access and disclosure of protected health information

Subdomain II.C.1
Create policies and procedures to manage access and disclosure of personal health information

1. Assess the following authorization form against the Privacy Rule criteria and determine if any element(s) is/are missing. Modify the document by adding language to incorporate any element(s) found missing.

PINE VALLEY COMMUNITY HOSPITAL
AUTHORIZATION TO RELEASE HEALTH INFORMATION

Patient's Name: _____ Date of Birth: _____

Patient's Social Security Number: _____

I hereby authorize Pine Valley Medical Center to release to the following:

Name: _____

Address: _____

Documents to be released are: _____

From Date of Service: _____

Purpose for record request is: _____

I understand that applicable laws may prohibit redisclosure of this information, but that PVMC will not be liable or responsible for any redisclosure that takes place after the information has been released.

I understand that I will not be denied treatment if I refuse to sign this authorization.

I understand that I am entitled to a copy of this authorization.

I understand that the information will be handled confidentially in compliance with applicable state and federal laws.

I have read and understand the nature of this release.

_____   _____
Patient's Signature/Legal Representative   Date

_____   _____
Witness   Date

Figure 2.2. Pine Valley Community Hospital authorization to release health information

References

Brodnik, M. S., L. A. Rinehart-Thompson, and R. B. Reynolds. 2012. *Fundamentals of Law for Health Informatics and Information Management*, 2nd ed., revised reprint. Chicago: AHIMA.

2.3

Subpoena preparation

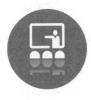

Subdomain II.A.3
Apply legal concepts and principles to the practice of HIM

As the HIM director, you have been served with a subpoena to produce records for an upcoming court case. Your release of information (ROI) clerk is new and when you direct her to the procedure to follow for prepping records in response to a subpoena, you find there isn't one. Select the steps to include in the procedure and outline them.

References

Brodnik, M. S., L. A. Rinehart-Thompson, and R. B. Reynolds. 2012. *Fundamentals of Law for Health Informatics and Information Management*, 2nd ed., revised reprint. Chicago: AHIMA.

2.4

Security policy—HIM student practicum

Subdomain II.B.1
Apply confidentiality, privacy, and security measures and policies and procedures for internal and external use and exchange to protect electronic health information.

Subdomain II.B.3
Apply system security policies according to departmental and organizational data/information standards

Subdomain II.B.5
Develop educational programs for employees in privacy, security, and confidentiality

Your HIM department is going to begin taking students as part of their Professional Practice Experience (PPE). The HIM director has asked you to create a short educational program on privacy, security, and confidentiality for the students to complete before they start their PPE. Create a PowerPoint presentation of no more than 12 slides that covers the following elements:

- Differentiate between privacy, security, and confidentiality
- Access to be based on minimum necessary standard
- Release of information requires authorization
- Use and protection of passwords and security codes
- Duty to report breaches

Further Student Reading

AHIMA. 2014. Professional Practice Experience Guide Version IV. http://www.ahima.org/~/media/AHIMA/Files/PPE/FINAL%20FINAL%20PPE%20GUIDE%20VERSION%20II.ashx?la=en

AHIMA. 2010. Information Security—An Overview (Updated). http://library.ahima.org/xpedio/groups/public/documents/ahima/bok1_048962.hcsp?dDocName=bok1_048962

2.5

Information access

Subdomain II.C.1
Apply policies and procedures surrounding issues of access and disclosure of protected health information

Analyze the following scenarios to determine who can appropriately access health information.

1. Mrs. John Smith is requesting the emergency room records from last week of her daughter, Katy. Mrs. Smith is the noncustodial parent of Katy, who lives with her dad. Should you release the records to her? Why or why not?

2. Mr. Fred Mitchell is requesting the birth record for Amy, his birth daughter. Mr. and Mrs. Mitchell gave Amy up for adoption four years ago. Should you release the records to him? Why or why not?

3. Mrs. Lynn Olsen is requesting the lab results of her husband, Tim. She has a note, signed by him, giving his permission for her to have the records. Should you release the records to her? Why or why not?

4. An investigator from the Health and Human Services department is conducting an audit of patient records and has provided a list of records that they want to review. Should you release the information to the investigator? Why or why not?

5. Dr. Rex Harrison is requesting the medical records of Martha Flynn. He states he is a family friend and has been asked by Mrs. Flynn's son to review her last inpatient admission for appropriateness of care. Should you release the records to Dr. Harrison? Why or why not?

References

Brodnik, M. S., L. A. Rinehart-Thompson, and R. B. Reynolds. 2012. *Fundamentals of Law for Health Informatics and Information Management*, 2nd ed., revised reprint. Chicago: AHIMA.

2.6

Legal document conundrum

Subdomain II.A.2
Identify the use of legal documents

Correctly identify the appropriate legal document required for each scenario below.

1. After serious consideration, Harry has decided to undergo a new and extremely delicate heart procedure. At 56, his hypertrophic cardiomyopathy has required him to adopt a sedentary lifestyle. Medication no longer manages his disease, so surgery is the option of last resort. After much thought, Harry has decided that if he should suffer a cardiac or respiratory arrest, he does not want any cardiopulmonary resuscitation. What specific legal document should Harry complete and share with his healthcare providers?

2. Prior to Harry's heart surgery, his physician will discuss Harry's diagnosis and the procedure in detail. He will share any alternatives to the surgery, outline the benefits of the procedure, and discuss the risks associated with the procedure. Harry will have the opportunity to ask any questions he may have regarding the surgery. The physician will then complete what legal document that certifies that the patient has been made aware of this information?

3. Early onset familial Alzheimer's disease runs in Ruth's family. Her mother had the disease, and Ruth has just had genetic testing, which indicates that she will have the disease as well. After her initial shock, Ruth has decided to be proactive with her healthcare and to that end, has decided to appoint her daughter to make healthcare decisions for her once she is unable to make them for herself. Ruth needs to complete what legal document to ensure that her daughter is legally empowered to make those decisions?

4. Martha has learned that she has metastatic breast cancer. Her physicians have indicated that she will need a mastectomy, along with both chemotherapy and radiation therapy. She recognizes that there could be many obstacles and setbacks as she fights this disease and that there could come a time that she would be unable to make her own decisions. To that end, Martha has decided to complete a legal document outlining her wishes for treatment if she is ever unable to communicate them for herself. What legal document should Martha complete?

5. George is an eighty year-old man in relatively good health. However, he sees many of his friends dealing with healthcare issues and how sometimes, families bicker over the healthcare decisions of a loved one who is incapacitated. George would like to be confident that no issues like that would arise in the event of a decline in his mental function so he is going to issue what type of legal document(s) that will be effective in the event he becomes incapacitated?.

References

Brodnik, M. S., L. A. Rinehart-Thompson, and R. B. Reynolds. 2012. *Fundamentals of Law for Health Informatics and Information Management*, 2nd ed., revised reprint. Chicago: AHIMA.

2.7

Legal health record maintenance

Subdomain II.A.3
Apply legal concepts and principles to the practice of HIM

Subdomain II.A.2
Analyze legal concepts and principles to the practice of HIM

Judge each scenario below to determine if the documentation practice presented would be legally defensible, meaning does it meet regulatory, accreditation, legal, and professional practice standards? Defend your answer.

1. Discharge summary dictated on 11/24/15 for a patient discharged on 9/30/15.

2. Process whereby emergency room transcribed reports are considered approved and signed if no corrections are made to the transcription within 48 hours of posting.

3. A faxed order and signature for a patient to receive physical therapy.

4. The following order handwritten in pencil:

   Turn patient every 2 hours to prevent decubitus ulcers.

   Dr. Timothy Reynolds 12/2/15 11:15 a.m.

5. The correction shown here:

   Administer two units of ~~fresh frozen plasma~~. ERROR –wrong blood product TR 12/18/15, 5:27 p.m.

   Dr. Timothy Reynolds 12/18/15 5:25 p.m.

   Administer two units of packed red cells.

   Dr. Timothy Reynolds 12/18/15 5:30 p.m.

6. In a patient's EHR for their last inpatient admission, a coder notices that the operative report is located under the discharge summary tab and brings it to your attention. You have it moved to the correct location within the account without annotation.

7. Nursing documentation for 10/31/15:

   3:00 p.m.- 11:00 p.m. Administered dose of antibiotic. Walked patient in hallway. Sat patient up in chair. Performed vitals. Assisted patient back to bed. Checked on patient-resting comfortably, no pain. Walked patient in hallway and assisted to bathroom. Checked vitals. Administered antibiotic and pain medication.

8. Physician order:

   Give Lotensin 20mg. daily

   Dr. Gregory Marshall *10/26/15 2:55p.m.*

9. A physician copies and pastes his progress note from two days ago into his most current note, adding a brief comment that there is no change in the patient's condition.

   Progress note 11/4/15
   Patient showing improvement in breathing. Responding well to antibiotic. Able to get out of bed and move around with assistance. Performed a bedside debridement of a lower leg ulcer, excisional, subcutaneous.

Progress note 11/6/15

Patient showing improvement in breathing. Responding well to antibiotic. Able to get out of bed and move around with assistance. Performed a bedside debridement of a lower leg ulcer, excisional, subcutaneous.

No change. Continued improvement.

10. An organization has a policy for record retention that states hard copies are kept for 7 years. In 2015, records purged for destruction included the following list:

MR #	YEAR
0015698	2006
0051482	2005
0742412	2007
0089364	2005
0009332	2006
0041127	2005
0065435	2008
0126525	2007
0039254	2006
0001153	2006
0248761	2007
0044879	2007
0964578	2006
0676766	2005
0037526	2004

References

AHIMA e-HIM Work Group on Maintaining the Legal EHR. 2005. Update: Maintaining a Legally Sound Health Record—Paper and Electronic. *Journal of AHIMA* 76(10):64A-L.

Brodnik, M. S., L. A. Rinehart-Thompson, and R. B. Reynolds. 2012. *Fundamentals of Law for Health Informatics and Information Management,* 2nd ed., revised reprint. Chicago: AHIMA.

2.8

Potential privacy violation

Subdomain II.B.2
Recommend elements included in the design of audit trails and data quality monitoring programs

On 11/23/15, the female mayor of your town was seen in your ER and subsequently admitted with injuries that included an orbital floor blow-out fracture and multiple bruises. Past rumors have hinted that the mayor is in an abusive relationship and speculation is rampant that these injuries are a result of abuse. Local papers have printed health information that should not be available to them. To address a potential privacy breach, the IT department ran an audit trail to see who had accessed the patient's records. Five employees in the HIM department accessed the record, and you are tasked with determining if any of those violated privacy policy.

(At this facility, records are still hybrid.)

The employees are:

- N. Northwest,-coder
- L. Easton,-coder
- S. Southward,-transcriptionist
- E. Downey,-file clerk
- W. Upton,-file clerk

Below is the audit trail you were given from IT. You call IT recommending them to include what other relevant elements in the audit trail?

Audit Trail for MR#655966	
User	Date
N. Northwest	11/28/15
S. Southward	11/27/2015
L. Easton	11/26/2015
E. Downey	11/24/2015
W. Upton	11/29/2015

References

AHIMA. 2011. Security Audits of Electronic Health Information (Updated). *Journal of AHIMA* 82(3):46–50.

Rinehart-Thompson, L.A. 2016.Data Security. Chapter 10 in *Health Information Management Technology: An Applied Approach*, 5th ed. Sayles, N.B. and L. Gordon, eds. Chicago: AHIMA.

2.9

HIM staff privacy and security education

Subdomain II.A.5
Develop educational programs for employees in privacy, security, and confidentiality

Subdomain VI.H.4
Create programs and policies that support a culture of diversity.

You want to provide ongoing privacy and security training for your 25 HIM staff. The HIM department is diverse: workers range in age from 25–62; three men; four Latinos, two African-Americans, and the remainder Caucasian; four of your older staff still struggle with computer literacy; 11 are college graduates (seven baccalaureate degrees, four associate degrees); one staff member is in a wheelchair; and 12 work from home.

1. From this information theorize at least 3 delivery methods that might be considered in order to have a successful privacy and security education.

2. Identify at least 5 cultural or diversity issues that could raise barriers during the training.

3. Formulate a plan for educating your HIM staff on privacy and security. The focus of this portion of the assignment is not the content of the education but the delivery method(s) to be used.

References

AHIMA. 2003. Think salad, not stew: managing cultural differences in your HIM department. *AHIMA Advantage.* 7:1.

Patena, K. 2016. Employee Training and Development. Chapter 24 in *Health Information Management: Concepts, Principles, and Practice*, 5th ed. Oachs, P. and A. Watters, eds. Chicago: AHIMA.

2.10

Privacy and security education

Subdomain II.A.5
Develop educational programs for employees in privacy, security, and confidentiality

As the HIM director at Pine Valley Community Hospital, a critical access hospital, you are also the Privacy and Security officer for the organization. You are preparing an annual privacy and security training for non-clinical staff.

Create a PowerPoint presentation (minimum of 20 slides) to be provided at an in-service along with a short post-test (10 questions). Make sure to cover the relevant HIPAA and HITECH information for these non-clinical staff including a distinction between privacy, security, and confidentiality.

References

AHIMA. 2010. Information Security—An Overview (Updated). http://library.ahima.org/xpedio/groups/public/documents/ahima/bok1_048962.hcsp?dDocName=bok1_048962

2.11

Legal terminology II

Subdomain II.A.1
Apply healthcare legal terminology

Subdomain II.A.1
Identify laws and regulations applicable to healthcare

Distinguish the two types of defamation of character. Identify the best defenses against these types of claims. Research the internet to find an article related to one of these types of healthcare defamation and provide a short synopsis. Provide the plaintiff, the defendant, and settlement in the case.

References

Brodnik, M. S., L. A. Rinehart-Thompson, and R. B. Reynolds. 2012. *Fundamentals of Law for Health Informatics and Information Management,* 2nd ed., revised reprint. Chicago: AHIMA.

Samples of recent articles

Counsel Financial. Ex-Employee's Defamation Claims Yield Sizable $855,600 Settlement.

http://attorneylending.com/?litigation_post=ex-employees-defamation-claims-yield-sizable-855600-settlement

Variety. 'American Sniper' Libel Case: MPAA, Media Companies Back Chris Kyle Estate in Appeal. http://variety.com/2015/biz/news/american-sniper-libel-case-mpaa-media-companies-back-chris-kyle-estate-in-appeal-1201450729/

2.12

HIM department breach

Subdomain II.C.2
Protect electronic health information through confidentiality and security measures, policies, and procedures

On 10/14/15, a well-known local politician died in your ER from injuries sustained in a motor vehicle accident. As part of the normal course of business, the IT department ran an audit trail to see who had accessed the patient's records. Five employees in the HIM department accessed the record, and you are tasked with determining if any of those violated privacy policy.

(At this facility, records are still hybrid.)

The employees are:

    N. Northwest-coder

    L. Easton-coder

    S. Southward-transcriptionist

    E. Downey-file clerk

    W. Upton-file clerk

1. Based on the audit trail below, formulate an opinion on whether or not any of these employees may have violated the privacy policy. Support your decision.

Audit Trail for MR#655966				
User	**Date**	**Workstation**	**Application Accessed**	**Action**
N. Northwest	10/16/2015	Home workstation 12	EHR, encoder, lab, radiology	R, M, R, R
S. Southward	10/15/2015	Home workstation 18	EHR, transcription system, radiology	R, M, M
L. Easton	10/17/2015	Home workstation 9	EHR, lab, radiology	R, R, R
E. Downey	10/15/2015	8th floor nurse's station	EHR, lab, radiology	R, R, R
W. Upton	10/15/2015	HIM department workstation 3	EHR, Chart tracking system	R, M
R=Read				
M=Modified				

2. Propose the next steps to take if there was a concern that one or more the employees violated the privacy policy.

Further Student Reading

AHIMA. 2011. Security Audits of Electronic Health Information (Updated). *Journal of AHIMA* 82(3):46–50.

Oachs, P. and A. Watters, eds. *Health Information Management: Concepts, Principles, and Practice*, 5th ed. Chicago: AHIMA.

2.13

Subpoenas and documentation

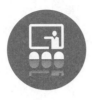

Subdomain II.A.3
Apply legal concepts and principles to the practice of HIM

While conducting the preparation of a record in response to a subpoena received on 12/10/15, you realize that there is a potential legal issue with the discharge summary. Give your opinion about the discharge summary that follows and what issue(s) it presents.

PATIENT: Jane Johnson

MR#: 1026336

DISCHARGE DATE: 9/24/15

DISCHARGE DIAGNOSIS: Infection right hip prosthesis

ADDITIONAL DISCHARGE DIAGNOSES:
1. Hypertension
2. Type II diabetes
3. Tobacco use
4. Chronic renal failure
5. Restless leg syndrome

REASON FOR ADMISSION: 74-year-old white female admitted with an infected right hip prosthesis. The patient presented to my office with low-grade fever, and slight redness, accompanied by warmth over the previous incision. She directly admitted to the hospital.

HOSPITAL COURSE: The patient was admitted on 9/19/15 and was immediately started on IV antibiotics. She was encouraged to keep the extremity elevated. A wound culture was taken and returned as MRSA. I then changed the antibiotic to Vancomycin. Daily wound care was provided. During the stay, the patient's smoking was addressed, and I indicated that continued smoking will delay healing and strongly urged the patient to quit smoking. On day one, the patient's hypertension was extremely elevated at 165-110. Cardene was administered and the blood pressure responded, eventually maintaining at 130-90. Edema of her lower extremities was reported and consult obtained. Concern was that her chronic hepatitis C was causing the edema, but consultant felt it was secondary to chronic venous stasis. The patient's progress was slow but steady. Compression was added to the treatment and by 09/24/15 her wound had only minimal redness and swelling was down with compression. The patient was discharged home to self care.

DISCHARGE INSTRUCTIONS: The patient was discharged on doxycycline 100 mg p.o. b.i.d. x10 days along with pain medication of OxyContin. She was instructed how to perform daily wound care with followup in my office in two weeks.

DISCHARGE CONDITION: Stable.

Dr. Stephen Williams
Dr. Stephen Williams
Dictated: 12/3/15
Electronically signed: 12/4/15

Further Student Reading

Brodnik, M. S., L. A. Rinehart-Thompson, and R. B. Reynolds. 2012. Civil Procedure. Chapter 3 in *Fundamentals of Law for Health Informatics and Information Management,* 2nd ed., revised reprint. Chicago: AHIMA.

2.14

Subpoenas and testifying

Subdomain II.A.3
Apply legal concepts and principles to the practice of HIM

Assume that you have now been called to testify regarding the record discussed in 2.13. Study the following questions and decide whether or not these should be answered in your role as HIM director. Provide the rationale for your answer.

1. How long have you been in your position as HIM director and custodian of health records?
2. Was this record prepared in the normal course of business?
3. Can you read the progress note dated XX/XX/XXXX?

   Discuss the points you must bear in mind if asked to read an excerpt from the record entered into evidence.
4. In your opinion, was the delay in ordering a chest x-ray warranted?
5. There is an ER record from a transferring facility that was supplied with your documents as it was used in decision making for the patient. The attorney wants to know if this was created in the normal course of business. How would you respond?

Reference

Brodnik, M.S., L.A. Rinehart-Thompson, and R.B. Reynolds. 2012. *Fundamentals of Law for Health Informatics and Information Management*. 2nd ed. revised reprint. Chicago: AHIMA.

2.15

Back-ups and e-discovery

Subdomain II.B.2
Apply retention and destruction policies for health information

You are the recently hired health information manager for a very large physician group practice. You are reviewing policies and procedures related to e-Discovery and notice that there is no mention of a policy related to back-up media. You contact the information technology manager who says that she tried to address this issue a year ago, but the prior HIM manager did not feel it was important, stating it was covered under HIM policies related to retention and destruction. You decide to hold a meeting to reintroduce the topic.

1. Determine who should take part in the meeting.
2. Assume that you will get pushback for addressing this topic again. Offer insight to the group on why this topic must be addressed.

References

AHIMA. 2013. E- Discovery Litigation and Regulatory Investigation Response Planning: Crucial Components of Your Organization's Information and Data Governance Processes. *Journal of AHIMA* 84(11): expanded web version.

Brodnik, M. S., L. A. Rinehart-Thompson, and R. B. Reynolds. 2012. *Fundamentals of Law for Health Informatics and Information Management,* 2nd ed., revised reprint. Chicago: AHIMA.

2.16

ROI cost

Subdomain II.C.1
Apply policies and procedures surrounding issues of access and disclosure of protected health information

Mrs. A. Smith has requested records from her last inpatient stay in the hospital and states that she will pick the records up when they are ready. Her stay was a result of a motor vehicle accident and she is requesting the films of her head CT and leg MRI (5 films total) be specifically included; additionally, there are 47 total pages that will need to be printed from the EHR. Your state imposes restrictions on what can be charged for production of medical record requests. Using the information below, calculate the cost to Mrs. Smith for her records.

For requests made by patients or their representatives, hospitals may charge:

$3.40 per page for the first 10 pages,
68 cents per page for pages 11-50,
30 cents per page for pages numbering more than 50.

With respect to data resulting from an x-ray, MRI, or CAT scan, recorded on paper or film:

$3.15 per film

The actual cost of postage may be charged.

For a requests made by someone other than the patient or patient's representative, hospitals may charge:

An initial fee of $25.00 to compensate for the records search.

$1.75 per page for the first 10 pages,
68 cents per page for pages 11 through 50,
30 cents per page for pages numbering more than 50.

With respect to data resulting from an x-ray, MRI, or CAT scan, recorded on paper or film:

$3.15 per film

The actual cost of postage may be charged.

References

Brodnik, M. S., L. A. Rinehart-Thompson, and R. B. Reynolds. 2012. *Fundamentals of Law for Health Informatics and Information Management*, 2nd ed., revised reprint. Chicago: AHIMA.

2.17

ROI error

Subdomain II.B.1
Analyze privacy, security, and confidentiality policies and procedures for internal and external use and exchange of health information

Martha, a new release of information clerk is being trained. She has been given a copy of the ROI procedure to follow, which is (in part) as follows:

<u>Walk-in requests</u>

1. Validate authorization
2. Process the request
3. Enter the request in the ROI database

On Friday morning, at the end of Martha's first week, a woman stating she was Mrs. Turner walked in requesting records. Joyce, Martha's trainer, had been called to the HIM director's office, so Martha was on her own. She presented Mrs. Turner with an authorization form, and then once it was completed, she printed the records requested. These were lab tests which included pregnancy results. Martha presented the records to Mrs. Turner, and then proceeded to enter the information into the ROI database as per protocol. When Joyce returned to the office, she reviewed Martha's handling of the request. Joyce became concerned about the request because Mrs. Turner was well known to her and her review of the authorization identified a concern with the signature. When she asked Martha for a description of the woman, her fears were confirmed as it was not Mrs. Turner who had requested the records.

What changes could be recommended to the ROI procedure to ensure that this type of release error would be less likely to happen in the future?

References

Brodnik, M. S., L. A. Rinehart-Thompson, and R. B. Reynolds. 2012. *Fundamentals of Law for Health Informatics and Information Management*, 2nd ed., revised reprint. Chicago: AHIMA.

2.18

Mobile health technology security

Subdomain II.B.4
Analyze the security and privacy implications of mobile health technologies

Your organization's director of home health services wants to equip her staff with laptops to record patient data. She has done a work study that proves there is a significant amount of staff time spent in duplication of work, as they collect patient information on paper in the home and then must transfer it into the information system back at the office. The IT director has concerns about the privacy and security of information that would be collected on the laptops. Strategize at least four ways to minimize privacy and security concerns.

References

AHIMA. 2012. Mobile Device Security (Updated). *Journal of AHIMA* 83(4):50–55.

Brodnik, M. S., L. A. Rinehart-Thompson, and R. B. Reynolds. 2012. *Fundamentals of Law for Health Informatics and Information Management*, 2nd ed., revised reprint. Chicago: AHIMA.

2.19

Mobile health technology security II

Subdomain II.B.4
Analyze the security and privacy implications of mobile health technologies

Next month, Three River Home Health nursing staff are going to receive laptops to record patient data while at the patient's home. As Three River's privacy and security consultant you are well aware that stolen laptops often result in a breach of privacy and security. Design a set of standards (at least four) for off-site laptop use that can prevent theft.

References

AHIMA. 2012. Mobile Device Security (Updated). *Journal of AHIMA* 83(4):50–55.

2.20

Disaster recovery planning

Subdomain II.B.2
Recommend elements included in the design of audit trails and data quality monitoring programs

You have been hired as the privacy and security director of a rural community hospital in southern Maine with 45 beds. You decide to begin by reviewing the policies and procedures already in place against what is required under HIPAA. You are dismayed to find that although there are a number of policies and procedures in effect, a security risk assessment was never performed. Create a 9-step plan for conducting the security risk assessment.

References

Brodnik, M. S., L. A. Rinehart-Thompson, and R. B. Reynolds. 2012. *Fundamentals of Law for Health Informatics and Information Management,* 2nd ed., revised reprint. Chicago: AHIMA.

Walsh, T. 2011. Security Risk Analysis and Management: an Overview (Updated). (AHIMA Practice Brief).

2.21

Security audit

Subdomain II.C.2
Protect electronic health information through confidentiality and security measures, policies, and procedures

Last month, your information system was hacked. As part of the ongoing root cause analysis, it was apparent that the IT department was not auditing the system unless there was a VIP receiving care.

Discover the best practices for security auditing. Determine under what circumstances audits should be taken and when should they take place?

References

AHIMA. 2011. Security Audits of Electronic Health Information (Updated). *Journal of AHIMA* 82(3):46–50.

Brodnik, M. S., L. A. Rinehart-Thompson, and R. B. Reynolds. 2012. *Fundamentals of Law for Health Informatics and Information Management,* 2nd ed., revised reprint. Chicago: AHIMA.

2.22

Patient mix up

Subdomain II.B.1
Analyze privacy, security, and confidentiality policies and procedures for internal and external use and exchange of health information

In the group family practice where you are the administrator for six participating physicians, patients share a waiting room. Patients are called by first name to go to their respective physician's exam room. The third patient of the day was Ted Jones, Jr. He sees Dr. Williams, but his father, Ted Jones, Sr. sees Dr. Morrison. When he is called back to the exam room, he is placed in one for Dr. Morrison. Twenty minutes later, when Dr. Morrison comes in, they realize he was placed in the wrong room. He now has to wait another thirty minutes to see the correct physician and is very irate when he leaves. Later that same day, Karen Smith is registered to see Dr. Cole. She steps out to the restroom and the newly hired medical assistant calls for Karen. Karen Maxwell gets up and goes in for her first visit with Dr. Cole and it isn't until the medical assistant asks about her response to the medication that was prescribed at the last visit that they realize the patient is not Karen Smith. You recommend that the practice implement a patient verification policy to prevent these types of errors in the future. What criteria would you include in the policy at registration and in the examination room?

References

AHIMA. 2014. Managing the Integrity of Patient Identity in Health Information Exchange (Updated). *Journal of AHIMA* 85(5):60–65.

2.23

E-Discovery preservation

Subdomain II.B.1
Analyze privacy, security, and confidentiality policies and procedures
for internal and external use and exchange of health information

Your organization is in the process of creating an e-discovery policy and procedure. You
have been asked to recommend the methods of preservation that should be outlined in the
procedure section. Research and present at least four recommendations.

References

AHIMA e-Discovery Task Force. 2008. Litigation Response Planning and Policies for E-Discovery.
AHIMA Model E-Discovery Policies: Preservation and Legal Hold for Health Information and
Records. *Journal of AHIMA* 79(2): BoK Extras.

Brodnik, M. S., L. A. Rinehart-Thompson, and R. B. Reynolds. 2012. *Fundamentals of Law for Health
Informatics and Information Management,* 2nd ed., revised reprint. Chicago: AHIMA.

2.24

E-Discovery policy review

Subdomain II.B.1
Analyze privacy, security, and confidentiality policies and procedures for internal and external use and exchange of health information

Your organization is reviewing their policy and procedure for e-discovery after an issue with a recent lawsuit highlighted some problems. One issue was that by the time the notice for the lawsuit was received, some documentation had already been destroyed even though weeks earlier a charge nurse had been told that by a family that they intended to sue. Review the following policy and procedure and suggest modifications that could help prevent future issues.

Community Hospital
Legal Hold Policy and Procedure

Purpose: To prevent spoliation of evidence in the event or anticipation of litigation, this policy addresses the process for retention and preservation of health records.

Policy: It is the policy of Community Hospital to preserve all forms of health information (paper or electronic) when litigation is anticipated and to initiate a legal hold process that prevents destruction of said information until the legal hold is lifted to prevent spoliation.

Procedure:

Legal hold is issued
Appropriate data stewards are notified of legal hold
Preservation process initiated
Review and update legal hold notices as appropriate
Assign responsibility for oversight of legal hold notices
Audit and track compliance with legal holds
Release legal hold when no longer needed
    Review other legal holds to ensure no overlap
    Via written notice alert data stewards of lifting of the legal hold
    Commence normal retention and destruction schedule
        If information on hold would have been destroyed during the legal hold process, proceed with destruction

References

AHIMA e-Discovery Task Force. 2008. Litigation Response Planning and Policies for E-Discovery. AHIMA Model E-Discovery Policies: Preservation and Legal Hold for Health Information and Records. *Journal of AHIMA* 79(2): BoK Extras.

Brodnik, M. S., L. A. Rinehart-Thompson, and R. B. Reynolds. 2012. *Fundamentals of Law for Health Informatics and Information Management*, 2nd ed., revised reprint. Chicago: AHIMA.

2.25

Security access controls

Subdomain II.B.3
Apply system security policies according to departmental and organizational data/information standards

You are the HIM director at a brand new long-term care facility. You are working with IT to develop access controls for your staff which will consist of two coders, one scanner tech, one chart analyzer, one clerk who will handle release of information and incomplete records, and three transcriptionists.

1. Analyze the three different types of access controls noting the differences.
2. Recommend which type of access control to assign to each staff member.

References

Brodnik, M. S., L. A. Rinehart-Thompson, and R. B. Reynolds. 2012. *Fundamentals of Law for Health Informatics and Information Management,* 2nd ed., revised reprint. Chicago: AHIMA.

2.26

Remote access controls

Subdomain II.B.3
Apply system security policies according to departmental and organizational data/information standards

Subdomain II.B.1
Analyze privacy, security, and confidentiality policies and procedures for internal and external use and exchange of health information

As the HIM coding supervisor, you would like to migrate your in-house coding to home-based. In anticipation of concerns that IT might raise about remote access, you have been evaluating best practices for remote security. Your recommendation would be to provide each coder with a laptop for remote access to your organization's information.

1. Explain why this is your choice in view of HIPAA security provisions.
2. Make at least four other recommendations that would control remote access and promote security.

References

AHIMA Privacy and Security Practice Council. 2007. Safeguards for Remote Access. *Journal of AHIMA* 78(7):68–70.

Brodnik, M. S., L. A. Rinehart-Thompson, and R. B. Reynolds. 2012. *Fundamentals of Law for Health Informatics and Information Management,* 2nd ed., revised reprint. Chicago: AHIMA.

Fulmer, K. October 11, 2010. Securing Remote Access to EHRs. *For the Record.* 22(18):6.

Legal terminology III

Subdomain II.A.1
Apply healthcare legal terminology

Subdomain II.A.1
Identify laws and regulations applicable to healthcare

Susan R. went to the Reynolds Medical Imaging Pavilion for her first ever mammogram. She signed in, presented her information and order, and then took a seat in the waiting room. 10 minutes later, the technician called for Susan and she went back to the room. She was told to remove her blouse and bra, put on the gown with the opening in the front, and then lie on the table face down. Slightly confused, but thinking this must be a new method for mammograms, she did as she was told. Five minutes later, a physician came into the room and performed a breast biopsy on her.

The patient was shocked when the procedure began and attempted to explain to the physician that there was a mistake but the physician proceeded with the biopsy. Afterwards, it was determined that Susan B. was the patient who was scheduled for a biopsy, not Susan R.

Susan R. began having nightmares after the procedure. This was accompanied by extreme anxiety when anyone came too close to her. After a conversation with her husband, she contacted a lawyer to initiate a lawsuit.

Apply the concept of torts to this scenario and distinguish which type of tort is depicted.

References

Brodnik, M. S., L. A. Rinehart-Thompson, and R. B. Reynolds. 2012. *Fundamentals of Law for Health Informatics and Information Management*, 2nd ed., revised reprint. Chicago: AHIMA.

2.28

Medical identity theft and PHRs

 Subdomain II.B.1
Apply confidentiality, privacy and security measures, and policies and procedures for internal and external use and exchange to protect electronic health information

Assume that your parents have decided to create individual PHRs. They found a vendor, PHRs-R-Us, online and want your advice, as an HIM student, about using their service. They are quick to tell you the vendor is HIPAA-compliant. Offer your opinion on using that vendor and be sure to address your concern about medical identity theft in your response.

References

Brodnik, M. S., L. A. Rinehart-Thompson, and R. B. Reynolds. 2012. *Fundamentals of Law for Health Informatics and Information Management,* 2nd ed., revised reprint. Chicago: AHIMA.

Rinehart-Thompson, L. A. 2008. Raising Awareness of Medical Identity Theft: For Consumers, Prevention Starts with Guarding, Monitoring Health Information. *Journal of AHIMA* 79(10):74–75, 81.

2.29

Medical identity theft

 Subdomain II.B.1
Apply confidentiality, privacy and security measures and policies and procedures for internal and external use and exchange to protect electronic health information

For each of the following scenarios determine if the situation is identity theft, medical identity theft, or neither.

1. A billing clerk takes a patient's account payment by credit card over the phone. She then uses the credit card number and patient information to make an online purchase.

2. George gives his unemployed twin brother his insurance card so he can go to the local express care for treatment for the flu.

3. Dr. Morehouse employs a janitorial service that supplies him with discarded patient information from other facilities where they work. He then uses the information to submit claims for psychiatric services.

4. A hacker enters your IT system and changes the blood type for every patient.

References

Brodnik, M. S., L. A. Rinehart-Thompson, and R. B. Reynolds. 2012. *Fundamentals of Law for Health Informatics and Information Management,* 2nd ed., revised reprint. Chicago: AHIMA.

Rinehart-Thompson, L. A. 2008. Raising Awareness of Medical Identity Theft: For Consumers, Prevention Starts with Guarding, Monitoring Health Information. *Journal of AHIMA* 79(10):74–75, 81.

2.30

Consent

Subdomain II.A.2
Identify the use of legal documents

Last week, a 26-year-old, 36-week pregnant female showed up at the ER. As she was walking into the building alone, she grabbed her head and fell to the ground. Staff rushed her to the ER where it was discovered that she had accelerated hypertension of 225/140. She suffered a seizure, lapsing into a coma, and severe stroke was diagnosed. Vital signs were not able to be stabilized and the decision was made to perform an emergency c-section to save the baby. Shortly after the surgery, the woman died as a result of the stroke. Staff had been unable to contact a family member as the woman did not have a purse, wallet, or phone on her person when she came in.

1. What type(s) of consent can be applied to this scenario?
2. How might the lack of consent(s) obtained in this scenario impact the physician and/or organization?

References

Brodnik, M. S., L. A. Rinehart-Thompson, and R. B. Reynolds. 2012. *Fundamentals of Law for Health Informatics and Information Management*, 2nd ed., revised reprint. Chicago: AHIMA.

2.31

Confidentiality statement

Subdomain II.B.1
Apply confidentiality, privacy, and security measures and policies and procedures for internal and external use and exchange to protect electronic health information.

Subdomain II.B.3
Apply system security policies according to departmental and organizational data/information standards

Subdomain II.B.5
Develop educational programs for employees in privacy, security, and confidentiality

Your HIM department is going to begin taking students as part of their Professional Practice Experience (PPE). Your HIM Director wants to have a confidentiality statement signed by the students before they begin their PPE. She has asked you to compose a draft for her approval.

References

AHIMA. 2014. Professional Practice Experience Guide. Version IV.

AHIMA. 2010. Information Security—An Overview (Updated).

2.32

Encryption

Subdomain II.B.3
Collaborate in the design and implementation of risk assessment, contingency planning, and data recovery procedures

Compare and contrast symmetric and asymmetric encryption. If you are looking for the most secure type of encryption for your organization which would you choose and why?

References

Sandefer, R. 2016. Health Information Technologies. Chapter 12 in *Health Information Management: Concepts, Principles, and Practice*, 5th ed. Oachs, P. and A. Watters, eds. Chicago: AHIMA.

Sayles, N. B. and K. C. Trawick. 2014. *Introduction to Computer Systems for Health Information Technology*, 2nd ed. Chicago: AHIMA.

2.33

Authentication

 Subdomain II.B.3
Collaborate in the design and implementation of risk assessment, contingency planning, and data recovery procedures

You have outsourced your emergency room coding to an independent contractor. Your IT department is requiring a two-factor authentication method for that contractor as an added layer of security. Evaluate the options that you have (use of tokens, biometrics, or telephone call back) and make a method recommendation supporting your choice.

References

Brinda, D. and A. Watters. 2016. Data Privacy, Confidentiality, and Security. Chapter 11 in *Health Information Management: Concepts, Principles, and Practice*, 5th ed. Oachs, P. and A. Watters, eds. Chicago: AHIMA.

Sandefer, R. 2016. Health Information Technologies. Chapter 12 in *Health Information Management: Concepts, Principles, and Practice*, 5th ed. Oachs, P. and A. Watters, eds. Chicago: AHIMA.

Sayles, N. B. and K. C. Trawick. 2014. *Introduction to Computer Systems for Health Information Technology*, 2nd ed. Chicago: AHIMA.

2.34

Release of information policy

Subdomain II.C.1
Create policies and procedures to manage access and disclosure of personal health information

In recent weeks, there have been several questions emerge about releasing information of minors.

You have been asked to compose a procedure that addresses a minor's release of information to adoptive parents, biological parents of adopted minors, noncustodial parents, foster parents, and to an emancipated minor. Create that procedure for each type of release and note whether or not releasing information is appropriate.

References

Brodnik, M. S., L. A. Rinehart-Thompson, and R. B. Reynolds. 2012. *Fundamentals of Law for Health Informatics and Information Management,* 2nd ed., revised reprint. Chicago: AHIMA.

2.35

Retention and destruction

Subdomain II.B.2
Apply retention and destruction policies for health information

Below are several scenarios related to health record retention and destruction. Draw a conclusion for each scenario, based on health information guidelines, regulations, or best practices.

1. Your organization keeps paper records for ten years, and you are purging records for destruction. What concern do you have with staff pulling records strictly based on that ten year indicator?

2. Your HIM department is moving to a new office. In the moving process, in the back of a storage closet, a box of old registries is found. These contain records of births at the organization 50 years ago. What should be done with those records?

3. There has been debate in your HIM department about how long fetal monitoring strips must be retained. They are considered part of the mother's health record. What is your recommendation?

4. You have just taken a new job at a tertiary care facility after working in a small community hospital. At your previous employment, records were retained for 15 years and then destroyed. At this new facility, records are maintained permanently. What inference can you draw from this difference in procedure?

5. You have just become HIM director at a small critical access hospital. The hospital purges records for destruction quarterly, and the staff has all the records boxed and ready to go. The destruction company workers arrive to collect the records and load them into the truck. They are preparing to leave, but you stop them. Why?

References

Brodnik, M. S., L. A. Rinehart-Thompson, and R. B. Reynolds. 2012. *Fundamentals of Law for Health Informatics and Information Management,* 2nd ed., revised reprint. Chicago: AHIMA.

CHAPTER 3

Domain III: Informatics, Analytics, and Data Use

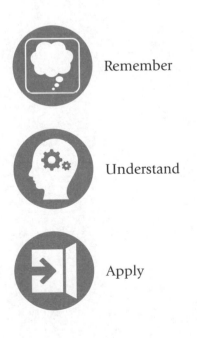 Remember

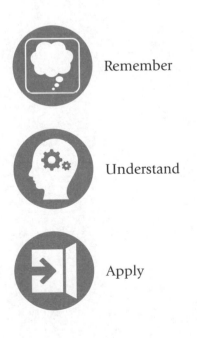 Understand

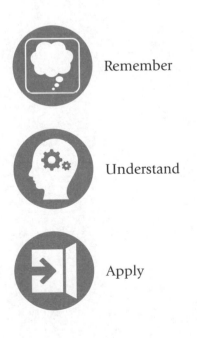 Apply

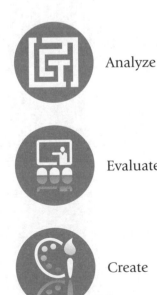 Analyze

 Evaluate

 Create

3.0

Inpatient census days

Subdomain III.D.1
Utilize basic descriptive, institutional, and healthcare statistics

Subdomain III.C.2
Apply data extraction methodologies

The HIM director for Pine Valley Community Hospital, which is a critical access hospital, verifies the inpatient service day calculations done by the nursing staff daily.

On Thursday, the census began with 17 inpatients. Of those patients, two were discharged, and one died. Then, four patients were admitted, with one transferred to another facility.

The nursing staff reported 17 inpatient service days. The HIM director is reporting 18. Compare nursing staff and HIM director reporting. Based on this comparison, who is correct and why?

References

Horton, L. A. 2016. *Calculating and Reporting Healthcare Statistics*, 5th ed. Chicago: AHIMA.

3.1

Average daily census

Subdomain III.D.1
Utilize basic descriptive, institutional, and healthcare statistics

Subdomain III.C.2
Apply data extraction methodologies

As HIM director of West General Hospital, you have been asked to supply the following statistics based on the inpatient service days for the first quarter of this year (non-leap year). Your facility has 150 adult beds, 15 pediatric beds, and 20 bassinets.

Table 3.1 West General Community Hospital Inpatient Service Days 1st Quarter 20xx

West General Community Hospital Inpatient Service Days 1st Quarter 20xx	
Type of Service	Service Days
Adult	10430
Pediatric	1077
Newbom	1505

1. What was the average daily census for newborns in the first quarter? (Round to nearest whole number)
2. What was the average daily census for adults and children in the first quarter? (Round to the nearest whole number)

References

Horton, L. A. 2016. *Calculating and Reporting Healthcare Statistics,* 5th ed. Chicago: AHIMA.

3.2

Bed occupancy rate and change

Subdomain III.D.1
Utilize basic descriptive, institutional, and healthcare statistics

Subdomain III.C.2
Apply data extraction methodologies

The Chief of Pediatrics at West General Hospital is interested in the bed occupancy rate for the pediatric unit for the first quarter of the year.

1. Use the information from exercise 3.1 to supply the data requested, and round to one decimal point.

2. How does the bed occupancy rate for the pediatric unit alone compare with the overall (adults and pediatric patients) bed occupancy rate for the facility?

    Again, use the data from exercise 3.1 to make the comparison. (Round to one decimal point)

3. Calculate the change in the pediatric bed occupancy rate if the bed count changed on February first from 10 beds to 15 beds and stayed at that level throughout the remainder of the first quarter.

    Use the information from exercise 3.1 and above to supply the data requested.

References

Horton, L. A. 2016. *Calculating and Reporting Healthcare Statistics*, 5th ed. Chicago: AHIMA.

3.3

Length of Stay/ALOS

Subdomain III.D.1
Utilize basic descriptive, institutional, and healthcare statistics

Subdomain III.C.2
Apply data extraction methodologies

The HIM director for Pine Valley Community Hospital, a critical access hospital, was reviewing the length of stay for recently discharged patients. Below, this table lists the discharges for the last two weeks of May.

- Calculate the length of stay for each discharge.
- Calculate the total length of all the stays.
- Calculate the average length of stay for all discharges. PVCH LOS

Pine Valley Community Hospital Length of Stay		
Date admitted	**Date discharged**	**Length of Stay**
5/14	5/14 (died)	
5/14	5/17	
5/14	5/21	
5/15	5/21	
5/15	5/18	
5/16	5/21 (died)	
5/16	5/21	
5/17	5/21	
5/17	5/21	
5/18	5/28	
5/18	5/22	
5/18	5/22	
5/19	5/19	
5/19	5/21	
5/20	5/28	
5/21	5/22	
5/22	5/28	
5/23	5/28	
5/23	5/28	
5/24	6/4	
Total		

References

Horton, L. A. 2016. *Calculating and Reporting Healthcare Statistics,* 5th ed. Chicago: AHIMA.

3.4

Average daily census/ALOS

Subdomain III.D.1
Utilize basic descriptive, institutional, and healthcare statistics

Subdomain III.C.2
Apply data extraction methodologies

Based on the data supplied below, solve for the answer to the following questions.

Round answers to two decimal places unless otherwise directed.

1. What is the inpatient nosocomial infection rate for the hospital?
2. What was the anesthetic death rate?
3. What is the maternal death rate?
4. What is the fetal death rate?
5. What is the post-operative infection rate?

References

Horton, L. A. 2016. *Calculating and Reporting Healthcare Statistics,* 5th ed. Chicago: AHIMA.

3.5

IT audit

Subdomain III.A.4
Take part in the development of networks, including intranet and internet applications

Random IT audits have been showing an increase in the number of non-work related websites that are being accessed, such as Facebook, Ticketmaster, QVC, etc.

- Propose a simple IT solution that could prevent this access and discuss the variety of different ways that the solution is effective.

References

Sayles, N. B. and K. C. Trawick. 2014. *Introduction to Computer Systems for Health Information Technology*, 2nd ed. Chicago: AHIMA.

3.6

Electronic signature

Subdomain III.A.2
Assess systems capabilities to meet regulatory requirements

A physician has asked your opinion regarding electronically signing his reports. He knows that his EHR will support digital, digitized, and electronic signatures, but he needs clarification about the differences. Give your opinion about which type of signature to use and justify your selection.

References

Sayles, N. B. and K. C. Trawick. 2014. *Introduction to Computer Systems for Health Information Technology*, 2nd ed. Chicago: AHIMA.

3.7

Information management plan

Subdomain III.B.1
Take part in the development of information management plans that support the organization's current and future strategy and goals

Your organization's strategic plan incorporates the following tenets:

- Excel in quality patient care
- Provide exceptional service
- Enhance the patient care environment and facility infrastructure
- Foster partnership
  - Internally-staff, physicians, leadership
  - Externally-community
- Maintain financial stability through efficiency and growth

The information management plan needs to be updated to espouse those principles. Determine an objective that would fit each of these tenets to incorporate in the information management plan and supply the rationale(s) for each objectives inclusion.

References

Gordon, L. and M. Gordon. 2016. Management. Chapter 19 in *Health Information Management Technology: An Applied Approach*, 5th ed. Sayles, N.B. and L. Gordon, eds. Chicago: AHIMA

3.8

HIM department strategic plan

 Subdomain III.B.1
Take part in the development of information management plans that support the organization's current and future strategy and goals

Your organization's strategic plan incorporates the following tenets:
- Excel in quality patient care
- Provide exceptional service
- Enhance the patient care environment and facility infrastructure
- Foster partnership
  - Internally-staff, physicians, leadership
  - Externally-community
- Maintain financial stability through efficiency and growth

Create an HIM mission and vision statement that promotes those principles.

References

Gordon, L. and M. Gordon. 2016. *Health Information Management Technology: An Applied Approach*, 5th ed. Sayles, N.B. and L. Gordon, eds. Chicago: AHIMA.

3.9

Coding intranet

Subdomain III.A.4
Take part in the development of networks, including intranet and Internet applications

As Coding Supervisor you have requested and received permission to establish an intranet specifically for coding staff. Recommend elements to include on the site.

Create a screen design for the items you have selected.

References

Sayles, N. B. and K. C. Trawick. 2014. *Introduction to Computer Systems for Health Information Technology*, 2nd ed. Chicago: AHIMA.

3.10

Password management

Subdomain III.H.2
Implement policies and procedures to ensure data integrity internal and external to the enterprise

1. At Pine Valley Community Hospital (PVCH), passwords are required to be a minimum of five characters and must contain one number. HIM clerk Julie was hired more than a year ago and has yet to be prompted to change her password. This gave her concern, as she recalled password-management best practices from her recent studies.

   • What recommendations might Julie make to improve password management at PVCH? Create an example of a secure password and justify the selection.

2. Determine if this password would meet the requirements you provided and justify your response.

References

Sayles, N. B. and K. C. Trawick. 2014. *Introduction to Computer Systems for Health Information Technology*, 2nd ed. Chicago: AHIMA.

3.11

Research methodology

Subdomain III.E.1
Explain common research methodologies and why they are used in healthcare

A classmate is struggling to understand the concepts of qualitative, quantitative, and mixed methods as they relate to research methodologies. Explain these concepts to help him better understand.

References

Forrestal, E. 2016. Research Methods. Chapter 19 in *Health Information Management: Concepts, Principles, and Practice*, 5th ed. Oachs, P. and A. Watters, eds. Chicago: AHIMA.

3.12

Literature review (Medline)

 Subdomain III.E.1
Apply principles of research and clinical literature evaluation to improve outcomes

The chief of obstetrics and gynecology has requested your help with some research. She is hoping to initiate single-site robotic hysterectomies at your hospital. However, administration is requesting details about the procedure, including its safety, and how it compares with standard laparoscopic hysterectomy.

- Make use of Medline to find at least five relevant articles that will assist the OB-GYN chief in making her case with administration. Present your answers in the preferred bibliographic format.

Further Student Reading

Oachs, P. and A. Watters. 2016. *Health Information Management: Concepts, Principles, and Practice*, 5th ed. Chicago: AHIMA.

3.13

Informed consent IRB

Subdomain III.E.2
Plan adherence to Institutional Review Board (IRB) processes and policies

Because of your HIM background, your pregnant cousin has e-mailed you a copy of the informed consent that she received regarding participation in a research study on gestational diabetes.. Assess the document based on the criteria for research informed consents and provide her with your opinion. Be sure to defend your judgment.

Research on the topic of Gestational Diabetes Management

You are invited to participate in a research study examining the effects of Metformin in the treatment of gestational diabetes. The decision to engage in participation or not is strictly yours. This study plans to address the correlation between the use of Metformin and the effect it may have on the fetus.

Participants will engage in a double-blind research study. You will take a medication to treat your gestational diabetes, and will have regular follow-up appointments with our team of physicians, as will your infant after birth. This study will begin at the onset of the gestational diabetes diagnosis and follow you through the first year of the infant's life.

Your participation in the study may be terminated at the discretion of the investigators without your consent.

Risks that may be associated with the study include:

- Adverse effects of the medications

The benefit from this research may include control of your gestational diabetes, but there is no guarantee. Women who become pregnant in the future and their children may benefit from the information obtained from this study.

Medications will be provided free of charge while participating in this study. Physician visits for the infant will be covered monthly after delivery. Mileage to these visits will be paid.

Your participation in this research study is voluntary. There is no requirement to participate or to continue participation once you have started. You will incur no penalty nor lose any benefits that you are entitled to if you decide to terminate your participation. Your relationship with our health network will not suffer as a result of termination.

You may call J. Jackson at 999-999-9999 or e-mail J. Jackson at J.Jackson@health.hlt with any questions that you have. This includes questions regarding the study, or questions regarding physical or psychological issues that are developing which you believe to be unusual or unexpected.

CONSENT OF SUBJECT
(or Legally Authorized Representative)

_____   _____
Signature of Subject or Representative   Date

References

Watzlaf, V. 2016. Biomedical and Research Support. Chapter 20 in *Health Information Management: Concepts, Principles, and Practice*, 5th ed. Oachs, P. and A. Watters, eds. Chicago: AHIMA.

3.14

AHIMA Foundation research

Subdomain III.E.1
Explain common research methodologies and why they are used in healthcare

Subdomain III.E.1
Apply principles of research and clinical literature evaluation to improve outcomes

1. Locate the article, "The Growth in the Clinical Documentation Specialist Profession" from the AHIMA Foundation's online research journal, *Educational Perspectives in Health Informatics and Information Management*. Determine the research methodology used for the data collection on this topic. Defend this choice of methodology.

2. Interpret the response rate for this data collection and give your opinion regarding its significance, include factors that impact response rate.

References

Barnhouse, T. and W. Rudman. 2013. The growth in the clinical documentation specialist profession. *Educational Perspectives in Health Informatics and Information Management*. 1–7.

Forrestal, E. 2016. Research Methods. Chapter 19 in *Health Information Management: Concepts, Principles, and Practice*, 5th ed. Oachs, P. and A. Watters, eds. Chicago: AHIMA.

3.15

PHR choices

Subdomain III.F.1
Explain usability and accessibility of health information by patients, including current trends and future challenges

Subdomain III.F.1
Educate consumers on patient-centered health information

Your 70-year-old retired grandfather is very computer-literate. He also has multiple health issues and sees a number of different specialists. He recently heard about personal health records and would like you to explain the various options to him. Provide your grandfather with the requested information and advise him on which selection might best suit his needs.

References

AHIMA Personal Health Record Practice Council. 2006. Helping consumers select PHRs: questions and considerations for navigating an emerging market. *Journal of AHIMA* 77(10):50–56.

3.16

Patient-centered medical home

Subdomain III.F.1
Explain usability and accessibility of health information by patients, including current trends and future challenges

Subdomain III.F.1
Educate consumers on patient-centered health information

1. Explain the concept of patient-centered medical home (PCMH).
2. Discover how information technology will foster PCMH.

References

Casto, A. B. and E. Forrestal. 2013. *Principles of Healthcare Reimbursement*, 4th ed. Chicago: AHIMA.

Dimick, C. 2008. Home sweet medical home: can a new care model save family medicine? *Journal of AHIMA* 79(8):24–28.

3.17

IRB vulnerable populations

Subdomain III.E.2
Plan adherence to Institutional Review Board (IRB) processes and policies

As the new director of HIM for Oak Ridge Regional Hospital, one of your duties is to serve as a resource for the Institutional Review Board (IRB). You are reviewing their policies and procedures to familiarize yourself with the IRB's functions, and are concerned when you do not find any mention of "vulnerable subjects." As you prepare for a meeting with the IRB, what recommendations will you make in regards to addressing vulnerable subjects, and how will you defend your position?

References

Watzlaf, V. 2016. Biomedical and Research Support. Chapter 20 in *Health Information Management: Concepts, Principles, and Practice*, 5th ed. Oachs, P. and A. Watters, eds. Chicago: AHIMA.

3.18

HIE models

Subdomain III.G.3
Differentiate between various models for health information exchange

1. Evaluate the three different models of health information exchanges (HIEs): centralized, federated, and hybrid, and include how privacy and security practices will determine which model is implemented.

2. Evaluate the opt-in and opt-out selections for patients as they relate to HIEs and justify your opinion on which selection has the better chance for success and why.

References

AHIMA Thought Leadership Series. 2012. Ensuring Data Integrity in Health Information Exchange. http://library.ahima.org/xpedio/groups/public/documents/ahima/bok1_049675.pdf.

AHIMA. 2010. Understanding the HIE landscape. *Journal of AHIMA* 81(9):60–65.

3.19

HIE policies and procedures

 Subdomain III.G.1
Collaborate in the development of operational policies and procedures for health information exchange

A health information exchange (HIE) is being established in your area and there are openings for individuals with an HIM background. You learn that one of the primary tasks will be writing policies and procedures. Discover at least five policy topics that an HIM professional could contribute to in an HIE setting.

References

AHIMA. 2011. HIE management and operational considerations. *Journal of AHIMA* 82(5):56–61.

3.20

HIE challenges

Subdomain III.G.1
Explain current trends and future challenges in health information exchange

As an HIM professional, you have been asked to take part in an open community forum regarding health information exchanges (HIEs). You are anticipating that there will be questions about the challenges that face HIE adoption. Prepare for these questions by identifying at least three HIE challenges.

References

Berry, K. 2013. HIE quality check. *Journal of AHIMA* 84(2):28–32.

3.21

HIE and data integrity

Subdomain III.G.2
Conduct system testing to ensure data integrity and quality of health information exchange

Suppose you are an HIM professional employed at a health information exchange with 25 component organizations and you see the following report. Discuss these results relative to data integrity.

- Propose at least five steps to remediate the issue.

MRN	SSN	Last Name	First Name	Middle	DOB	Payment
47233	546-23-XXXX	Baker Sr.	Louis	Howard	5/18/1954	Medicaid
158237	315-24-XXXX	Watson	Michelle	Lee	7/22/1942	Medicare
520613	588-32-XXXX	Jones	Lynn	Tara	10/12/1963	Commercial
723341	213-22-XXXX	Harris	Ann	Marie	9/10/1952	Self
894231	588-32-XXXX	Jones	Tara	Lynn	10/21/1963	Commercial
189011	533-44-XXXX	Marshall	Tucker	B.	11/4/1961	Commercial
218220	151-24-XXXX	Leonard	Timothy	Allen	6/17/1943	Medicare
797536	213-22-XXXX	Harris-Smythe	Ann	Marie	9/10/1952	Commercial
36524	315-24-XXXX	Watson	Michelle	Lee	7/22/1924	Medicare
466100	546-23-XXXX	Baker	Louis	Howard	5/18/1945	Medicare
744183	626-26-XXXX	Baker	Louis	Howard	4/18/1965	Commercial
118231	641-58-XXXX	Thomas	Paul	Carlson	1/16/1971	Self
237352	641-58-XXXX	Carlson	Thomas	Paul	1/16/1971	Self
898233	213-22-XXXX	HarrisSmythe	Ann	Marie	9/1/1952	Commercial
789321	151-24-XXXX	Allen	Timothy	Leonard	6/17/1934	Medicare
664455	213-22-XXXX	SmytheHarris	Ann	Marie	9/1/1925	Commercial
98723	315-42-XXXX	Watson	Michelle	Lee	7/22/1924	Medicare
587532	546-23-XXXX	Baker	Howard	Louis	5/18/1954	Medicaid

References

Landsbach, G. and B. Just. 2013. Five risky HIE practices that threaten data integrity. *Journal of AHIMA* 84(11):40–42.

3.22

System testing

Your information technology department has several system applications due to go live at the same time. They have asked you as the coding supervisor to move up the installation of your encoder to help them free up some time. No testing has been done yet with the new encoder. Defend your position to wait until the testing is complete to proceed with the installation.

References

Sayles, N. B. and K. C. Trawick. 2014. *Introduction to Computer Systems for Health Information Technology*, 2nd ed. Chicago: AHIMA.

3.23

Data normalization

Subdomain III.C.5
Apply knowledge of database querying and data exploration and mining techniques to facilitate information retrieval

1. Illustrate how you would apply normalization to the following patient demographic data.

   Margaret C. Whitfield (Johnson)

   123 North West Street, Pine Valley, OH 44444

   62 years old, 10/13/52

   Blue Cross/Blue Shield 123 East Market St., Lansing, MI 55555

2. What is an organization's motivation for ensuring the normalization of data?

References

Sayles, N. B. and K. C. Trawick. 2014. *Introduction to Computer Systems for Health Information Technology*, 2nd ed. Chicago: AHIMA.

3.24

Data quality model

Subdomain III.H.5
Model policy initiatives that influence data integrity

Select three data elements from AHIMA's Data Quality Model and identify how an HIM director would factor them into running reports for quality management.

References

Sayles, N. B. and K. C. Trawick. 2014. *Introduction to Computer Systems for Health Information Technology*, 2nd ed. Chicago: AHIMA.

3.25

Data integrity

Subdomain III.H.5
Model policy initiatives that influence data integrity

1. In your current electronic health record (EHR), registration clerks often bypass the diagnosis field. This is a problem, since coders work from a list which pulls that information to be coded. What initiative can you request with your next update to eliminate that problem?

2. If you implement the initiative you identified, will the problem be totally eliminated? Explain your answer.

References

Sayles, N. B. and K. C. Trawick. 2014. *Introduction to Computer Systems for Health Information Technology*, 2nd ed. Chicago: AHIMA.

3.26

PDA vs. Laptop

 Subdomain III.A.3
Recommend device selection based on workflow, ergonomic, and human factors

As office manager for the new Oakmont Physician Group, you are trying to get all physicians to utilize laptops for office use to facilitate care and reduce costs. Two of the group's physicians are concerned about laptop security. Defend your recommendation by supplying at least five security features that can be undertaken with laptops to heighten security.

References

AHIMA. 2012. Mobile Device Security (2012 update). *Journal of AHIMA* 83(4):50–55.

3.27

Thin client

Subdomain III.A.I
Utilize technology for data collection, storage, analysis, and reporting of information

At a morning meeting, Joe, the information technology manager of the newly formed Oakmont Physician Group, announced that he wants to initiate a thin client/server network for the practice. One of the physicians approaches you after the meeting and asks for you to educate her on what that means. Provide an explanation to help her understand that concept.

References

Sayles, N. B. and K. C. Trawick. 2014. *Introduction to Computer Systems for Health Information Technology*, 2nd ed. Chicago: AHIMA.

3.28

Denial dashboard

Subdomain III.C.I
Apply analytical results to facilitate decision-making

The denial management coordinator at Pine Valley Community Hospital provides administration with the following dashboard information monthly. As the revenue cycle manager for the facility, you also receive a copy of this dashboard. Formulate four questions that you would have as a result of studying this dashboard and provide the rationale for your question.

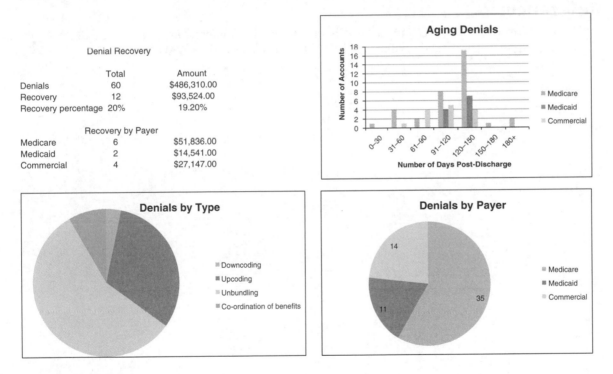

Denial Recovery

	Total	Amount
Denials	60	$486,310.00
Recovery	12	$93,524.00
Recovery percentage	20%	19.20%

Recovery by Payer

Medicare	6	$51,836.00
Medicaid	2	$14,541.00
Commercial	4	$27,147.00

References

Swenson, D. X. 2016. Managing and Leading During Organizational Change. Chapter 22 in *Health Information Management: Concepts, Principles, and Practice*, 5th ed. Chicago: AHIMA.

3.29

Intrusion detection

Subdomain III.H.I
Discover threats to data integrity and validity

As the information technology manager for a large physician practice, you are concerned about unauthorized system access. You want to invest in an intrusion detection system (IDS) to monitor the IT system in real-time. Defend this choice to the practice physicians who are reluctant to invest in an IDS.

References

Rinehart-Thompson, L. 2016. Data Security. Chapter 10 in *Health Information Management Technology: An Applied Approach*, 5th ed. Sayles, N.B. and L. Gordon, eds. Chicago: AHIMA.

3.30

Quality management tools

Subdomain III.H.3
Apply quality management tools

Choose the appropriate quality management tool for each scenario presented below and defend your selection.

1. Your multi-disciplinary performance improvement team is working on solutions to bed turnaround time. You have collected data on the issue and there are seven main problems. Recommend the quality management tool to use to prioritize the problems by identifying those most responsible for them.

2. Unfortunately, your healthcare organization has experienced a sentinel event, which is an unexpected death or serious physical injury. You will be part of the team that works on the root cause analysis. What quality management tool is most often used in this process?

3. The chief of staff is helping the HIM department reduce the number of delinquent charts. He has asked for an illustration that shows the various medical departments (orthopedics, dermatology, ophthalmology, urology, respiratory) and the percentage of the overall delinquencies for which they are responsible. What quality management tool will show this information appropriately?

4. Your performance improvement team has been tracking a key process improvement for the past year. What quality management tool will be of assistance in tracking any variances?

5. A process improvement team is collecting data to determine if there is a correlation between medication errors and pharmacy tech overtime. What is the best tool to plot this data?

References

Shaw, P. L. and D. Carter. 2015. *Quality and Performance Improvement in Healthcare, A Tool for Programmed Learning,* 6th ed. Chicago: AHIMA.

Watzlaf, V. 2016. Research and Data Analysis. Chapter 13 in *Health Information Management Technology: An Applied Approach*, 5th ed. Sayles, N.B. and L. Gordon, eds. Chicago: AHIMA.

3.31

Database structure

Subdomain III.A.6
Create the electronic structure of health data to meet a variety of end user needs

Elaborate on the ability of the relational database structure to meet user needs.

References

Sayles, N. B. and K. C. Trawick. 2014. *Introduction to Computer Systems for Health Information Technology*, 2nd ed. Chicago: AHIMA.

Sharp, M. 2016. Secondary Data Sources. Chapter 7 in *Health Information Management: Concepts, Principles, and Practice*, 5th ed. Oachs, P. and A. Watters, eds. Chicago: AHIMA.

3.32

Delivery statistics

Subdomain I.D.5
Evaluate data from varying sources to create meaningful presentations

Subdomain III.C.3
Recommend organizational action based on knowledge obtained from data exploration and mining

Subdomain III.C.4
Analyze clinical data to identify trends that demonstrate quality, safety, and effectiveness of healthcare

Subdomain III.D.1
Interpret inferential statistics

1. In 2010, the chief of obstetrics became concerned about the c-section rate at Oakwood Memorial Hospital. The national rate for c-section delivery at that time was 32.8 percent. A report at that time provided the following data.

Oakwood Memorial Births	
	2010
Vaginal	332
Cesarean	179
Total	511

- Determine if his concern is warranted.
- Predict the next course of action by the Chief of Obstetrics based on this information.

2. In the early months of 2016, the new chief of obstetrics asked for a report from the past six years that shows the vaginal and cesarean births. You supply the following information.

Oakwood Memorial Births						
	2010	2011	2012	2013	2014	2015
Vaginal	332	350	356	388	391	369
Cesarean	179	206	178	183	168	155
Total	511	556	534	571	559	524

- The chief of obstetrics wants to know how her department performs against the current national c-section rate of 32.7 percent. Compile the data to answer her question.
- Create a graph to show the C-section rate trend over the past six years.

3. The chief now wants to know if there is any correlation between the number of c-sections and maternal deaths versus those that occur after a vaginal delivery. You take the information from 2015 and compile this Chi square.

	Maternal death	No maternal death	Total
Vaginal delivery	1	368	369
C-section delivery	4	151	155
Total	5	519	524

If our null hypothesis is that there is no correlation between delivery method and maternal death, and the result of our Chi square is $p = 0.013$, what interpretation do you give the chief of obstetrics?

References

Horton, L. A. 2016. *Calculating and Reporting Healthcare Statistics*, 5th ed. Chicago: AHIMA.

3.33

Critical access hospital LOS

Subdomain I.D.5
Evaluate data from varying sources to create meaningful presentations

Subdomain III.C.3
Recommend organizational action based on knowledge obtained from data exploration and mining

Subdomain III.C.4
Analyze clinical data to identify trends that demonstrate quality, safety, and effectiveness of healthcare

Subdomain III.D.2
Analyze statistical data for decision making

As HIM director for a critical access hospital (CAH), you track the average length of stay for the facility. This is a critical piece of information since CMS requires that a CAH have an annual average length of stay of 96 hours or less per patient.

1. Using the data below, solve for the ALOS for the month of February 2015 and test if it meets the ALOS goal.

2. Calculate the standard deviation for this data.

Length of stay (in days)	Number of patients
1	5
2	13
3	23
4	21
5	9
6	3
7	1
8	1
10	1
12	1

3. Using the data below, determine if the facility met the goal for the month of August.

4. Based on the data below, what further action would you propose?

Length of stay (in days)	Number of patients
2	6
3	12
4	14
5	10
6	7
7	8
8	16
9	10
10	4
11	2
12	3
15	3
18	4
19	1
20	1

5. Create a control chart to show the ALOS by physician using the data below.

Physician	Number of patients	Length of stay (in days)
Dr. Mellendorf	14	75
Dr. Snodgrass	15	82
Dr. Gunion	20	137
Dr. Oliver	38	342
Dr. Joyce	14	88
Total		

6. Theorize at least three reasons that the ALOS requirement was not met.

7. Based on the results illustrated on the control chart, predict which actions, if any, should be taken by the organization?

8. Create a control chart to depict the 2015 annual ALOS based on the following information.

Jan	4.12
Feb	3.64
March	3.39
April	4.79
May	5.23
June	3.21
July	3.03
Aug	7.17
Sept	3.77
Oct	4.18
Nov	3.54
Dec	3.89

9. What deductions can you make based on this control chart?

10. The control chart does not indicate if the hospital met the annual goal of an ALOS of four days (96 hours) or less. Using the data given, solve for that answer.

Further Student Reading

Horton, L. A. 2016. *Calculating and Reporting Healthcare Statistics,* 5th ed. Chicago: AHIMA.

3.34

Strategic planning

Subdomain III.B.2
Utilize health information to support enterprise-wide decision support for strategic planning

Subdomain III.C.2
Apply report generation technologies to facilitate decision-making

Subdomain III.C.6
Evaluate administrative reports using appropriate software

1. At a recent department head meeting, your organization's CEO indicated that there is discussion about purchasing a lithotripsy machine. What can you assume will be HIM's role in these discussions?

2. You asked your assistant director to run a report for the CEO on the number of patients transferred out for open heart surgery. This is a preliminary investigation to determine if the organization should pursue the expansion of the heart center to include performing open heart surgery. Analyze the following section of the report to identify any errors before you send it on to the CEO.

Patient MRN	Patient Name	Physician	Date of Admission	Date of Discharge	Discharge Disposition
025124	James, T.	Smith	1/3/2015	1/3/2015	X-H
067481	Henderson, P.	Jones	7/22/2015	7/23/2015	X-H
129530	Lewis, J.	Baker	4/15/2015	4/19/2015	X-SNF
088352	Marigold, B.	Conrad	5/12/2015	5/15/2015	X-H
046721	Goodwin, D.	Heller	1/29/2015	1/30/2015	X-H
033799	Summers, T.	Peterson	2/28/2015	3/3/2015	X-NH
080808	Behringer, L.	McMurray	6/23/2015	7/2/2015	X-HO
163540	Lockhart, I.	Campbell	9/12/2015	9/16/2015	X-SNF
118912	Singh, O.	Smith	10/12/2015	10/14/2015	X-H
134577	Packer, W.	Heller	12/1/2015	12/1/2015	X-H
018297	Wade, H.	Jones	4/25/2015	5/1/2015	X-SNF
094722	Lawson, B.	Thompson	10/12/2015	10/13/2015	X-H
075831	Clinger, C.	Smith	11/7/2015	11/8/2015	X-H
039854	DiCesare, D.	Heller	2/3/2015	2/3/2015	X-H
064721	Watson, C.	Peterson	3/18/2015	3/21/2015	X-H

X-H	transfer to hospital			
X-NH	transfer to nursing home			
X-SNF	transfer to skilled nursing home			
X-HO	transfer to hospice			

3. What overall conclusion can you reach about the report?

4. The chief of staff requests a report from HIM on all the patients who have sepsis that died in 2015. Below is a sample of the criteria used to run the report. Evaluate it for accuracy and recommend changes if necessary, justifying your change(s).

Patient Medical Record Number	all
Patient Name	all
Discharge Date	01/01/15-12/13/15
Discharge Disposition	X=expired
MS-DRG	870, 871, 872

References

McClernon, S.E. 2016. Strategic Thinking and Management. Chapter 29 in *Health Information Management: Concepts, Principles, and Practice*, 5th ed. Oachs, P. and A. Watters. Chicago: AHIMA.

3.35

ROI tracking log

Subdomain III.A.1
Utilize health information to support enterprise-wide decision support for strategic planning

You have been hired as a release of information (ROI) clerk at Pine Valley Community Hospital, which is a small critical access hospital. They keep a manual log of all the requests for patient information. Take part in a discussion with your HIM director regarding the benefits of an automated ROI tracking system.

References

Rinehart-Thompson, L. A. 2016. Data Privacy and Confidentiality. Chapter 9 in *Health Information Management Technology: An Applied Approach*, 5th ed. Sayles, N.B. and L. Gordon, eds. Chicago: AHIMA.

Bock, L. J., B. Demster, A. Dinh, E. Gorton, J. Lantis. 2008. Management Practices for the Release of Information. *Journal of AHIMA* 79(11): 77-80.

3.36

Network security procedures

Subdomain III.A.2
Explain policies and procedures of networks, including intranet and Internet to facilitate clinical and administrative applications

Compare and contrast firewalls and intrusion detection systems.

References

Sayles, N. B. and K. C. Trawick. 2014. *Introduction to Computer Systems for Health Information Technology*, 2nd ed. Chicago: AHIMA.

3.37

Best of....

Subdomain III.B.1
Explain the process used in the selection and implementation of health information management systems

There has been much discussion in your organization regarding the purchase of an EHR. Two factions are squaring off in the discussions: those that favor best of fit, and those that favor best of breed. Explain the difference between the two.

References

Sayles, N. B. and K. C. Trawick. 2014. *Introduction to Computer Systems for Health Information Technology*, 2nd ed. Chicago: AHIMA.

3.38

Data analytics—decision support

Subdomain III.C.1
Explain analytics and decision support

1. Explain the value of a decision-support system.
2. Relate how a dashboard is effective as part of a decision-support system.

References

Sayles, N. B. and K. C. Trawick. 2014. *Introduction to Computer Systems for Health Information Technology*, 2nd ed. Chicago: AHIMA.

3.39

Delivery analysis

Subdomain III.D.2
Analyze data to identify trends

The chief of obstetrics is asking for a six year trend of vaginal versus cesarean section deliveries.

You supply the following graph.

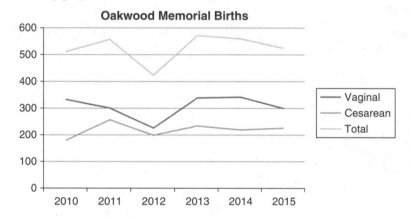

- Knowing that the national average of c-sections is running at 32.8 percent, what inferences can you make about the hospital's c-section rate based on analysis of this chart?

Using the national average and the hospital c-section rates, you now create this control chart.

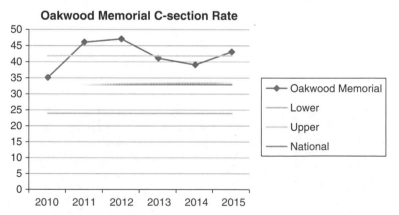

- What inferences can you make about the organization's cesarean section rate based on analysis of this chart?

Further Student Reading

Horton, L. A. 2016. *Calculating and Reporting Healthcare Statistics,* 5th ed. Chicago: AHIMA.

3.40

Corrections

Subdomain III.H.1
Apply policies and procedures to ensure the accuracy and integrity of health data both internal and external to the health system

You are the coding manager for a large city hospital. You outsource some overflow coding to a vendor. As the contact person for those coders, you sometimes get e-mails asking for discharge dates or dispositions to be entered so the account can be finalized. You would like those coders to be able to enter that information themselves to save you time. Your HIM director has a differing opinion. What explanations would lead you to support her position?

References

Sayles, N. B. 2016. Health Information Functions, Purposes, and Users. Chapter 3 in *Health Information Management Technology: An Applied Approach*, 5th ed. Sayles, N.B. and L. Gordon, eds. Chicago: AHIMA.

CHAPTER 4

Domain IV: Revenue Management

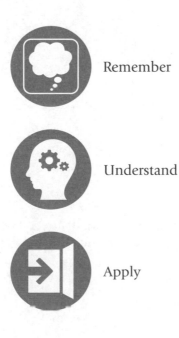

Remember

Analyze

Understand

Evaluate

Apply

Create

Revenue Cycle and Reimbursement

4.0

Case mix issue

Subdomain IV.A.1
Manage the use of clinical data required by various payment and reimbursement systems

Last year when you were hired as the HIM director at a small community hospital, the CEO wanted you to focus on increasing the case mix index. The hospital base rate is $7,862. At the time you came onboard, there were three coders; only one of whom was certified as a Certified Coding Specialist (CCS). You began by reviewing the number of MS-DRGs submitted over the past year. The MS-DRG that jumped out was: MS-DRG 304, which is hypertension with an MCC. There were 53 submissions of this MS-DRG. As you reviewed the data for 10 of those submissions you began to notice a trend. Evaluate the data below to identify the issue.

Chart	Codes submitted
1	I10, J44.9, N18.6, E11.9
2	I10, N18.6, E10.9, E03.9, G47.33
3	I10, G20, I25.10, N18.5
4	I10, F17.210, I70.213, N18.6, E11.9
5	I10, N18.6, I25.5, I25.10
6	I10, E08.22, N18.6
7	I10, E66.01, E03.9, N18.6, F17.210
8	I10, E87.6, J45.909, N18.6
9	I10, E11.9, E66.9, E78.5, N18.5
10	I10, I25.10, N18.6, R33.9, N18.G, E10.9

Further Student Reading

Centers for Medicare and Medicaid Services. 2016. Draft ICD-10-CM/PCS MS-DRGv28 Definitions Manual. List of MS-DRGs Version 28.0. https://www.cms.gov/icd10manual/fullcode_cms/P0368.html

Oachs, P. and A. Watters. 2016. *Health Information Management: Concepts, Principles, and Practice*, 5th ed. Chicago: AHIMA.

4.1

Case mix issue (Continued)

Subdomain IV.A.1
Manage the use of clinical data required by various payment and reimbursement systems

Continue using the same information from exercise 4.0.

After review of all 53 cases in MS-DRG 304, you determined that 46 of them had the same error.

Correcting the errors results in reassignment of those cases to a different MS-DRG. Calculate the impact this has on reimbursement by determining the relative weight of the two MS-DRGs and performing the calculations to determine the reimbursement difference.

Further Student Reading

Centers for Medicare and Medicaid Services. 2016. Draft ICD-10-CM/PCS MS-DRGv28 Definitions Manual. List of MS-DRGs Version 28.0. https://www.cms.gov/icd10manual/fullcode_cms/P0368.html

Oachs, P. and A. Watters. 2016. *Health Information Management: Concepts, Principles, and Practice*, 5th ed. Chicago: AHIMA.

4.2

Compliance and case mix

Subdomain IV.A.4
Implement processes for revenue cycle management and reporting

Subdomain V.A.2
Determine processes for compliance with current laws and standards related to health information initiatives and revenue cycle

Determine the aspects of a compliance plan that need to be addressed following the identification of coding errors such as those that were found in exercise 4.0, and explain why they must be tackled.

References

Casto, A. B. and E. Forrestal. 2015. *Principles of Healthcare Reimbursement*, 5th ed. Chicago: AHIMA.

4.3

Inpatient-only procedure denials

Subdomain IV.A.1
Apply policies and procedures for the use of data required in healthcare reimbursement

Subdomain III.H.4
Perform quality assessment, including quality management, data quality, and identification of best practices for health information systems

Subdomain IV.A.1
Manage the use of clinical data required by various payment and reimbursement systems

Your organization just opened a new service line: outpatient spinal fusions. The first cervical spinal fusions were done last week, and your coders have coded 10 of them. Unfortunately, several weeks and another 25 procedures later, you get a memo from the business office stating that there are denials on the Medicare fusions (17 to date). The billing manager states that it is something about a status indicator "C." She would like you to review the CPT code assignments and help determine what the problem is and how it can be resolved because the charges for these procedures exceed $35,000 per case.

After reviewing the cases, the CPT codes assigned are correct.
22551–arthrodesis cervical
*22845–anterior instrumentation
22851-use of biomechanical device (cage)
*20936-autograft of bone from same site
*denotes a status indicator of C for that CPT code

1. Explain to the billing manager what status indicator C means.

2. In order to facilitate a prompt resolution to this issue, you and the billing manager decide to create a process improvement team. Decide what hospital departments should be part of the team.

3. Brainstorm at least three possible solutions to the problem.

References

Hazelwood, A. and C. Venable. 2016. Reimbursement Methodologies. Chapter 7 in *Health Information Management: Concepts, Principles, and Practice*, 5th ed. Oachs, P. and A. Watters, eds. Chicago: AHIMA.

Shaw, P. L. and D. Carter. 2015. *Quality and Performance Improvement in Healthcare*, 6th ed. Chicago: AHIMA.

4.4

Chargemaster process

 Subdomain IV.A.2
Take part in selection and development of applications and processes for chargemaster and claims management

As the new HIM director at Pine Valley Community Hospital, a small critical access hospital, you are surprised to learn that there is no formal process in place for chargemaster maintenance. Requests for additions are supplied by individual departments directly to IT for entry into the chargemaster. No one has deleted any codes for years, and there has never been a systemic review of the chargemaster. You decide to design an improved process for chargemaster maintenance to present to the CEO. Present your newly formulated process below.

References

American Health Information Management Association. 2010. Care and maintenance of chargemasters (updated). http://library.ahima.org/xpedio/groups/public/documents/ahima/bok1_047258.hcsp?dDocName=bok1_047258

Malmgren, C. and C. J. Solberg. 2016. Revenue Cycle Management. Chapter 8 in *Health Information Management: Concepts, Principles, and Practice*, 5th ed. Oachs, P. and A. Watters, eds. Chicago: AHIMA.

4.5

Case management—discharge disposition

Subdomain IV.A.1
Apply policies and procedures for the use of data required in healthcare reimbursement

Your coding staff has been reporting an increase in the number of discharge dispositions that are incorrectly entered in the patients' records in the EHR. They have to take the time to investigate the correct disposition and make the change, which is causing a decrease in productivity and a corresponding increase in the discharged not final billed total. You have the staff complete a data collection over the next two weeks.

1. Using CMS information, determine the correct discharge status for the seven error types identified based on the information below.

2. Prepare an interpretation of the information and offer recommendations for error reduction to the case manager director.

Coding staff identified the following on review of 198 discharged charts in the two-week period:

Pine Valley Community Hospital–critical access hospital
Valley High Children's Hospital–children's hospital
Valley View Hospital–long-term care hospital
Big Valley VA Hospital–veteran's affairs hospital
Valley Vista–inpatient psychiatric hospital

Errors found were:

12 transfers to Pine Valley Community Hospital listed as "04."
5 transfers to Valley High Children's Hospital listed as "02."
7 patients listed as expired "41."
3 transfers to Pine Valley Community Hospital swing bed listed as "66."
2 patients discharged to jail listed as "10."
4 transfers to Valley View Hospital listed as "04."
1 transfer to Big Valley VA Hospital inpatient psych unit listed as "65."

Errors by case manager:

25 errors by GNF
3 errors by MJF
6 errors by SWT

References

Casto, A. B. and E. Forrestal. 2015. *Principles of Healthcare Reimbursement*, 5th ed. Chicago: AHIMA.

Centers for Medicare and Medicaid Services. 2014. Clarification of patient discharge status codes and hospital transfer policies. https://www.cms.gov/Outreach-and-Education/Medicare-Learning-Network-MLN/MLNMattersArticles/downloads/SE0801.pdf

O'Dell, R. M. 2016. Clinical Quality Management. Chapter 21 in *Health Information Management: Concepts, Principles, and Practice*, 5th ed. Oachs, P. and A. Watters, eds. Chicago: AHIMA.

4.6

UR—two-midnight rule

Subdomain IV.A.1
Apply policies and procedures for the use of data required in healthcare reimbursement

As HIM director, you have been approached by the utilization review director, to collaborate with her on a presentation for physicians regarding the two-midnight rule as initiated by the Centers for Medicare and Medicaid Services. Review the rule and recommend important information that should be included in the presentation.

References

Centers for Medicare and Medicaid Services. (2015). Fact Sheet: Two-midnight Rule. https://www.cms.gov/Newsroom/MediaReleaseDatabase/Fact-sheets/2015-Fact-sheets-items/2015-07-01-2.html

Harris, S. L and J. Kelly. 2015. Building clarity on the two-midnight rule. *Journal of AHIMA* 86(10):68–70.

4.7

ABN process

Subdomain IV.A.2
Evaluate the revenue cycle management processes

At a small critical access hospital, individual departments (laboratory, radiology, respiratory therapy) are responsible for issuing an Advance Beneficiary Notice for any tests that Medicare may not cover. Give your opinion on this practice and defend your position.

References

Centers for Medicare and Medicaid Services. 2014. Medical Learning Network: Advance Beneficiary Notice of Noncoverage. 4th ed. https://www.cms.gov/Outreach-and-Education/Medicare-Learning-Network-MLN/MLNProducts/downloads/ABN_Booklet_ICN006266.pdf

Malmgren, C. and C.J. Solberg. 2016. Revenue Cycle Management. Chapter 8 in *Health Information Management: Concepts, Principles, and Practice*, 5th ed. Oachs, P. and A. Watters, eds. Chicago: AHIMA.

4.8

RBRVS

Subdomain IV.A.1
Apply policies and procedures for the use of data required in healthcare reimbursement

1. Calculate the RBRVS payment for a lumbar hemilaminectomy—discectomy performed in each of the cities below using the physician fee schedule search on the CMS website to collect the necessary values. Use the 2015B fee schedule. Show your work.
   - Dallas
   - Chicago
   - San Francisco

2. Which city has the highest rate? Explain.

References

Casto, A. B. and E. Forrestal. 2015. *Principles of Healthcare Reimbursement,* 5th ed. Chicago: AHIMA.

Centers for Medicare and Medicaid Services. 2016. Physician Fee Schedule Search. https://www.cms.gov/apps/physician-fee-schedule/search/search-criteria.aspx

4.9

Patient-centered medical home

Subdomain IV.A.1
Apply policies and procedures for the use of data required in healthcare reimbursement

Assess the relationship of health information management professionals to the concept of patient-centered medical homes (PCMH), a model of value-based purchasing.

References

Casto, A. B. and E. Forrestal. 2015. *Principles of Healthcare Reimbursement*, 5th ed. Chicago: AHIMA.

Dimick, C. 2008. Home Sweet Medical Home: Can a New Care Model Save Family Medicine? *Journal of AHIMA* 79(8):24–28.

4.10

PCMH II

Subdomain IV.A.1
Apply policies and procedures for the use of data required in healthcare reimbursement

1. Compare the similarities and differences between reimbursement for PCMH and capitation.
2. Justify the position that a PCMH model will save money.

References

Casto, A. B. and E. Forrestal. 2015. *Principles of Healthcare Reimbursement,* 5th ed. Chicago: AHIMA.

Dimick, C. 2008. Home Sweet Medical Home: Can a New Care Model Save Family Medicine? *Journal of AHIMA* 79(8):24–28.

4.11

A/R days

Subdomain IV.A.2
Evaluate the revenue cycle management processes

Subdomain IV.A.4
Implement processes for revenue cycle management and reporting

1. As revenue cycle manager, you oversee the all revenue processes. You just received the report below and need to determine if the patient accounting department is meeting the goal of having less than 20 percent of the accounts receivable older than 90 days.

2. Decide what other information may be relevant to resolving the outstanding accounts below.

Pine Valley Community Hospital A/R Report March 31, 2015

Account Number	Patient Name	Current	Days Outstanding 30-60	61-90	91-120	121-150	151-180	+180	Total
0013424	Jones		$58.75			$212.15			$270.90
0054261	Williams	$678.50						$6,351.12	$7,029.62
0023789	Matthews	$478.65							$478.65
0052113	Colson			$1,425.97					$1,425.97
0016732	Smith				$653.26				$653.26
0044304	Reynolds		$7,369.82						$7,369.82
0022115	Foster	$682.15		$11,659.72					$12,341.87
0038458	Bell		$5,364.66						$5,364.66
0030071	Brown						$8,416.65		$8,416.65
0021631	Miller		$4,652.31						$4,652.31
0019578	Lockwood	$115.80			$713.48				$829.28
0029824	Johnson		$112.53						$112.53
0043754	Carson	$12,865.40							$12,865.40
0052111	Davis					$311.52			$311.52
0018423	Lawson	$8,789.65							$8,789.65
Totals									
Percentage									

References

Casto, A. B. and E. Forrestal. 2015. *Principles of Healthcare Reimbursement,* 5th ed. Chicago: AHIMA.

Malmgren, C. and C. J. Solberg. 2016. Revenue Cycle Management. Chapter 8 in *Health Information Management: Concepts, Principles, and Practice,* 5th ed. Oachs, P. and A. Watters, eds. Chicago: AHIMA.

4.12

Payroll variance

Subdomain VI.G.3
Explain budget variances

Subdomain IV.A.3
Apply principles of healthcare finance for revenue management

In anticipation of ICD-10 implementation, you plan to contract with a coding consultant to provide coding services for your outpatient endoscopy and heart-center procedures and have included this in your annual budget. It is expected that this service will be needed for two months while staff become familiar with ICD-10 coding, but you reserve the right to shorten or extend the contract based on circumstances at the time. Payment will be at the rate of $3.50 per chart. The projected volume for the period is 365 charts per week.

Two weeks after ICD-10 is implemented, you realize that the coding staff can take on the outpatient and heart center procedures earlier than originally anticipated. You give the consultant two weeks' notice that you will be returning the workload to in-house staff.

At the conclusion of the consultant's service you receive this invoice.

Week 1 377 charts coded
Week 2 363 charts coded
Week 3 358 charts coded
Week 4 372 charts coded
Total 1,470 charts coded @ $3.50 per chart = $5,145.00

- Classify and explain the type of budget variance depicted in this scenario.

References

Revoir, R. and N. Davis. 2016. Financial Management. Chapter 26 in *Health Information Management: Concepts, Principles, and Practice*, 5th ed. Oachs, P. and A Watters, eds. Chicago: AHIMA.

4.13

OCE audit

Subdomain IV.A.2
Evaluate the revenue cycle management processes

Subdomain IV.A.4
Implement processes for revenue cycle management and reporting

Two months ago, your organization initiated pain management services. In recent weeks, you have watched the accounts receivable for Medicare slowly climbing. You begin to audit the accounts that are outstanding, and realize the reason for the increase is pain management operative procedures, specifically sacroiliac joint injections. These were all billed with CPT code 27096 at approximately $410.00 per case with an average of 5 cases per day over the past two months. They all have an Outpatient Code Editor (OCE) edit of 28. Determine what your next steps should be to resolve this issue and reduce the accounts receivable.

References

Casto, A. B. and E. Forrestal. 2015. *Principles of Healthcare Reimbursement*, 5th ed. Chicago: AHIMA.

Malmgren, C. and C. J. Solberg. 2016. Revenue Cycle Management. Chapter 8 in *Health Information Management: Concepts, Principles, and Practice*, 5th ed. Oachs, P. and A. Watters, eds. Chicago: AHIMA.

4.14

Chargemaster issue

Subdomain IV.A.2
Evaluate the revenue cycle management processes

Subdomain IV.A.2
Take part in selection and development of applications and processes for chargemaster and claims management

Billing has indicated that they are receiving rejections (OCE edit 28) on Medicare vaccination claims. As the new physician practice manager, you have decided to review the chargemaster for influenza, pneumonia, and hepatitis B vaccination charges to identify the issue, since these claims would be hard-coded. The practice sees only adult patients, with a significant portion of them having Medicare as their payer, so it is important to resolve the error quickly. Review the relevant portion of the chargemaster below and revise as necessary.

Revenue Code	Charge Number	Charge Description	Charge	HCPCS Code	Modifier	CPT code	Status
0252	0682475135	Vaccine-influenza preservative-free IM 6-35 months	$1.79			90655	Active
0252	0682475136	Vaccine-influenza preservative-free IM 3 yrs.+	$2.37			90656	Active
0252	0682475137	Vaccine-influenza IM 6-35 months	$0.83			90657	Active
0252	0682475138	Vaccine-influenza IM 3 yrs. +	$1.32			90658	Active
0252	0693381421	Vaccine-pneumococcal conjugate 7 IM	$5.64			90669	Active
0252	0693381422	Vaccine-pneumococcal conjugate 13 IM	$15.96			90670	Active
0252	0693381423	Vaccine-pneumococcal polysaccharide 23 IM/SQ	$7.89			90732	Active

0771	0753215465	Admin of flu vaccine	$21.75			90471	Active
0771	0753215466	Admin of pneumococcal vaccine	$16.85			90471	Active
0771	0753215467	Admin of hep B vaccine	$19.20			90471	Active

References

Casto, A. B. and E. Forrestal. 2015. *Principles of Healthcare Reimbursement*, 5th ed. Chicago: AHIMA.

Centers for Medicare and Medicaid Services. 2015. Medicare Part B Immunization Billing. https://www.cms.gov/Outreach-and-Education/Medicare-Learning-Network-MLN/MLNProducts/downloads/qr_immun_bill.pdf

Malmgren, C. and C. J. Solberg. 2016. Revenue Cycle Management. Chapter 8 in *Health Information Management: Concepts, Principles, and Practice*, 5th ed. Oachs, P. and A. Watters, eds. Chicago: AHIMA.

4.15

Budgeting process

Subdomain IV.A.3
Apply principles of healthcare finance for revenue management

It is time to prepare the annual departmental operating budget for fiscal year 2015–2016. In your organization, the fiscal year runs from July 1–June 30. At this point in time, medical records are hybrid. Build a list of at least three organizational and three departmental budget assumptions that will need clarified in order to prepare the budget.

References

Gordon, L. and M. Gordon. 2016. Management. Chapter 19 in *Health Information Management Technology: An Applied Approach*, 5th ed. Sayles, N.B. and L. Gordon, eds. Chicago; AHIMA.

Revoir, R. and N. Davis. 2016. Financial Management. Chapter 26 in *Health Information Management: Concepts, Principles, and Practice*, 5th ed. Oachs, P. and A Watters, eds. Chicago: AHIMA.

4.16

Cost reporting

Subdomain IV.A.3
Apply principles of healthcare finance for revenue management

Analyze the function of cost reports. Include in your analysis a comparison of the four methods of allocating overhead costs.

References

Gordon, L. and M. Gordon. 2016. Management. Chapter 19 in *Health Information Management Technology: An Applied Approach*, 5th ed. Sayles, N.B. and L. Gordon, eds. Chicago: AHIMA.

Revoir, R. and N. Davis. 2016. Financial Management. Chapter 26 in *Health Information Management: Concepts, Principles, and Practice*, 5th ed. Oachs, P. and A Watters, eds. Chicago: AHIMA.

4.17

Chargemaster composition

Subdomain IV.A.2
Take part in selection and development of applications and processes for chargemaster and claims management

Examine the portion of a chargemaster illustrated below. Identify the missing elements that should be included for a complete chargemaster and explain their necessity.

Charge Number	Charge Description	Charge	CPT code
0042364527	Chest x-ray, single view	$89.75	71010
0042364528	Chest x-ray, two views	$110.85	71020
0049533561	CT scan, thorax w/o contrast	$450.25	71250
0049533562	CT scan, thorax w/contrast	$525.60	71260
0049533563	CT scan, thorax w/o and w/ contrast	$611.20	71270
0059781213	MRI chest, w/o contrast	$985.00	71550
0059781214	MRI chest, w/contrast	$1,062.65	71551
0059781215	MRI chest, w/o and w/contrast	$1,145.70	71552

References

American Health Information Management Association. 2010. Care and maintenance of chargemasters (updated). http://library.ahima.org/xpedio/groups/public/documents/ahima/bok1_047258.hcsp?dDocName=bok1_047258

Malmgren, C. and C. J. Solberg. 2016. Revenue Cycle Management. Chapter 8 in *Health Information Management: Concepts, Principles, and Practice*, 5th ed. Oachs, P. and A. Watters, eds. Chicago: AHIMA.

4.18

Chargemaster requisition form

Subdomain IV.A.2
Take part in selection and development of applications and processes for chargemaster and claims management

Create a form to be used for chargemaster requisitions.

References

American Health Information Management Association. 2010. Care and maintenance of chargemasters (updated). http://library.ahima.org/xpedio/groups/public/documents/ahima/bok1_047258.hcsp?dDocName=bok1_047258

Malmgren, C. and C. J. Solberg. 2016. Revenue Cycle Management. Chapter 8 in *Health Information Management: Concepts, Principles, and Practice*, 5th ed. Oachs, P. and A. Watters, eds. Chicago: AHIMA.

Richey, J. 2001. A new approach to chargemaster management. *Journal of AHIMA* 72(1): 51–55.

4.19

Remittance advice

Subdomain IV.A.2
Evaluate the revenue cycle management processes

Subdomain IV.A.1
Manage the use of clinical data required by various payment and reimbursement systems

The claim for S. Smith, a 10-year-old that had a tonsillectomy on 5/8/15, was billed with the following information on May 12, 2015.

S. Smith
123 New Road
Bridgeville, OH 44556
DOB 6/12/1950

CPT code 42825
Claim adjustment reason code (CARC) 6 returned on the remittance advice to indicate the procedure was not paid.

* Determine the issue that the CARC identifies and what steps must be taken to correct it.

References

Casto, A. B. and E. Forrestal. 2015. *Principles of Healthcare Reimbursement,* 5th ed. Chicago: AHIMA.

Washington Publishing Company. 2015. Claim Adjustment Reason Codes. http://www.wpc-edi.com/reference/codelists/healthcare/claim-adjustment-reason-codes/

4.20

Claim reconciliation

Subdomain IV.A.2
Evaluate the revenue cycle management processes

Subdomain IV.A.1
Manage the use of clinical data required by various payment and reimbursement systems

Mrs. Jones had an arthroscopic shoulder procedure on 7/8/15. Her physician performed a subacromial decompression. The coder assigned CPT 29826 to the encounter. The bill dropped on 7/12/15. On 7/22/15, the patient accounting department was processing the latest remittance advice and remark code N122 was attributed to the CPT code for this claim.

1. Determine what the remittance advice remark code (RARC) N122 signifies.

2. Determine the steps needed to correct the claim.

References

Casto, A. B. and E. Forrestal. 2015. *Principles of Healthcare Reimbursement*, 5th ed. Chicago: AHIMA.

Washington Publishing Company. 2015. Claim Adjustment Reason Codes. http://www.wpc-edi.com/reference/codelists/healthcare/claim-adjustment-reason-codes/

4.21

EDI

Subdomain IV.A.2
Evaluate the revenue cycle management processes

Subdomain IV.A.4
Implement processes for revenue cycle management and reporting

1. Explain in detail HIPAA's influence on electronic data interchange.

2. Elaborate on the eight claims and billing transactions with emphasis on their benefits.

References

Moynihan, J. 2010. Preparing for 5010: Internal testing of HIPAA Transaction Upgrades recommended by December 31. *Journal of AHIMA* 81(1):22–26.

Murphy, G. and M. Brandt. 2001. Practice Brief: Health informatics standards and information transfer: exploring the HIM role. *Journal of AHIMA* 72(1):68A-D.

Sandefer, R. 2016. Health Information Technologies. Chapter 12 in *Health Information Management: Concepts, Principles, and Practice*, 5th ed. Oachs, P. and A. Watters, eds. Chicago: AHIMA.

ubdomain IV.A.1
pply policies and procedures for the use of data required in
ealthcare reimbursement

ubdomain IV.A.1
Manage the use of clinical data required by various payment and
reimbursement systems

morbidly obese white male, was admitted to the facility with an acute
of COPD. He is a previous smoker, but has not smoked for the past year
breathing issues have continued to worsen. He was started on oxygen and
n an oral corticosteroid with prophylactic antibiotics administered. The progress
note of day two states that the pressure ulcer of his right heel (stage 4) was non-excisionally
debrided at the bedside.

As an auditor, you review the POA status, code assignment, and DRG assignment shown
below for this patient's stay. You conclude there is an error.

1. What is the error, and what impact does it have on reimbursement?
2. What action might need to be taken to justify your conclusion of a coding error?

[handwritten: should be → Yes]

POA status	ICD-10-CM codes assigned	DRG assignment 192
Y	J44.1 *COPD*	
N	L89.614 *ulcer*	
Y	E66.01 *morbid obese*	
E	Z87.891 *smoking*	

[handwritten margin notes: 672349 3617.00 ; DRG 190 weight 1.1481 5174.50]

References

Casto, A. B. and E. Forrestal. 2015. *Principles of Healthcare Reimbursement,* 5th ed. Chicago: AHIMA.

Hunt, T. J. 2016. Clinical Documentation Improvement and Coding Compliance. Chapter 9 in *Health Information Management: Concepts, Principles, and Practice,* 5th ed. Oachs, P. and A. Watters, eds. Chicago: AHIMA.

[handwritten:]
- Acute Exacerbation of COPD
- History of Smoking

[handwritten:] Need to query about the pressure ulcer if it was present on admission

4.23

Budget variance

Subdomain VI.G.3
Explain budget variances

Subdomain IV.A.3
Apply principles of healthcare finance for revenue management

Your organization is in the process of microfilming all the old records in storage. The budget for this process is $500,000 dollars over 3 years. You have contracted with a company to perform the microfilm services at $0.09 per page and have estimated that there are about 5.5 million pages to be converted. At the end of the first year, you review the invoice and see that you have been billed for converting 2,083,333 pages.

1. Determine your budget variance and what type it is.
2. Provide a short explanation that can be given to administration regarding the variance.

References

Revoir, R. and N. Davis. 2016. Financial Management. Chapter 26 in *Health Information Management: Concepts, Principles, and Practice*, 5th ed. Oachs, P. and A Watters, eds. Chicago: AHIMA.

4.24

APC audit

Subdomain IV.A.2
Evaluate the revenue cycle management processes

Subdomain IV.A.4
Implement processes for revenue cycle management and reporting

Subdomain V.A.2
Determine processes for compliance with current laws and standards related to health information initiatives and revenue cycle

As the physician practice manager, you have run the report with the results depicted in the graph below which shows the distribution of E&M codes billed for established patients over the previous six months.

1. What conclusions can you draw from the graph?
2. Recommend four steps that should be taken as a result of your conclusions.

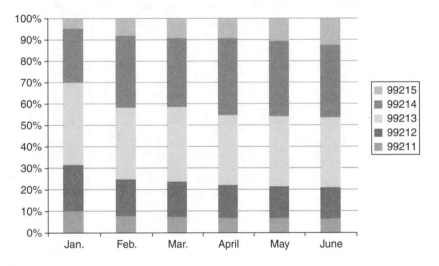

References

Casto, A. B. and E. Forrestal. 2015. *Principles of Healthcare Reimbursement*, 5th ed. Chicago: AHIMA.

Hazelwood, A. and C. Venable. 2016. Reimbursement Methodologies. Chapter 7 in *Health Information Management: Concepts, Principles, and Practice*, 5th ed. Oachs, P. and A. Watters, eds. Chicago: AHIMA.

4.25

Claim denial

Subdomain IV.A.2
Evaluate the revenue cycle management processes

Subdomain IV.A.2
Take part in selection and development of applications and processes for chargemaster and claims management

A patient had a right-posterior subcapsular cataract extraction done with phacoemulsification. An anterior chamber intraocular lens was inserted during the same operative session. The claim is returned with OCE edit 71.

- Create a line item for the chargemaster that will resolve this issue in the future.

References

Casto, A. B. and E. Forrestal. 2015. *Principles of Healthcare Reimbursement*, 5th ed. Chicago: AHIMA.

Malmgren, C. and C. J. Solberg. 2016. Revenue Cycle Management. Chapter 8 in *Health Information Management: Concepts, Principles, and Practice*, 5th ed. Oachs, P. and A. Watters, eds. Chicago: AHIMA.

CHAPTER 5

Domain V: Compliance

 Remember

Understand

 Apply

 Analyze

 Evaluate

 Create

5.0

Notice of privacy practices

Subdomain V.A.1
Analyze policies and procedures to ensure organizational compliance with regulations and standards

Subdomain V.A.1
Appraise current laws and standards related to health information initiatives

1. Compare the Notice of Privacy Practices (NPP) provided in figure 5.0 against the HIPAA and ARRA related elements that must be present in an NPP. Determine if elements are missing and revise the document to include those elements.

2. Why are all the elements necessary?

Your Information. Your Rights. Our Responsibilities.

Your Rights

You have the right to:

- Get a copy of your paper or electronic medical record
- Request confidential communication
- Ask us to limit the information we share
- Get a list of those with whom we've shared your information
- Get a copy of this privacy notice
- Choose someone to act for you
- File a complaint if you believe your privacy rights have been violated

Your Choices

You have some choices in the way that we use and share information as we:

- Tell family and friends about your condition
- Provide disaster relief
- Include you in a hospital directory
- Provide mental health care
- Market our services and sell your information
- Raise funds

Figure 5.0. Notice of Privacy Practices (NPP)
Source: HHS 2016.

Our Uses and Disclosures

We may use and share your information as we:

- Treat you
- Run our organization
- Bill for your services
- Help with public health and safety issues
- Do research
- Comply with the law
- Respond to organ and tissue donation requests
- Work with a medical examiner or funeral director
- Address workers' compensation, law enforcement, and other government requests
- Respond to lawsuits and legal actions

Your Rights

When it comes to your health information, you have certain rights. This section explains your rights and some of our responsibilities to help you.

Get an electronic or paper copy of your medical record

- You can ask to see or get an electronic or paper copy of your medical record and other health information we have about you. Ask us how to do this.
- We will provide a copy or a summary of your health information, usually within 30 days of your request. We may charge a reasonable, cost-based fee.

Request confidential communications

- You can ask us to contact you in a specific way (for example, home or office phone) or to send mail to a different address.
- We will say "yes" to all reasonable requests.

Ask us to limit what we use or share

- You can ask us not to use or share certain health information for treatment, payment, or our operations. We are not required to agree to your request, and we may say "no" if it would affect your care.

Get a list of those with whom we've shared information

- You can ask for a list (accounting) of the times we've shared your health information for six years prior to the date you ask, who we shared it with, and why.
- We will include all the disclosures except for those about treatment, payment, and health care operations, and certain other disclosures (such as any you asked us to make). We'll provide one accounting a year for free but will charge a reasonable, cost-based fee if you ask for another one within 12 months.

Get a copy of this privacy notice

You can ask for a paper copy of this notice at any time, even if you have agreed to receive the notice electronically. We will provide you with a paper copy promptly.

Choose someone to act for you

- If you have given someone medical power of attorney or if someone is your legal guardian, that person can exercise your rights and make choices about your health information.
- We will make sure the person has this authority and can act for you before we take any action.

File a complaint if you feel your rights are violated

- You can complain if you feel we have violated your rights by contacting us using the information on page 1.
- You can file a complaint with the U.S. Department of Health and Human Services Office for Civil Rights by sending a letter to 200 Independence Avenue, S.W., Washington, D.C. 20201, calling 1-877-696-6775, or visiting **www.hhs.gov/ocr/privacy/hipaa/complaints/.**
- We will not retaliate against you for filing a complaint.

Your Choices

For certain health information, you can tell us your choices about what we share. If you have a clear preference for how we share your information in the situations described below, talk to us. Tell us what you want us to do, and we will follow your instructions.

In these cases, you have both the right and choice to tell us to:

- Share information with your family, close friends, or others involved in your care
- Share information in a disaster relief situation
- Include your information in a hospital directory

If you are not able to tell us your preference, for example if you are unconscious, we may go ahead and share your information if we believe it is in your best interest. We may also share your information when needed to lessen a serious and imminent threat to health or safety.

In these cases we never share your information unless you give us written permission:

- Marketing purposes
- Sale of your information
- Most sharing of psychotherapy notes

In the case of fundraising:

- We may contact you for fundraising efforts, but you can tell us not to contact you again.

Our Uses and Disclosures

How do we typically use or share your health information?

We typically use or share your health information in the following ways.

Treat you

> We can use your health information and share it with other professionals who are treating you.
>
> *Example: A doctor treating you for an injury asks another doctor about your overall health condition.*

Run our organization

> We can use and share your health information to run our practice, improve your care, and contact you when necessary.
>
> *Example: We use health information about you to manage your treatment and services.*

Bill for your services

> We can use and share your health information to bill and get payment from health plans or other entities.
>
> *Example: We give information about you to your health insurance plan so it will pay for your services.*

How else can we use or share your health information?

We are allowed or required to share your information in other ways – usually in ways that contribute to the public good, such as public health and research. We have to meet many conditions in the law before we can share your information for these purposes. For more information see: www.hhs.gov/ocr/privacy/hipaa/understanding/consumers/index.html.

Help with public health and safety issues

> We can share health information about you for certain situations such as:

- Preventing disease
- Helping with product recalls
- Reporting adverse reactions to medications
- Reporting suspected abuse, neglect, or domestic violence
- Preventing or reducing a serious threat to anyone's health or safety

Do research

> We can use or share your information for health research.

Comply with the law

We will share information about you if state or federal laws require it, including with the Department of Health and Human Services if it wants to see that we're complying with federal privacy law.

Respond to organ and tissue donation requests

We can share health information about you with organ procurement organizations.

Work with a medical examiner or funeral director

We can share health information with a coroner, medical examiner, or funeral director when an individual dies.

Address workers' compensation, law enforcement, and other government requests

We can use or share health information about you:

- For workers' compensation claims
- For law enforcement purposes or with a law enforcement official
- With health oversight agencies for activities authorized by law
- For special government functions such as military, national security, and presidential protective services

Respond to lawsuits and legal actions

We can share health information about you in response to a court or administrative order, or in response to a subpoena.

Our Responsibilities

- We are required by law to maintain the privacy and security of your protected health information.
- We will let you know promptly if a breach occurs that may have compromised the privacy or security of your information.
- We must follow the duties and privacy practices described in this notice and give you a copy of it.
- We will not use or share your information other than as described here unless you tell us we can in writing. If you tell us we can, you may change your mind at any time. Let us know in writing if you change your mind.

For more information see: www.hhs.gov/ocr/privacy/hipaa/understanding/consumers/noticepp.html.

Changes to the Terms of this Notice

We can change the terms of this notice, and the changes will apply to all information we have about you. The new notice will be available upon request, in our office, and on our web site.

References

Brodnik, M. S., L. A. Rinehart-Thompson, and R. B. Reynolds. 2012. *Fundamentals of Law for Health Informatics and Information Management*, 2nd ed., revised reprint. Chicago: AHIMA.

US Department of Health and Human Services. 2016. Model Notices of Privacy Practices. http://www.hhs.gov/ocr/privacy/hipaa/modelnotices.html

5.1

Joint Commission—Do Not Use abbreviations

Subdomain V.A.1
Analyze policies and procedures to ensure organizational compliance with regulations and standards

Subdomain VI.F.1
Identify departmental and organizational survey readiness for accreditation, licensing, and/or certification processes

Locate a copy of The Joint Commission's Do Not Use Abbreviation (DNUA) list. Examine the sample transcription reports and compare them with the DNUA list. Determine any error(s) found that conflict with the DNUA list and recommend the necessary corrections.

Report 1
Procedure:	Trigger Point Injection
Anesthesia:	Local and MAC
Complications:	None

Procedure: The 48-year-old white female was brought to the procedure suite. After reviewing the risks, benefits, and alternatives to the procedure, she decided to procedure with the trigger point injection. Her upper back was sterilely prepped. I isolated the muscle in spasm and used a 25-gauge 5-inch needle to perform an aspiration of the area, which was negative. Then 4.0 cc of Marcaine .5 percent was injected into three trigger points. She tolerated the procedure very well.

Report 2
Procedure:	Right prepatellar bursal injection
Anesthesia:	MAC
Complications:	None

This 57-year-old black male has acute prepatellar bursitis. The right knee is swollen and warm to the touch. He has had similar symptoms in the past, responded well to Aristospan injection, and is here today for an injection.

I reviewed the risks, benefits, and alternatives to the procedure with the patient, who expressed his understanding and agreed to proceed with the injection. MAC sedation was initiated and I prepped the knee with a sterile alcohol wipe. I then injected 20.0 mg of Artistospan into the right prepatellar bursa. No complications from the injection were noted. Discharge after criteria met. Instructed patient it was okay to continue his Novolog 100 U before each meal for his type I diabetes.

References

Brodnik, M. S., L. A. Rinehart-Thompson, and R. B. Reynolds. 2012. *Fundamentals of Law for Health Informatics and Information Management*, 2nd ed., revised reprint. Chicago: AHIMA.

Shaw, P. L. and D. Carter. 2015. *Quality and Performance Improvement in Healthcare, A Tool for Programmed Learning*, 6th ed. Chicago: AHIMA.

5.2

Joint Commission—Do Not Use abbreviations

Subdomain V.A.2
Determine processes for compliance with current laws and standards related to health information initiatives and revenue cycle

As the HIM director for Riverdale Medical Center, you co-chair the medical records committee with Dr. Taylor, an internal medicine doctor. Dr. Taylor has presented an agenda item for the next meeting to discuss additions to Riverdale's do-not-use abbreviation list. She is proposing the addition of two new abbreviations to the current list which include the original list from The Joint Commission plus the three organization-specific additions which were required. You are against adding any more abbreviations to the current list. Defend your position by creating bullet points of the key reasons for leaving the list as is.

References

Brodnik, M. S., L. A. Rinehart-Thompson, and R. B. Reynolds. 2012. *Fundamentals of Law for Health Informatics and Information Management*, 2nd ed., revised reprint. Chicago: AHIMA.

The Joint Commission. 2015. Facts about the Official "Do Not Use" List of Abbreviations. http://www.jointcommission.org/facts_about_do_not_use_list/

5.3

POA

Subdomain V.B.1
Analyze current regulations and established guidelines in clinical classification systems

You have just taken a job as an inpatient coder at Pine Valley Community Hospital, a critical access hospital, after previously working at a large teaching facility in the same role. During your training at PVCH, you are surprised that the trainer stated that you do not have to assign the POA status on inpatient discharges. You decide to research this practice. After research, prove the trainer's state is correct. To prove this statement, provide reasons and at least two references used in your research.

References

Centers for Medicare and Medicaid Services. 2014a. Medicare Learning Network: Critical Access Hospitals. https://www.cms.gov/Outreach-and-Education/Medicare-Learning-Network-MLN/MLNProducts/downloads/critaccesshospfctsht.pdf

Centers for Medicare and Medicaid Services. 2014b. Medicare Learning Network: Hospital-Acquired Conditions and Present on Admission Indicator Reporting Provision. https://www.cms.gov/Outreach-and-Education/Medicare-Learning-Network-MLN/MLNProducts/Downloads/wPOA-Fact-Sheet.pdf

5.4

POA analysis

Subdomain V.B.1
Analyze current regulations and established guidelines in clinical classification systems

1. Determine the POA status for the following scenarios.

- A newborn suffers a dislocated shoulder during delivery. What is the POA status for the shoulder dislocation? *Y*

- A child fell from the jungle gym at the school playground and was taken to the emergency room for treatment since she was complaining of pain in her elbow. She was diagnosed with a supracondylar fracture of the humerus and taken to the operating room. After surgery she experienced severe postoperative nausea and vomiting and was admitted for rehydration. Assign the POA status for the:
  - Supracondylar fracture *Y*
  - Post-op nausea and vomiting *Y*
  - Fall from jungle gym *Y*

2. Determine if the following POA status assignments are correct. If the assigned POA is not correct, indicate what change should be made to correct the assignment.

- Physician notes genetic susceptibility for breast malignancy in patient's record

  Code assigned was Z15.01   POA assigned was Y   *CORRECT*

- Patient admitted with chest pain. In the progress note of the second day, the physician states the patient had a mild NSTEMI (non-ST elevation myocardial infarction).

  Code assigned was I21.4   POA assigned was N   *WRONG Y*

- Three days after hip replacement surgery, the physician documents "Rule out pneumonia" in a progress note after noting fever and cough upon examination. At discharge, the physician documents pneumonia as one of the discharge diagnoses.

  Code assigned was J18.9   POA assigned was Y   *WRONG N*

References

Optum 360°. 2016. *ICD-10-CM Expert for Hospitals*. Appendix I. Present on Admission Reporting Guidelines. Salt Lake City: Optum.

5.5

Anemia query

Subdomain V.D.2
Develop appropriate physician queries to resolve data and coding discrepancies

Create a physician query for the following scenario.

A 79-year-old female, Mrs. Carmichael, is admitted on June 15, 2015 with a right hip fracture. Prior to surgery, her attending physician, Dr. Fellows, orders blood work to check her hemoglobin and hematocrit levels because she is borderline anemic. The patient is cleared for surgery with hemoglobin of 12 and hematocrit of 44 percent. Post-surgery, levels are checked again with drop in both to 8 and 32 percents, respectively. The physician orders a blood transfusion of 3 units of packed red cells. In the discharge summary the physician only notes anemia, along with the patient's hip fracture.

References

AHIMA. 2013. Guidelines for achieving a compliant query practice. *Journal of AHIMA* 84(2):50–53.

AHIMA. 2008. Managing an effective query process. *Journal of AHIMA* 79(10):83–88.

5.6

Coding error

Subdomain V.D.1
Identify discrepancies between supporting documentation and coded data

As the coding manager at a facility in Ohio, you receive accounts from the billing department with potential coding issues prior to billing. It is your job to investigate the account and ensure the proper codes have been assigned. Today, there is a medical necessity edit that has not been cleared concerning Epoetin administration. The codes assigned to this outpatient account were:

I10
N18.6
D64.9
E10.9
T82.868A

1. Read the following information from this chart and determine what the coding error(s) is or are.

2. Identify if you will be able to clear the medical necessity edit based on the documentation.

Patient Name: Joe Smith
MR#3654777
Acct. # 0000325414
DOS: 10/28/15
Discharge date: 10/29/15

Mr. Smith arrives today with thrombosis of his AV graft. He was unable to receive his dialysis treatment today and will undergo a thrombectomy procedure to restore graft function. He is a 54 year-old with hypertension and diabetes taken to the OR and prepped and draped in the usual sterile fashion. An incision was made permitting access to the graft. A graftotomy was done and Fogarty catheter inserted to pull back the thrombosis. After successful removal of the thrombosis, an injection was performed of the anastomotic area to ensure that the graft was functional. Incision into the graft was then closed, as was the access incision. Patient was taken to the recovery room in stable condition. He will be observed overnight, and receive his dialysis tomorrow prior to discharge. He is also to receive an injection of Epoetin for his anemia.

References

Centers for Medicare and Medicaid Services. 2016. Local Coverage Determinations by State Index. https://www.cms.gov/medicare-coverage-database/indexes/lcd-state-index.aspx?bc=AgAAAAAAAAAA

Optum360°. 2016. *ICD-10-CM Expert for Hospitals*. Official Coding Guidelines. Salt Lake City: Optum.

5.7

Coding and UHDDS

Subdomain V.B.1
Analyze current regulations and established guidelines in clinical classification systems

You have agreed to accept an HIM student for their professional practice experience at your facility. Today you are working on coding. You are giving feedback on the codes that the student assigned for the following scenario. Explain in detail, by tying your feedback to the Uniform Hospital Discharge Data Set and reimbursement, justify what the correct coding should be.

Patient: John Smith   MR#121212   Acct. # 000633553

Patient came to ER complaining of chest pain. EKG and labs, including troponin levels, were performed. Nitroglycerin was administered and oxygen therapy initiated. Results of the tests indicated the patient was having an anterior wall myocardial infarction. Patient was taken to the cath lab for immediate single vessel angioplasty. Following the percutaneous coronary intervention, the patient was admitted to the floor. He was monitored continuously. Beta blockers and Coumadin therapy were begun. The patient's hypertension was addressed and he received medication for low potassium levels as well. His diabetes was managed by medication and diet with no significant issues during the admission. After four days the patient was discharged home to continue his medication regime and begin cardiac rehab.

Codes assigned by student:
Px Dx: R07.9 - chest pain, unspecified
          I10 - Essential (primary) Hypertension
          E87.6 - Hypokalemia
          I21.09 - ST elevation myocardial infarction involving other coronary artery of anterior wall
          E11.9 - Type 2 diabetes mellitus w/o complications
PX Px 02703ZZ

References

Optum 360°. 2016. ICD-10-CM Expert for Hospitals. Official Coding Guidelines: Section II Selection of Principal Diagnosis. Salt Lake City: Optum.

Sayles, N. B. and L. Gordon. 2016. *Health Information Management Technology: An Applied Approach*, 5th ed. Chicago: AHIMA.

5.8

Tracer methodology

Subdomain V.A.2
Collaborate with staff in preparing the organization for accreditation, licensure, and/or certification

Subdomain VI.F.1
Identify departmental and organizational survey readiness for accreditation, licensing, and/or certification processes

Consider the role that health information management has on preparation for tracer methodology surveys. Determine at least three ways that HIM can assist in tracer preparation.

References

HcPro. 2004 (January). *HIM-HIPAA Insider*. Preparing for Tracer Methodology. http://www.hcpro.com/HIM-37036-865/Preparing-for-Tracer-Methodology.html

Shaw, P. L. and D. Carter. 2015. *Quality and Performance Improvement in Healthcare, A Tool for Programmed Learning*, 6th ed. Chicago: AHIMA.

5.9

Delinquent medical records

Subdomain V.A.2
Collaborate with staff in preparing the organization for accreditation, licensure, and/or certification

When you came on board as HIM director, an issue needing immediate attention was the high delinquency rate of medical record completion. In fact, at the last The Joint Commission survey, the organization received a zero (0) for insufficient compliance with this standard.

The organization's current practice is that a letter is sent to physicians once charts have become delinquent at 30 days post-discharge. Follow-up letters continue weekly, and if charts weren't completed, the previous director would call the physician office. Strategize solutions to the high delinquency rate.

1. Recommend a minimum of four options that could be implemented easily and have a positive impact on the record completion process.

2. Note three options that will take longer to implement and assess the pros and cons of implementing those options.

References

Medical Staff Briefing. 2007 (July). Knock out Medical Record Delinquencies. http://healthleadersmedia.com/content/HOM-90847/Knock-out-medical-record-delinquencies.html

Reynolds, R. 2016. Health Record Content and Documentation. Chapter 4 in *Health Information Management: Concepts, Principles, and Practice*, 5th ed. Oachs, P. and A. Watters, eds. Chicago: AHIMA.

5.10

CAC and fraud detection

Subdomain V.C.1
Determine policies and procedures to monitor abuse or fraudulent trends

As a coding supervisor, you would like to see computer-assisted coding (CAC) implemented in your organization. You recognize that you will have to convince administration of the merit of investing in this technology that goes beyond coding. Knowing that compliance has been a major focus of the organization, create a memo to the chief financial officer, Ms. Moneybags, which proposes the use of CAC to assist with fraud detection and prevention.

References

American Health Information Management Association. 2005. Automated coding software: Development and use to enhance anti-fraud activities. http://bok.ahima.org/PdfView?oid=65240

Eramo, Lisa A. 2011. Stopping fraud: Detecting and preventing fraud in the e-Health era. *Journal of AHIMA* 82(3):28–30.

5.11

Struggling CDI process

Subdomain V.D.2
Develop appropriate physician queries to resolve data and coding discrepancies

Subdomain V.D.2
Create method to manage present on admission, hospital-acquired conditions, and other CDI components

There is one physician at your organization that has seven outstanding queries over the past month, several more than three weeks old. These are all regarding the clinical validity of an acute blood anemia diagnosis that he has listed on the chart. As revenue cycle manager, you want to get these issues resolved as quickly as possible so you propose an internal escalation policy. Formulate a proposal to share with your CDI and HIM directors for feedback.

References

AHIMA. 2013. Guidance on a compliant query: internal escalation policy. *Journal of AHIMA* http://journal.ahima.org/2013/05/01/guidance-on-a-compliant-query-internal-escalation-policy/

Brinda, D. 2016. Data Management. Chapter 6 in *Health Information Management Technology: An Applied Approach*, 5th ed. Sayles, N. B. and L. Gordon, eds. Chicago: AHIMA.

5.12

Fraud and abuse focus

Subdomain V.C.1
Identify potential abuse or fraudulent trends through data analysis

Subdomain V.C.1
Determine policies and procedures to monitor abuse or fraudulent trends

New to your role as revenue cycle manager, you are nonetheless surprised to learn that there is no formal process in place for isolating potential areas of compliance concern. You recognize that this would generate a focused approach for internal or external auditing, leading to identification of coding compliance concerns and opportunities for coder education. Recommend to the coding supervisor a minimum of four best practices for determining focus areas for auditing and monitoring of coding compliance.

References

AHIMA. 2008. Benchmarking Coding Quality. http://campus.ahima.org/audio/2008/RB072408.pdf

Hunt, T. J. 2016. Clinical Documentation Improvement and Coding Compliance. Chapter 9 in *Health Information Management: Concepts, Principles, and Practice*, 5th ed. Oachs, P. and A. Watters, eds. Chicago: AHIMA.

5.13

Stark anti-kickback

Subdomain V.C.1
Identify potential abuse or fraudulent trends through data analysis

1. Distinguish the differences between the Stark Law and anti-kickback Statute.

2. President Bush's call for widespread adoption of electronic health records (EHR) by 2014 impacted both of these rules. What term describes the subsequent action taken to facilitate EHR adoption within the rules?

3. Provide a short synopsis of the answer in question 2, noting the exceptions for promoting EHR adoption.

References

Brodnik, M. S., L. A. Rinehart-Thompson, and R. B. Reynolds. 2012. *Fundamentals of Law for Health Informatics and Information Management*, 2nd ed., revised reprint. Chicago: AHIMA.

Further Student Reading

Edelstein, S. A. 2007. Implementing the new Stark Law exceptions and anti-kickback safe harbors for electronic prescribing and electronic health records. AHIMA's 79th National Convention and Exhibit Proceedings. Philadelphia, PA.

5.14

Query retention

Subdomain V.D.2
Develop appropriate physician queries to resolve data and coding discrepancies

Subdomain V.D.1
Implement provider querying techniques to resolve coding discrepancies

Your organization is in the process of implementing a clinical documentation improvement program. The newly appointed CDI director has made it clear that she is not interested in having input from the HIM department on the program's development. However, in your role as HIM director, someone has made you aware of a CDI policy stating that once a query is answered and the information passed on to the coder, the query form will not be retained.

Consider how to approach the CDI director with your differing opinion on this policy. Be sure to justify the position that you take.

References

AHIMA. 2013. Guidelines for achieving a compliant query practice. *Journal of AHIMA* 84(2):50–53.

AHIMA. 2008. Managing an effective query process. *Journal of AHIMA* 79(10):83–88.

Sharp, M. 2016. Secondary Data Sources. Chapter 7 in *Health Information Management Technology: An Applied Approach*, 5th ed. Sayles, N. B. and L. Gordon, eds. Chicago: AHIMA.

5.15

Query format

Subdomain V.D.2
Develop appropriate physician queries to resolve data and coding discrepancies

Subdomain V.D.1
Implement provider querying techniques to resolve coding discrepancies

Decide if the following is an acceptably-formatted physician query and defend your response.

Dr. Hightower

Mrs. Smith was admitted on 8/25, and two days later you mention in a progress note a stage three pressure ulcer of her heel that you debrided at the bedside. Can you clarify was the stage three heel pressure ulcer present on admission?

_____Yes
_____No
C. Coder 9/2
Ext. 2112

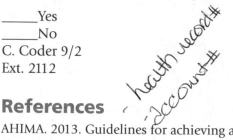

References

AHIMA. 2013. Guidelines for achieving a compliant query process. *Journal of AHIMA* 84(2):50–53.

AHIMA. 2008. Managing an effective query process. *Journal of AHIMA* 79(10):83–88.

Sharp, M. 2016. Secondary Data Sources. Chapter 7 in *Health Information Management Technology: An Applied Approach*, 5th ed. Sayles, N. B. and L. Gordon, eds. Chicago: AHIMA.

5.16

Coding audit

Subdomain V.B.2
Manage coding audits

A coding manager conducted an internal audit of cases in MS-DRG 195 Simple pneumonia without an MCC/CC. There were 619 discharges in this MS-DRG in the previous six months coded by one of five inpatient coders. Twenty-five charts were pulled at random and the coding reviewed with the results noted below.

	# of Charts reviewed	MS-DRG change?
Martha	7	1
John	3	0
Samantha	1	1
Karen	12	4
Tom	2	2
Total	25	8

- Evaluate the audit **process** used.

References

Gordon, L. and M. Gordon. 2016. Management. Chapter 19 in *Health Information Management Technology: An Applied Approach*, 5th ed. Sayles, N. B. and L. Gordon, eds. Chicago: AHIMA

Hunt, T. J. 2016. Clinical Documentation Improvement and Coding Compliance. Chapter 9 in *Health Information Management: Concepts, Principles, and Practice*, 5th ed. Oachs, P. and A. Watters, eds. Chicago: AHIMA.

5.17

Coding audit, Part II

 Subdomain V.B.2
Manage coding audits

A coding manager conducted an internal audit of cases in MS-DRG 195 Simple pneumonia without an MCC/CC. There were 619 discharges in this MS-DRG in the previous six months coded by one of five inpatient coders. Twenty-five charts were pulled at random and the coding reviewed with the results noted below.

	# of Charts reviewed	MS-DRG change?
Martha	7	1
John	3	0
Samantha	1	1
Karen	12	4
Tom	2	2
Total	25	8

- Evaluate the audit **results** and recommend next steps.

References

Gordon, L. and M. Gordon.2016. Management. Chapter 19 in *Health Information Management Technology: An Applied Approach*, 5th ed. Sayles, N. B. and L. Gordon, eds. Chicago: AHIMA

Hunt, T. J. 2016. Clinical Documentation Improvement and Coding Compliance. Chapter 9 in *Health Information Management: Concepts, Principles, and Practice*, 5th ed. Oachs, P. and A. Watters, eds. Chicago: AHIMA.

5.18

Whistleblower

Subdomain V.C.1
Identify potential abuse or fraudulent trends through data analysis

Subdomain V.A.1
Appraise current laws and standards related to health information initiatives

As an inpatient coder, you have been instructed by your coding supervisor to code all debridements as excisional. You are not comfortable with this practice, and tried to discuss it with her, but she stated that you were to follow her instructions and not issue queries. You went to the HIM director who only half-listened to your concerns, saying that the coding supervisor must have a good reason for the instruction. The other coders are following her instructions without question.

You are reluctant to get into trouble for not following the instructions and equally worried that the coding supervisor will retaliate against you in some manner if you report this practice.

1. Assess your options in this situation.
2. Appraise the impact of the False Claims Act as it relates to this situation.

References

Casto, A. B. and E. Forrestal. 2015. *Principles of Healthcare Reimbursement*, 5th ed. Chicago: AHIMA.

5.19

New staff physician

Subdomain V.B.3
Identify severity of illness and its impact on healthcare payment systems

Your organization just hired a new pulmonologist on staff. He has an established practice and many of his patients are geriatric with advanced COPD, severe asthma, emphysema, or lung cancer. What influence do you expect to see in the organization's case mix index as a result of his hiring and why?

References

Edgerton, C. G. 2016. Healthcare Statistics. Chapter 16 in *Health Information Management: Concepts, Principles, and Practice*, 5th ed. Oachs, P. and A. Watters, eds. Chicago: AHIMA.

Shaw, P. L. and D. Carter. 2015. *Quality and Performance Improvement in Healthcare, A Tool for Programmed Learning*, 6th ed. Chicago: AHIMA.

5.20

CDI monitoring

Subdomain V.D.2
Develop appropriate physician queries to resolve data and coding discrepancies

Subdomain V.D.2
Create methods to manage Present on Admission, hospital acquired conditions, and other CDI components

In July of 2012, your organization implemented a clinical documentation improvement program. Below is information regarding the quarterly case mix index over the past several years. Discuss the results, theorizing about the fluctuations.

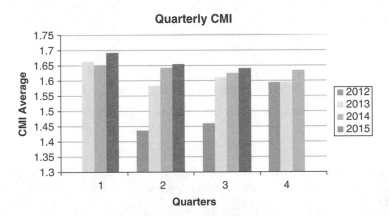

Quarterly Case Mix Index				
	1st quarter	2nd quarter	3rd quarter	4th quarter
2012		1.4362	1.4587	1.5941
2013	1.6627	1.5829	1.6101	1.5955
2014	1.6518	1.6425	1.6247	1.6340
2015	1.6921	1.6543	1.6401	

References

Horton, L. 2016. Healthcare Statistics. Chapter 14 in *Health Information Management Technology: An Applied Approach*, 5th ed. Sayles, N. B. and L. Gordon, eds. Chicago: AHIMA.

Further Student Reading

American Health Information Management Association. 2010. *CDI Toolkit*. Chicago: AHIMA.

5.21

Compliance policy

Subdomain V.A.1
Analyze policies and procedures to ensure organizational compliance with regulations and standards

Subdomain V.A.3
Adhere to the legal and regulatory requirements related to the health information management

Subdomain V.A.1
Appraise current laws and standards related to health information initiatives

Subdomain V.A.2
Determine processes for compliance with current laws and standards related to health information initiatives and revenue cycle

1. Formulate a series of considerations that should be covered in a policy regarding an external coding audit by a consultant. (Provide at least five considerations.)
2. Elaborate on the importance of having such a policy in place.

References

Foltz, D. A., K. Lankisch, and N. Sayles. 2016. Fraud and Abuse Compliance. Chapter 16 in *Health Information Management Technology: An Applied Approach*, 5th ed. Sayles, N. B. and L. Gordon, eds. Chicago: AHIMA.

Hunt, T. J. 2016. Clinical Documentation Improvement and Coding Compliance. Chapter 9 in *Health Information Management: Concepts, Principles, and Practice*, 5th ed. Oachs, P. and A. Watters, eds. Chicago: AHIMA.

Further Student Reading

Prophet, S. 1998. Coding compliance: practical strategies for success. *Journal of AHIMA* 69(1):50–61.

5.22

Bilateral reporting

Subdomain V.A.3
Adhere to the legal and regulatory requirements related to the health information management

Subdomain V.B.1
Construct and maintain processes, policies, and procedures to ensure the accuracy of coded data based on established guidelines

A recent audit of hospital accounts with bilateral cataract procedures coded showed the following:

35 accounts coded	66984-RT Unit of service 1
	66984-LT Unit of service 1
172 accounts coded	66984-50 Unit of service 1
7 accounts coded	66984 Unit of service 1
	66984-50 Unit of service 1
2 accounts coded	66984 Unit of service 2

- Develop a coding procedure for bilateral cataract procedures that will meet compliance under the National Correct Coding Initiative.

References

Centers for Medicare and Medicaid Services. 2015. *NCCI Policy Manual for Medicare Services.* https://www.cms.gov/Medicare/Coding/NationalCorrectCodInitEd/index.html?redirect=/nationalcorrectcodinited/

Hazelwood, A. and C. Venable. 2016. Reimbursement Methodologies. Chapter 7 in *Health Information Management: Concepts, Principles, and Practice*, 5th ed. Oachs, P. and A. Watters, eds. Chicago: AHIMA.

5.23

Coding review

Subdomain V.D.1
Identify discrepancies between supporting documentation and coded data

Analyze the scenario below and identify the errors in coding based on the documentation.

H&P

A 63-year-old woman is admitted with severe, unrelenting headache. CT scan in ER shows an area suspicious for a brain tumor. The woman is admitted to control pain and identify source of primary.

She is a diabetic with hypertension. She smokes a pack of cigarettes a day and has for the past forty years. There is a family history of breast cancer with her aunt and sister.

Patient will undergo an MRI of the brain and CT of chest and abdomen in hopes of identifying primary source of tumor.

Consult

This 63-year-old white female is complaining of numbness and tingling to her feet. She is diabetic, type I, with noncompliance with her insulin treatment. She states that she takes half of the required dosage as it is difficult for her to afford her medications. Examination of extremities is indicative of diabetic neuropathy. Have stressed with the patient the need for her to strictly follow her insulin regimen, and follow up for additional tests as an outpatient. Patient needs to have annual foot and eye exams.

Progress Note I

Patient having CT scans this morning. Will consult with radiology and proceed with recommendations once those results are read.

Progress Note II

Appreciate consult on diabetic management. Will echo consultant's call for compliance with medication.

CT scans showed a right breast lesion, suspicious for malignancy. Patient was informed and is willing to proceed to OR for mastectomy.

CT Report

Patient was given contrast material and CT of the chest performed. A density, consistent with a malignancy was identified in the lower-inner quadrant of the right breast. No abnormalities in the left breast or elsewhere in the chest.

OR Report

Patient was brought to the OR where she was prepped and draped in a sterile manner. She had previously been informed of the risks, benefits, and alternatives to the surgery and elected to proceed.

I made standard mastectomy incisions and dissected down to but not including the pectoral muscle. Bleeders were cauterized and hemostasis secured. The breast was lifted off the musculature. The patient did not want reconstruction at this time, so a primary closure was completed. The specimen was sent to pathology.

Blood loss was minimal and the patient tolerated the procedure well. She is sent to recovery and will be observed until she meets discharge criteria. I will have her follow up in the office in two weeks to discuss treatment of the brain cancer.

Pathology Report

Specimen is 0.3942 kgs. of breast tissue, right breast. Microscopic examination reveals adenocarcinoma.

Discharge Summary

An unfortunate woman who was found to have a breast malignancy (primary) after CT scan identified a metastasis to the brain. She underwent a mastectomy earlier today and is ready for discharge. She will follow up in two weeks to check the healing and discuss further treatment to focus on the brain. She is to follow her medication regimen for diabetes and hypertension. She has been counseled on smoking cessation.

Codes assigned:

C50.911
C71.9
E10.9
I10
F17.210
Z79.4
Z80.3
0HTT0ZZ

Further Student Reading

Hazelwood, A. and C. Venable. 2016. Reimbursement Methodologies. Chapter 7 in *Health Information Management: Concepts, Principles, and Practice*, 5th ed. Oachs, P. and A. Watters, eds. Chicago: AHIMA.

Optum360°. 2016. *ICD-10-CM Expert for Hospitals*. Official Coding Guidelines.

Optum360°. 2016. *ICD-10-PCS 2016 Official Code Set*.

5.24

Compliance policy II

Subdomain V.A.3
Adhere to the legal and regulatory requirements related to the health information management

Subdomain V.A.1
Appraise current laws and standards related to health information initiatives

1. Propose at least six policies and procedures that would be appropriate in a coding compliance plan.

2. Choose one and elaborate on its importance in being included in the coding compliance plan.

References

Hunt, T. J. 2016. Clinical Documentation Improvement and Coding Compliance. Chapter 9 in *Health Information Management: Concepts, Principles, and Practice*, 5th ed. Oachs, P. and A. Watters, eds. Chicago: AHIMA.

Further Student Reading

Prophet, S. 1998. Coding compliance: practical strategies for success. *Journal of AHIMA* 69(1):50–61.

5.25

Fraud trend analysis

Subdomain V.C.1
Identify potential abuse or fraudulent trends through data analysis

Subdomain V.C.1
Determine policies and procedures to monitor abuse or fraudulent trends

1. Create one graph to illustrate the comparison of three hospitals, with the state and national percentages for the distribution of MS-DRGs 190-192 using the data below.

2. Predict how each hospital might react to analysis of this graph.

MS-DRG 190 discharges
Hospital X	38
Hospital Y	112
Hospital Z	89
State	8300
Nation	315400

MS-DRG 191 discharges
Hospital X	23
Hospital Y	104
Hospital Z	31
State	7912
Nation	290565

MS-DRG 192 discharges
Hospital X	18
Hospital Y	67
Hospital Z	17
State	2214
Nation	93214

Further Student Reading

Casto, A. B. and E. Forrestal. 2015. *Principles of Healthcare Reimbursement,* 5th ed. Chicago: AHIMA.

Oachs, P. and A. Watters. 2016. *Health Information Management: Concepts, Principles, and Practice,* 5th ed. Chicago: AHIMA.

Sayles, N. B. and L. Gordon. 2016. *Health Information Management Technology: An Applied Approach,* 5th ed. Chicago: AHIMA.

5.26

NCCI guidelines

Subdomain V.B.1
Construct and maintain processes, policies, and procedures to ensure the accuracy of code data based on established guidelines

An internal audit of knee arthroscopy procedures has identified the following:

29880 and 29876 are being coded together for the same knee

1. Based on NCCI edits, elaborate on the appropriateness of this coding practice.
2. Develop a process to ensure that NCCI arthroscopy guidelines are followed.

References

Casto, A. B. and E. Forrestal. 2015. *Principles of Healthcare Reimbursement*, 5th ed. Chicago: AHIMA.

Centers for Medicare and Medicaid Services. (2015). *NCCI Policy Manual for Medicare Services.* https://www.cms.gov/Medicare/Coding/NationalCorrectCodInitEd/index.html?redirect=/nationalcorrectcodinited/

Hazelwood, A. and C. Venable. 2016. Reimbursement Methodologies. Chapter 7 in *Health Information Management: Concepts, Principles, and Practice*, 5th ed. Oachs, P. and A. Watters, eds. Chicago: AHIMA.

5.27

Severity of illness and DRGs

Subdomain V.B.3
Identify severity of illness and its impact on healthcare payment systems

1. Compare and contrast the MS-DRG and APR-DRG systems.
2. What inferences can you draw from the information you uncovered on these two payment systems in the context of paying for performance?

References

Casto, A. B. and E. Forrestal. 2015. *Principles of Healthcare Reimbursement*, 5th ed. Chicago: AHIMA.

Foltz, D. A., K. Lankisch, and N. Sayles. 2016. Fraud and Abuse Compliance. Chapter 16 in *Health Information Management Technology: An Applied Approach*, 5th ed. Sayles, N. B. and L. Gordon, eds. Chicago: AHIMA.

Further Student Reading

3M. *3M APR DRG Classification System and 3M APR DRG Software Fact Sheet*. http://multimedia.3m.com/mws/media/478415O/3m-apr-drg-fact-sheet.pdf?fn=aprdrg_fs.pdf

Sturgeon, J. 2013. APR-DRGs in the Medicaid population. *For The Record*. 25(5):6.

5.28

MS-DRGs

Subdomain V.B.3
Identify severity of illness and its impact on healthcare payment systems

1. Discover the motivation behind the evolution of the DRG payment system to MS-DRGs.
2. Examine the effect this change had on organizational reimbursement.

References

Casto, A. B. and E. Forrestal. 2015. *Principles of Healthcare Reimbursement,* 5th ed. Chicago: AHIMA.

5.29

Computer-assisted coding

Subdomain V.B.2
Determine accuracy of computer assisted coding assignment and recommend corrective action

Read the following excerpt from a patient record that has been processed with computer-assisted coding (CAC) software.

1. Determine any areas of inaccuracy in the CAC identification.
2. Recommend corrections to the code assignment.

Mr. Reynolds is a 57-year-old white male admitted with chest pain. He developed this pain while shoveling snow outside his home. He ranks it an 8 out of 10 on the pain scale. He has arm or jaw pain. He has hyperlipidemia, and hypertension, on medication for both conditions. Last year, he suffered an acute myocardial infarction and was treated with stents.

An EKG was performed and cardiac enzymes drawn. All results were normal. The patient exhibited the pain upon movement and palpation at the chondrosternal joint and a final diagnosis of sprain was determined.

Codes assigned by CAC:
R07.9
I21.3
R68.84
S23.421A
I10
E78.5

References

LaTour, K. M. and S. Eichenwald Maki. 2010. *Health Information Management: Concepts, Principles, and Practice*, 3rd ed. Chicago: AHIMA.

5.30

CAC roadblock

Subdomain V.B.2
Determine accuracy of computer assisted coding assignment and recommend corrective action

1. Explain the importance of a coder in an organization that utilizes computer-assisted coding (CAC) as it regards accuracy of codes assigned.

2. Discuss how coders will factor in corrective action regarding this automated coding process.

References

LaTour, K. M. and S. Eichenwald Maki. 2010. *Health Information Management: Concepts, Principles, and Practice*, 3rd ed. Chicago: AHIMA.

CHAPTER 6

Domain VI: Leadership

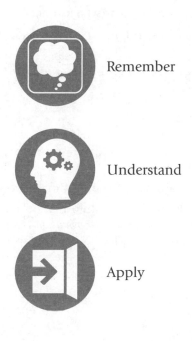 Remember

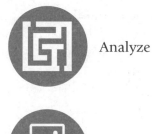 Analyze

Understand

 Evaluate

Apply

Create

Leadership Roles

6.0

Evolving leadership roles in HIM

Subdomain VI.A.1
Summarize health information related leadership roles

1. Increased adoption of health information technology is opening innovative leadership pathways for HIM professionals. Four areas of opportunity based on the HIT roadmap created by the Office of the National Coordinator for Health Information Technology include privacy and security, adoption of information technology, interoperability, and collaborative governance. Choose one of these to explore, listing the challenges and opportunities for HIM professionals.

2. Take one of the challenges you presented and address it by using the 3 I's Leadership Model for e-HIM that AHIMA adapted.

3. Postulate how earning an AHIMA credential can prepare you for leadership opportunity.

References

AHIMA. 2016a. e-HIM Overview and Instructions. AHIMA Leadership Model. http://library.ahima.org/xpedio/groups/public/documents/ahima/bok1_042565.pdf

AHIMA. 2016b. Why Get Certified. Certification. http://www.ahima.org/certification/whycertify

Zeng, X., Reynolds, R., and Sharp, M. 2009. Redefining the Roles of Health Information Management Professionals in Health Information Technology. *Perspectives in Health Information Management*. (6). http://perspectives.ahima.org/redefining-the-roles-of-health-information-management-professionals-in-health-information-technology/#.VfWxFNJVhBc

6.1

Labor and employment laws

Subdomain VI.D.2
Interpret compliance with local, state, federal labor regulations

Assess Pine Valley Hospital's compliance with the following laws based on these scenarios.

1. Equal Pay Act of 1963

Gertrude and Harry are both new coders at PVH. They have been hired at the entry level Coder 1 position which requires an associate degree, which they both recently earned. However, neither of them have previous HIM or coding experience. She will be working the first shift (day, 7 a.m.–3 p.m.), while he works second shift (evening, 3 p.m.–11 p.m.). Harry has achieved his CCS credential but Gertrude has not. The rate of pay for Gertrude is $14.21 per hour; Harry will be making $14.71. Is the pay difference a violation of Equal Pay Act of 1963?

2. Age Discrimination in Employment Act of 1967

Selena is the HIM director at a 200 bed hospital. She has had exemplary performance evaluations each of her 35 years (15 of which have been as director of HIM), and is a well-respected leader within the organization. Recent financial difficulties within the hospital have administration looking to cut costs. They have made a determination to dismiss Selena, and hire a new director at a reduced salary and fringe benefits.

References

LeBlanc, M. M. 2016. Human Resources Management. Chapter 23 in *Health Information Management: Concepts, Principles, and Practice*, 5th ed. Oachs, P. and A. Watters, eds. Chicago: AHIMA.

6.2

ROI for employee training and development

Subdomain VI.E.2
Explain return on investment for employee training/development

Martha, the HIM director for Richmond Medical Center, has lost her third release of information technician in the past year. It seems as though shortly after the new hire has passed the probationary period, they quit. Exit interviews have provided the following information:

- Job is too stressful (unfamiliar with HIPAA regulations, backlog high)
- Job is too much for one person
- Job is too confusing
- Lack of departmental training
- Lack of feedback

The last three ROI technicians have come from other departments in the hospital but none have had an HIM educational background. Martha has discovered that the HIM supervisor conducts one day of orientation and one day of training, but no feedback is provided, especially early in the new hire's service.

1. Decide what steps Martha could take to attract ROI candidates with stronger HIM backgrounds.

2. Identify at least four key areas where the HIM supervisor could positively impact retention and select methods for that improvement.

3. Identify two other steps that Martha and/or the supervisor could take to improve retention for ROI tech.

References

Prater, V. S. 2016. Human Resources Management and Professional Development. Chapter 20 in *Health Information Management Technology: An Applied Approach*, 5th ed. Sayles, N. B. and L. Gordon, eds. Chicago: AHIMA.

6.3

Committee consensus

Subdomain VI.A.5
Take part in enterprise-wide committees

Subdomain VI.A.6
Build effective teams

As HIM director of one of four acute care facilities under Norwood Health Services, you serve on the HIM ICD-10 transition committee. It is six months before ICD-10 implementation and recent discussion has centered on the use of ICD-10-PCS codes for outpatient coding. Two of the component hospitals have been dual-coding outpatient records with both ICD-10-CM and PCS codes, while the other two have not, including your facility. It is imperative to arrive at a consensus at today's meeting, as the Corporate HIM Director wants to develop a standardized corporate strategy. One of the sticking points has been report writing. One director is adamant that using the ICD-10-PCS codes will be the only way to capture the data for certain reports. Another director wants the benefit of cross-trained staff.

1. Provide at least three arguments can you present to influence those directors to join your position against training outpatient coders on ICD-10-PCS at this time?

2. Propose a plan of action that might achieve a consensus.

References

HCPro. 2013. Outpatient coding and ICD-10-PCS. *HIM-HIPAA Insider.* http://www.hcpro.com/HIM-298135-865/Outpatient-coding-and-ICD10PCS.html.

York, M. 2015. To code or not to code-PCS codes on outpatient claims. *Libman Education* blog. http://www.libmaneducation.com/to-code-or-not-to-code-pcs-codes-on-outpatient-claims/

6.4

Transcription PI

Subdomain VI.C.3
Utilize data for facility-wide outcomes reporting for quality management and performance improvement

As HIM director, concerns have been expressed to you from the head surgical nurse regarding the lack of H&Ps on patients' charts causing surgical delays. Since a patient is not permitted to go to surgery without an H&P on record, this is causing serious issues, including daily backlogs or cancellations. Patients are becoming angry and surgeons want something done to eliminate this issue.

1. Plan a data collection to assess the situation, selecting the relevant data elements to be included.

2. Identify any other information that may be pertinent to the evaluation of the data collection from the transcription standpoint.

3. Assume that the data collected identifies one particular physician who has this issue repeatedly. His surgeries are scheduled beginning at 6:00 a.m. and he routinely dictates the H&Ps starting at 5:50 a.m. What strategies can be developed to reduce the delays?

References

Shaw P. L. and D. Carter. 2015. *Quality and Performance Improvement in Healthcare: A Tool for Programmed Learning*, 6th ed. Chicago: AHIMA.

6.5

Ethical situation

Subdomain VI.H.1
Comply with ethical standards of practice

Subdomain VI.H.1
Comply with ethical standards of practice

Since May, you have been working with a recruiter to obtain a new position in HIM. Your experience includes over ten years in inpatient and outpatient coding, you are an AHIMA-approved ICD-10 trainer, and you have worked with your state association on coding projects over the past two years. Nothing the recruiter has presented to you has been a good fit, but in late September, the recruiter calls with positions open for coding auditor. You have never done that type of work before, but are confident you could learn, and the recruiter gets you a phone interview. During the conversation, the HIM manager for the organization says that she sees you have been an auditor since May. You immediately recognize that the HIM manager has the wrong impression of your experience.

Determine the appropriate course of action in response to the interviewer's statement. Provide justification based on the AHIMA Code of Ethics.

References

AHIMA. 2016. AHIMA Code of Ethics. http://library.ahima.org/xpedio/groups/public/documents/ahima/bok1_024277.hcsp?dDocName=bok1_024277

6.6

Ethics breach

 Subdomain VI.H.2
Evaluate the consequences of a breach of healthcare ethics

Your regional HIM association has enlisted a speaker on privacy and security based on the presentation experience listed on her resume. Immediately after the presentation, several members approach you to say they are certain that today's presentation was exactly the same one that they had attended at the state association meeting two years ago given by a different speaker. Assess the implications for this individual if she breached ethical standards by passing off someone else's work as her own.

References

AHIMA. 2016. AHIMA Code of Ethics. http://library.ahima.org/xpedio/groups/public/documents/ahima/bok1_024277.hcsp?dDocName=bok1_024277

Ethical dilemma

Subdomain VI.H.1
Comply with ethical standards of practice

Subdomain VI.H.2
Evaluate the consequences of a breach of healthcare ethics

Subdomain IV.A.2
Evaluate the revenue cycle management processes

Subdomain VI.H.1
Comply with ethical standards of practice

Subdomain IV.A.4
Implement processes for revenue cycle management and reporting

As HIM director of Pine Valley Community Hospital, a critical access hospital, you are concerned about a recent decision made by your CEO. He has decided that all patients will be issued an Advanced Beneficiary Notice for outpatient laboratory and radiology services. His rationalization is that by doing this, the hospital will be able to collect on all the tests performed that do not meet medical necessity. You know that is an unacceptable practice.

1. Defend your position.
2. Support your stance through the Code of Ethics as well.
3. Anticipate the consequences of continuing with the CEO's decision.

References

AHIMA. 2016. AHIMA Code of Ethics. http://library.ahima.org/xpedio/groups/public/documents/ahima/bok1_024277.hcsp?dDocName=bok1_024277

Centers for Medicare and Medicaid Services. 2015. Medicare Advance Beneficiary Notices. https://www.cms.gov/Outreach-and-Education/Medicare-Learning-Network-MLN/MLNProducts/downloads/abn_booklet_icn006266.pdf

6.8

Ethical decision-making

Subdomain VI.H.1
Comply with ethical standards of practice

Subdomain VI.H.2
Evaluate the consequences of a breach of healthcare ethics

Subdomain VI.H.1
Comply with ethical standards of practice

An inpatient coder has come to you as the Director of HIM concerned that she has been instructed by the coding supervisor to code all bedside debridements as excisional. In discussion with the coding supervisor, she explains that surgical trays are ordered for the bedside and that physicians have been ignoring the queries requesting clarification, instead, telling her verbally that those debridements are always excisional. Therefore, she issued the directive to the staff.

1. Use the ethical decision making process to determine if this is an unethical situation and if so, what AHIMA Code of Ethics or AHIMA's Standards of Ethical Coding it violates.

2. If it is a violation, give your opinion of what the implications might be to the coder, coding supervisor, yourself, and the organization.

References

AHIMA. 2011. AHIMA Code of Ethics. http://library.ahima.org/xpedio/groups/public/documents/ahima/bok1_024277.hcsp?dDocName=bok1_024277

AHIMA. 2008. AHIMA Standards of Ethical Coding. http://library.ahima.org/xpedio/groups/public/documents/ahima/bok2_001166.hcsp?dDocName=bok2_001166

Gordon, L. and M. Gordon. 2016. Ethical Issues in Health Information Management. *Health Information Management: Concepts, Principles, and Practice*, 5th ed. Oachs, P. and A. Watters, eds. Chicago: AHIMA.

Code of Ethics

★2.4

★ 4.1
★ 4.2
4.2
4.3
4.4
4.5
4.6
4.7
★ 4.8

Ethical coding

1 - 1.1 1.2 1.3 1.4 1.5 (ALL)
3 - 3.1 (ALL)
5 - 5.1, 5.2, 5.3, 5.4 (ALL)
10 - 10.3
11 - ALL
2 - 2.1 - 2.2 (ALL)

6.9

Preparing for an HIM job interview

Subdomain VI.D.2
Interpret compliance with local, state, federal labor regulations

Subdomain VI.D.2
Ensure compliance with employment laws

Imagine you are preparing for your first job interview in an HIM department. You are trying to prepare answers to likely interview questions. You are comfortable discussing everything on your resume, including your education, and previous non-HIM related work experience. You have thought about what strengths and weaknesses you have, and recalled a couple experiences that can illustrate your work ethic. You even role-play with a friend to reduce your anxiety, except you are thrown a curve when the first thing she asks you is "Tell me a little about yourself."

1. Make-up a response to this question.

2. Hypothesize why an HIM director might ask such a question.

References

LeBlanc, M. M. 2016. Human Resources Management. Chapter 23 in *Health Information Management: Concepts, Principles, and Practice*, 5th ed. Oachs, P. and A. Watters, eds. Chicago: AHIMA.

6.10

HIM job interview

Subdomain VI.D.2
Interpret compliance with local, state, federal labor regulations

Subdomain VI.D.2
Ensure compliance with employment laws

Evaluate the following interchange between an HIM Director and prospective employee. Critique the questions asked by the HIM Director and identify any that are inappropriate to ask during the interview process and explain why.

HIM Director: Welcome, Ms. Martin. I'm Sheila Reynolds, HIM Director. I see from your resume that you just completed the HIT program at Wentworth College. Tell me about your favorite class.

Ms. Martin: I really enjoyed the three coding classes that I took. I found them to be challenging but fun. Those classes had me utilizing my anatomy and physiology knowledge as well.

HIM Director: Indeed. As I reviewed your resume, I noticed there is a 10 year time lapse between your last job and returning to college. Can you explain that? Were you taking time to start a family?

Ms. Martin: Yes, now that my children are older, I am more comfortable getting back into the work force.

HIM Director: There are times throughout the year when our staff must put in overtime. Do you have after school childcare lined up?

Ms. Martin: There is an afterschool program at the school itself that they will attend. I think it will work out well.

HIM Director: Can you tell me what your greatest strength is?

Ms. Martin: I would say that I am a very conscientious person. I like to do a good job at whatever I do and work hard to learn when I have made a mistake.

HIM Director: Then what would be your greatest weakness?

Ms. Martin: I would have to say that I am impatient, however, the advantage to that is that I like to get things done quickly.

HIM Director: How are you with multi-tasking?

Ms. Martin: I worked part-time while going to school and raising my kids. I had to multi-task every day in order to keep everyone on schedule. I never was late for work, or turned in a late assignment.

HIM Director: Didn't your husband help out?

Ms. Martin: We are divorced.

HIM Director: Okay, well, tell me how you would handle a physician who comes into the department yelling about having to redictate several operative reports.

Ms. Martin: First, I would ask him to step into an office for a private discussion. Then I would listen to his complaints. I would tell him that I would investigate his concerns about the transcription system and explain that in the meantime, we really will have to ask him to dictate the reports again.

HIM Director: Thank you, Ms. Martin. I have a few more interviews and will be in touch by the end of the week with my decision.

Ms. Martin: Thank you, Ms. Reynolds. I appreciate the opportunity to interview for the coding position and look forward to hearing from you soon. Goodbye.

References

LeBlanc, M. M. 2016. Human Resources Management. Chapter 23 in *Health Information Management: Concepts, Principles, and Practice*, 5th ed. Oachs, P. and A. Watters, eds. Chicago: AHIMA.

6.11

Calculating ROI staffing levels

Subdomain VI.D.1
Report staffing levels and productivity standards for health information functions

Determine the number of full-time ROI staff that is needed for an HIM department based on the following information. Use a 7.5 hour work day for your calculation.

On average, ROI clerks process the following:

Open and log all the mail (average of 20 pieces of mail per day)

Of those 5 per day are attorney requests—35 minutes to complete and log

5 per week are subpoenas—2.5 hours to complete and log

9 per day are insurance requests—45 minutes to complete and log

1 miscellaneous request—30 minutes to complete and log

20 walk-in requests per day—10 minutes to complete and log requests

References

Horton, L. A. 2016. *Calculating and Reporting Healthcare Statistics,* 5th ed. Chicago: AHIMA.

6.12

Coder education

Subdomain VI.E.2
Explain return on investment for employee training/development

Budget planning is underway in your organization, and as HIM director, you are preparing the budgets for your department. A memo accompanied the annual worksheets for capital and operational budgets stating that all educational expenses were being cut this year. In past years, you have budgeted $2,500 for coding education which included sending two coders to your state association's annual meeting for the coding day presentations ($250 for both including travel), purchase of five AHIMA coding webinars ($750 total, $150 each), resource books ($250) and registration and travel for one person to the AHIMA annual meeting ($1,250). Draft a memo to your boss, Ms. Mary Winters, CFO and defend the necessity of keeping coding education in your budget.

References

Gordon, L. and M. Gordon. 2016. Management. Chapter 19 in *Health Information Management Technology: An Applied Approach*, 5th ed. Sayles, N. B. and L. Gordon, eds. Chicago: AHIMA.

Patena, K. 2016. Employee Training and Development. Chapter 24 in *Health Information Management: Concepts, Principles, and Practice*, 5th ed. Oachs, P. and A. Watters, eds. Chicago: AHIMA.

Prater, V. S. 2016. Human Resources Management and Professional Development. *Health Information Management Technology: An Applied Approach*, 5th ed. Sayles, N. B. and L. Gordon, eds. Chicago: AHIMA.

Revoir, R. and N. Davis. 2016. Financial Management. Chapter 26 in *Health Information Management: Concepts, Principles, and Practice*, 5th ed. Oachs, P. and A. Watters, eds. Chicago: AHIMA.

6.13

New service impact on coding staff levels

Subdomain VI.D.1
Report staffing levels and productivity standards for health information functions

In July, a new endoscopy suite will be opened in your organization. Projections are that 60 endoscopies will be performed per day. At the same time, an electrophysiology lab will be opening, with anticipation of 5 procedures being done there per day. You have done some preliminary work sampling to determine how much time it will take to code these types of cases and arrived at 5 minutes per endoscopy and 15 minutes per EP procedure. Calculate the number of FTEs that you will need to hire to cover the additional workload. Base your calculations on a 7.5-hour workday.

References

Horton, L. A. 2016. *Calculating and Reporting Healthcare Statistics*, 5th ed. Chicago: AHIMA.

6.14

New HIM roles

 Subdomain VI.A.2
Apply the fundamentals of team leadership

As a student, you recognize that the HIM profession is in a perpetual state of growth, with new opportunities on the horizon, and you are trying to decide what HIM niche is the right fit for you. Use the AHIMA career map to explore one of those emerging roles in HIM. Judge what additional skills and/or education you would need to qualify for the new role. Then compare the new role you have selected against the HIM Professional Core Model. Explain what functional area(s) the new role would fit in and why.

References

AHIMA. 2016a. Health Information Careers. http://hicareers.com/careermap/

AHIMA. 2016b. A new view of HIM: introducing the core model. http://library.ahima.org/xpedio/groups/public/documents/ahima/bok1_049283.pdf

6.15

HIM and the C-suite

Subdomain VI.A.2
Apply the fundamentals of team leadership

Subdomain VI.A.2
Discover personal leadership style using contemporary leadership theory and principles

Until recently, the healthcare C-suite did not have an HIM voice. Now, there are a variety of C-suite positions that an HIM professional with proper education could fill.

1. Identify at least five of these C-suite roles.
2. Determine what AHIMA credential(s) would correlate with the positions.

References

AHIMA. 2016a. Certification. http://www.ahima.org/certification

AHIMA. 2016b. Health Information Careers. http://hicareers.com/careermap/

Kellogg, D. W. 2016. Leadership. Chapter 17 in *Health Information Management Technology: An Applied Approach*, 5th ed. Sayles, N. B. and L. Gordon, eds. Chicago: AHIMA.

Sayles, N. B. 2016. Health Information Management Profession. Chapter 1 in *Health Information Management Technology: An Applied Approach*, 5th ed. Sayles, N. B. and L. Gordon, eds. Chicago: AHIMA.

6.16

HIM leadership roles

Subdomain VI.A.1
Summarize health information related leadership roles

1. Create an organizational chart for this HIM department.
2. Identify the leadership positions within the department and provide a brief summary of the responsibilities for each leadership role.

Melissa Reynolds: Coding Supervisor
Janet Jefferson: Transcriptionist
Margie Brown: Transcriptionist
Lois Evers: HIM Director
Mildred Cabot: Coder
Herman Goddard: Assistant HIM Director
Karen Marshall: Coder
Edna George: Lead Coder
Shirley Richards: Transcription Supervisor
Taylor Smith: ROI Clerk
Carol Fredrickson: Scanner Tech
Josh Maynor: Scanner Tech
Lisa Hubbard: Coder
Gloria Lawson: Transcriptionist
Denise Cavanaugh: Coder
Laura Benson: ROI Clerk
Delores Miles: Analyst
Kathy Jones: HIM Department Supervisor
Joyce Call: Analyst
Carla Wilson: Transcriptionist
Leah Carson: Coder
Beth McMahon: Analyst
Rebecca Morris: Lead Transcriptionist

Further Student Reading

Sayles, N. B. 2016. Health Information Functions, Purpose, and Users. Chapter 3 in *Health Information Management Technology: An Applied Approach*, 5th ed. Sayles, N. B. and L. Gordon, eds. Chicago: AHIMA.

6.17

Cultural awareness self-assessment

Subdomain VI.H.3
Assess how cultural issues affect health, healthcare quality, cost, and HIM

Subdomain VI.H.3
Assess how cultural issues affect health, healthcare quality, cost, and HIM

1. Locate an online cultural diversity self-assessment and complete it.
2. Provide the link for the on-line assessment that you complete.
3. Why did you choose this assessment?
4. Interpret the results and identify two areas for personal improvement.

Further Student Reading

AHIMA. 2003. Think salad, not stew: managing cultural differences in your HIM department. *AHIMA Advantage* 7:1.

Johns, M. 2013. Breaking the glass ceiling: structural, cultural, and organizational barriers preventing women from achieving senior and executive positions. *Perspectives in Health Information Management* 1(11).

6.18

ADA and HIM

Subdomain VI.H.4
Create programs and policies that support a culture of diversity

Subdomain VI.H.4
Create programs and policies that support a culture of diversity

1. Discuss the Americans with Disabilities Act.
2. Theorize when it would be appropriate as an HIM Director to refrain from hiring a person with a disability.

References

Oachs, P. and A. Watters. 2016. *Health Information Management: Concepts, Principles, and Practice*, 5th ed. Chicago: AHIMA.

6.19

HIM department diversity

Subdomain VI.H.2
Evaluate the culture of a department

A 60-year-old woman has just been hired as the HIM director at an organization where a majority of her staff is in their early 20s, with many of them being recent graduates. Assess the cultural diversity that you would expect to be evident in the department and the potential challenges that the director might face.

References

Dimick, C. 2007. HIM manager, non-HIM staff: managing staff with expertise beyond HIM. *Journal of AHIMA* 78(9).

Patena, K. 2016. Employee Training and Development. Chapter 24 in *Health Information Management: Concepts, Principles, and Practice*, 5th ed. Oachs, P. and A. Watters, eds. Chicago: AHIMA.

Swenson, D. X. 2016. Managing and Leading During Organization Change. Chapter 22 in *Health Information Management: Concepts, Principles, and Practice*, 5th ed. Oachs, P. and A. Watters, eds. Chicago: AHIMA.

6.20

Art of negotiating

Subdomain VI.A.1
Take part in effective negotiating and use influencing skills

You are training an assistant to participate in organizational performance improvement committees. After observing the interaction at a recent meeting, the assistant states that the committee seems divided in two on how best to proceed and both sides are entrenched in their positions. He is unsure how to proceed to get the committee back on track. Recommend at least four strategies for negotiation that the assistant can employ.

References

Dimick, C. 2007. HIM manager, non-HIM staff: managing staff with expertise beyond HIM. *Journal of AHIMA* 78(9).

Patena, K. 2016. Employee Training and Development. Chapter 24 in *Health Information Management: Concepts, Principles, and Practice*, 5th ed. Oachs, P. and A. Watters, eds. Chicago: AHIMA.

Swenson, D. X. 2016. Managing and Leading During Organization Change. Chapter 22 in *Health Information Management: Concepts, Principles, and Practice*, 5th ed. Oachs, P. and A. Watters, eds. Chicago: AHIMA.

6.21

Salary negotiation

Subdomain VI.A.1
Take part in effective negotiating and use influencing skills

For the past three weeks you have been in the application and interview process for an HIM director position. You currently work as an assistant director at another area hospital and have 15 years of HIM experience. Today you were offered the job, with a salary that is comparable to what you make now. The organization is roughly the same size as the one where you are currently employed. You think that you should make more for the upper level position. Develop a strategy to address your salary concern and then formulate your response to the offer.

References

Dimick, C. 2007. HIM Manager, non-HIM Staff: Managing Staff with Expertise Beyond HIM. *Journal of AHIMA* 78(9).

Kaplan-Quinn, G. 2003. New Job? More Money? Negotiating Pays Off. *Journal of AHIMA* 74(6):46.

LeBlanc, M. M. 2016. Human Resources Management. Chapter 23 in *Health Information Management: Concepts, Principles, and Practice*, 5th ed. Oachs, P. and A. Watters, eds. Chicago: AHIMA.

6.22

Identify types of budget variances

Subdomain VI.G.3
Explain budget variances

Subdomain IV.A.3
Apply principles of healthcare finance for revenue management

Identify the following types of budget variances by indicating if they are temporary/permanent and favorable/unfavorable.

1. $7,500.00 for outsourced coding services to address backlog
2. $12,500.00 as a result of Assistant Director laid off in November
3. $500 for new computer needed to replace one that quit and was not repairable
4. $4,000.00 1st quarter record destruction postponed a quarter due to staffing issues

References

Revoir, R. and N. Davis. 2016. Financial Management. Chapter 26 in *Health Information Management: Concepts, Principles, and Practice*, 5th ed. Oachs, P. and A. Watters, eds. Chicago: AHIMA.

6.23

Depreciation

Subdomain VI.G.2
Explain accounting methodologies

Calculate the straight line depreciation for $10,000 in office furniture with a residual value of $2,000. The useful life of the furniture is expected to be 10 years.

References

Revoir, R. and N. Davis. 2016. Financial Management. Chapter 26 in *Health Information Management: Concepts, Principles, and Practice*, 5th ed. Oachs, P. and A. Watters, eds. Chicago: AHIMA.

6.24

Hospital merger

Subdomain VI.B.1
Recognize the impact of change management on processes, people, and systems

Subdomain VI.B.1
Interpret concepts of change management theories, techniques, and leadership

Two local hospitals that are struggling financially have decided to merge. Consolidation of services, including HIM, will be taking place. Examine the two HIM department structures in place now and offer an opinion about how they could be restructured. Be sure to support your position.

Hospital 1	Hospital 2
Director	Director
Department Supervisor	Transcription Supervisor
Transcription Supervisor	4 coders
8 coders	5 transcriptionists
12 transcriptionists	2 assemblers/analysts
6 assemblers/analysts	1 ROI clerk
2 ROI clerks	1.5 scanner techs
3 scanner techs	1 incomplete records
2 incomplete records	4 file clerks
4 file clerks	1 cancer registrar
1 cancer registrar	

References

LeBlanc, M. M. 2016. Human Resources Management. Chapter 23 in *Health Information Management: Concepts, Principles, and Practice*, 5th ed. Oachs, P. and A. Watters, eds. Chicago: AHIMA.

Swenson, D. 2016. Managing and Leading During Organization Changes. Chapter 22 in *Health Information Management: Concepts, Principles, and Practice*, 5th ed. Oachs, P. and A. Watters, eds. Chicago: AHIMA.

6.25

Benchmarking performance

Subdomain VI.D.4
Benchmark staff performance data incorporating labor analytics

Subdomain VI.D.5
Evaluate staffing levels and productivity, and provide feedback to staff regarding performance

You have six scanner techs, three work first shift (D); three work second shift (A) and each is assigned to a specific scanner noted below. A scanning backlog is growing over the past week, so you have decided to evaluate their productivity. They each recorded their daily productivity over the past two weeks. Since they do not have other department responsibilities, all their time is spent on scanning. One staff member, Teresa, worked a half day on one of the days, and one person, John, had a personal day; otherwise the techs all worked their full 8-hour shift daily for the two-week period under study.

1. Calculate each tech's hourly productivity as well as an overall group productivity.

Scanner 1(D)	John	112,892
Scanner 2(D)	Teresa	160,588
Scanner 3(D)	Larry	193,248
Scanner 1(A)	Mary	138,800
Scanner 2(A)	Jenny	182,160
Scanner 3(A)	Tom	184,960

2. Determine if the individuals and group are meeting the benchmark of 1,200–2,400 scanned images per hour.

3. What conclusions can you draw from this study?

4. Recommend a new productivity standard based on the information gathered above in order to reduce the back log.

5. If your scanning backlog has been about 1,000 pages per day, will the new productivity standard erase that backlog?

6. Do you have enough staff to handle the current workload if there is no backlog?

References

Dunn, R. 2007. Benchmarking imaging: Making every image count in scanning programs. *Journal of AHIMA* 78(6):42–46.

Oachs, P. and A. Watters. 2016. *Health Information Management: Concepts, Principles, and Practice*, 5th ed. Chicago: AHIMA.

Further Student Reading

LeBlanc, M. M. 2016. Human Resources Management. Chapter 23 in *Health Information Management: Concepts, Principles, and Practice*, 5th ed. Oachs, P. and A. Watters, eds. Chicago: AHIMA.

Swenson, D. 2016. Managing and Leading During Organization Changes. Chapter 22 in *Health Information Management: Concepts, Principles, and Practice*, 5th ed. Oachs, P. and A. Watters, eds. Chicago: AHIMA.

6.26

IOM impact

Subdomain VI.F.4
Evaluate how healthcare policy-making both directly and indirectly impacts the national and global healthcare delivery systems

Assess at least four drivers of clinical quality that the Institute of Medicine's reports: *To Err is Human: Building a Safer Health System* and *Crossing the Quality Chasm: A New Health System for the 21st Century* fostered for patient safety.

References

O'Dell, R. 2016. Clinical Quality Management. Chapter 21 in *Health Information Management: Concepts, Principles, and Practice*, 5th ed. Oachs, P. and A. Watters, eds. Chicago: AHIMA.

6.27

Vendor selection

Subdomain VI.J.1
Explain Vendor/Contract Management

Your organization is going to implement a new EHR. During the vendor selection process, five vendors are recognized as potential suppliers. Three of the vendors are well-known companies; the other two are smaller companies.

1. Identify 5 criteria that you would expect to be used in the decision-making process.
2. Explain why cost should not be the determining factor when choosing an EHR vendor.

References

Amatayakul, M. K. 2013. *Electronic Health Records: A Practical Guide for Professionals and Organizations,* 5th ed. Chicago: AHIMA.

6.28

Project management life cycle

Subdomain VI.I.1
Summarize project management methodologies

Choose one aspect of the project management process group sequence and identify its importance. Include the repercussions that would ensue if that element was overlooked.

References

Olson, B. 2016. Project Management. Chapter 27 in *Health Information Management: Concepts, Principles, and Practice*, 5th ed. Oachs, P. and A. Watters. Chicago: AHIMA.

6.29

Healthcare policies

Subdomain VI.F.2
Understand the importance of healthcare policy-making as it relates to the healthcare delivery system

Choose a recent healthcare policy, legislation, or initiative and examine how it impacts access, cost, or quality in healthcare.

References

Shi, L. and D. Singh. 2013. *Essentials of the U. S. Health Care System*, 3rd ed. Burlington: Jones and Bartlett Learning.

6.30

Emergency plan training

Subdomain VI.E.1
Explain the methodology of training and development

The HIM director has asked you to train the HIM staff on departmental responsibilities when a Code Adam (missing child) is announced. Without getting into specifics, devise a plan that would appeal to each type of sensory learner (visual, auditory, and kinesthetic).

References

Patena, K. 2016. Employee Training and Development. Chapter 24 in *Health Information Management: Concepts, Principles, and Practice*, 5th ed. Oachs, P. and A. Watters, eds. Chicago: AHIMA.

Prater, V. S. 2016. Human Resources Management and Professional Development. *Health Information Management Technology: An Applied Approach*, 5th ed. Sayles, N. B. and L. Gordon, eds. Chicago: AHIMA.

6.31

Team facilitator

Subdomain VI.A.3
Organize and facilitate meetings

You have been asked to be a team facilitator for a process improvement project for the HIM department. Describe best practices for communication, interpersonal, and critical thinking skills in this role.

References

Shaw, P. L. and D. Carter. 2015. *Quality and Performance Improvement in Healthcare, A Tool for Programmed Learning,* 6th ed. Chicago: AHIMA.

6.32

Work redesign

Subdomain VI.A.3
Take part in effective communication through project reports, business reports, and professional communications

As coding supervisor, you want to institute remote coding at your facility. With an EHR in place, you feel this would be an opportune time to develop this program. Your Director has asked for a report on the work redesign that may need to be addressed in order for this transition to occur. Create a memo to director Margaret Smythe with the areas that will need to be addressed and predict the level of difficulty that could be associated with each.

References

Coplan-Gould, W., Carolan, K., and Friedman, B. 2011. Re-engineering the coding workflow: Assessing today with an Eye toward tomorrow. *Journal of AHIMA* 82(7):20–24.

Hunt, T. J. 2016. Clinical Documentation Improvement and Coding Compliance. Chapter 9 in *Health Information Management: Concepts, Principles, and Practice*, 5th ed. Oachs, P. and A. Watters, eds. Chicago: AHIMA.

Knight, B. and E. Lewis. 2004. *Three Steps to Remote Coding Success: The Sun Health Experience*. AHIMA Communities of Practice.

6.33

Mentor

Subdomain VI.A.4
Apply personnel management skills

As the coding supervisor at your organization, you have been approached by a file clerk who would like to become a coder. She has an associate degree in health information management, but she needs a mentor to help her reach her goal. Propose at least four steps that she can take to help her achieve her goal.

References

Patena, K. 2016. Employee Training and Development. Chapter 24 in *Health Information Management: Concepts, Principles, and Practice*, 5th ed. Oachs, P. and A. Watters, eds. Chicago: AHIMA.

Coding productivity standards

Subdomain VI.C.2
Construct performance management measures

As the newly hired coding manager at your 300-bed acute care facility, you are surprised that there are no coding productivity standards in place. Your organization outsources the same day surgery accounts, but everything else is coded internally with the number of charts per coder varying greatly. Unfortunately, the discharged not final billed amount is climbing at an alarming rate. In an effort to reduce the DNFB, you determine that coding productivity standards must be implemented. You benchmark against three local hospitals to set the standards. Their standards are:

	Inpatient	ER	Same day surgery	Ancillaries
Hospital A	30	150	60	265
Hospital B	18	90	40	250
Hospital C	27	120	50	275

1. Theorize at least four reasons why there is such a discrepancy in the productivity standards among these facilities.

Further Student Reading

Oachs, P. and A. Watters. 2016. *Health Information Management: Concepts, Principles, and Practice*, 5th ed. Chicago: AHIMA.

6.35

Workflow design

Subdomain VI.C.1
Analyze workflow processes and responsibilities to meet
organizational needs

Study the workflow illustrated below which shows the movement of discharged charts in
the HIM department once they are collected from patient floors on night shift. Recommend
changes to the workflow which would streamline the process.

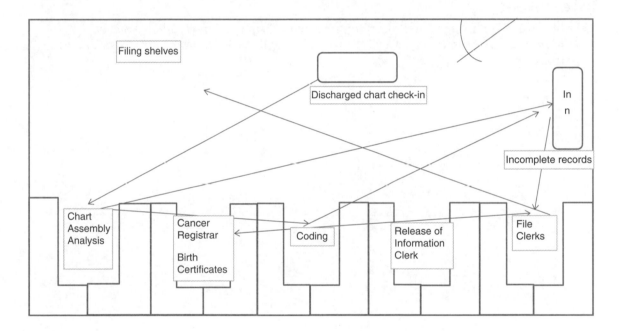

References

Oachs, P. 2016. Work Design and Process Improvement. Chapter 25 in *Health Information Management: Concepts, Principles, and Practice*, 5th ed. Oachs, P. and A. Watters, eds. Chicago: AHIMA.

6.36

Swimlane diagram

Subdomain VI.C.3
Demonstrate workflow concepts

Create a swimlane diagram for the revenue cycle process covering the basic steps from registration to closing the patient account.

References

Oachs, P. 2016. Work Design and Process Improvement. Chapter 25 in *Health Information Management: Concepts, Principles, and Practice*, 5th ed. Oachs, P. and A. Watters, eds. Chicago: AHIMA.

6.37

Disciplinary action

Subdomain VI.D.1
Manage human resources to facilitate staff recruitment, retention, and supervision

Assess the following situations and determine the disciplinary action that should be taken in each circumstance and justify your response.

1. One of your best inpatient coders was found to have violated HIPAA by looking at a physician's emergency room record. Investigation into that breach also found that he has accessed records of relatives and neighbors.

2. An audit of the file clerks has found that one clerk is making errors when filing loose sheets. They are not being incorporated into the correct chart. This same error was verbally addressed with the file clerk at her last performance evaluation two months ago.

3. On Saturday, your release of information clerk left the office open and unattended while she went to the restroom. This was reported to you by the nursing administrator on duty who had come to the office to request her recent lab results.

References

LeBlanc, M. M. 2016. Human Resources Management. Chapter 23 in *Health Information Management: Concepts, Principles, and Practice*, 5th ed. Oachs, P. and A. Watters, eds. Chicago: AHIMA.

6.38

Coder orientation

Subdomain VI.D.3
Create and implement staff orientation and training programs

1. Propose the topics that should be included in a department-specific orientation for new coding staff.

2. Choose one of the topics and suppose it was not covered during the orientation process, what would/could happen?

References

Patena, K. 2016. Employee Training and Development. Chapter 24 in *Health Information Management: Concepts, Principles, and Practice*, 5th ed. Oachs, P. and A. Watters, eds. Chicago: AHIMA.

6.39

RFI, FRP, budget

Subdomain VI.G.1
Evaluate capital, operating, and/or project budgets using basic accounting principles

Subdomain VI.G.2
Perform cost-benefit analysis for resource planning and allocation

Subdomain VI.G.3
Evaluate the stages of the procurement process

Subdomain VI.I.1
Take part in system selection processes

Your organization is considering outsourcing all of its coding services. Currently, coding staff use the 3M encoder and a computer-assisted coding program. The first step is to issue a request for information.

1. Evaluate the following results from your request for information and decide which three vendors to contact for a request for proposal.

	Turnaround time	Are coders certified? AHIMA/AAPC		Are coders familiar with 3M encoder?		Are coders familiar with computer assisted coding?		What coding services are provided?				Payment?	
		Yes	No	Yes	No	Yes	No	Inpatient	Outpatient	Emergency	Ancillary	Per chart	Per hour
Vendor 1	48 hrs.	X		X		X		X	X	X	X	X	
Vendor 2	48 hrs.		X	X			X	X	X	X	X		X
Vendor 3	24 hrs.		X	X		X		X	X	X	X	X	
Vendor 4	72 hrs.	X		X		X		X	X	X	X		X
Vendor 5	48 hrs.	X		X		X		X	X	X	X		X

2. Now determine eight items that should be included in the request for proposal that will be distributed.

3. Assume that you want to go with Vendor 1 after the RFPs are evaluated. Now you must perform a cost-benefit analysis to see if it is feasible to entirely outsource. Their pricing structure is $5 per inpatient chart, $3 per outpatient chart, $1.75 for each ER, and $1 per ancillary account. Base your calculations on the average daily accounts for each patient type listed below:

Inpatient   70
Outpatient   75
Emergency Room   185
Ancillary   360

4. Now calculate your coding budget for next year. All full-time staff will be getting a 2.5% raise; part-time staff will be getting 1%. In addition, you must also account for the fringe benefit costs associated with the coding staff which are 32% of their salary.

Coder	Current rate	This year's salary	Raise	Next year's salary
Inpatient Coder 1 FTE	24.00 per hr.			
Inpatient Coder 2 FTE	22.50 per hr.			
Inpatient Coder 3 FTE	21.85 per hr.			
Outpatient Coder 1 FTE	19.75 per hr.			
Outpatient Coder 2 FTE	19.75 per hr.			
ER Coder 1 FTE	18.25 per hr.			
ER Coder 2 PT	18.25 per hr.			
Ancillary Coder 1 FTE	17.50 per hr.			
Ancillary Coder 2 PT	17.50 per hr.			

5. Is it cost effective to consider outsourcing coding based on these results?

6. What would the outcome be if you considered Vendor 5 at $30.00 per hour?

References

Amatayakul, M. A. 2016. Health Information Systems Strategic Planning. Chapter 13 in *Health Information Management: Concepts, Principles, and Practice*, 5th ed. Oachs, P. and A Watters, eds. Chicago: AHIMA.

American Health Information Management Association. 2010. RFI/RFP Template (Updated). http://library.ahima.org/xpedio/groups/public/documents/ahima/bok1_047959. hcsp?dDocName=bok1_047959

Revoir, R. and N. Davis. 2016. Financial Management. Chapter 26 in *Health Information Management: Concepts, Principles, and Practice*, 5th ed. Oachs, P. and A Watters, eds. Chicago: AHIMA.

6.40

ACO, IG, and strategic planning

Subdomain VI.F.2
Implement a departmental strategic plan

Subdomain VI.F.5
Identify the different types of organizations, services, and personnel and their interrelationships across the healthcare delivery system

Subdomain VI.F.6
Collaborate in the development and implementation of information governance initiatives

Subdomain VI.F.7
Facilitate the use of enterprise-wide information assets to support organizational strategies and objectives

1. Identify the characteristics of an accountable care organization (ACO).

2. Explore the relationship of information governance (IG) to ACOs.

3. Which organizational stakeholders would you recommend be on the IG team/ council?

4. As HIM Director, you are revising your HIM department's strategic plan to include IG and ACOs. What goals would you include for those strategies?

5. Explain how the use of registries can facilitate an accountable care organization's strategies.

References

AHIMA. 2016. Information Governance Toolkit 2.0. http://bok.ahima.org/PdfView?oid=300993

AHIMA. 2014. Information Governance Offers a Strategic Approach for Healthcare. *Journal of AHIMA* 85(10):70–75.

AHIMA. Accountable Care: Implications for Managing Health Information. 2011. AHIMA Thought Leadership Series. http://library.ahima.org/xpedio/groups/public/documents/ahima/ bok1_049111.pdf

McClernon, S. E. 2016. Strategic Thinking and Management. Chapter 29 in *Health Information Management: Concepts, Principles, and Practice*, 5th ed. Oachs, P. and A. Watters, eds. Chicago: AHIMA.

White, S., Kallem, C., Viola, A., and Bronnert, J. 2011. An ACO primer: Reviewing the proposed rule on accountable care organizations. *Journal of AHIMA* 82(6):48–50.

6.41

CDI training

Subdomain VI.E.1
Evaluate initial and on-going training programs

A clinical documentation improvement (CDI) program has been up and running for six months. Initial training of the CDI staff covered the following:

Overview of the CDI program and goals
MS-DRGs including CCs and MCCs and their impact on MS-DRG assignment
The top 10 MS-DRGs for the organization
What documentation is used for code assignment and where to find in the paper and electronic record
Review of clinical indicators for specific diagnosis such as respiratory failure and protein calorie malnutrition

1. After reviewing the training program, recommend four additional topics that should be covered.

2. Why are these topics important to the CDI program?

References

AHIMA. 2013. Recruitment, selection, and orientation for CDI specialists. *Journal of AHIMA* 84(7):58–62 [expanded web version].

Patena, K. 2016. Employee Training and Development. Chapter 24 in *Health Information Management: Concepts, Principles, and Practice*, 5th ed. Oachs, P. and A. Watters, eds. Chicago: AHIMA.

6.42

Management principles

Subdomain VI.F.3
Apply general principles of management in the administration of health information services

AS HIM director, you have decided to bring the release of information services back in-house. For the last two years, you have outsourced that work, but continual complaints and an increasing backlog have made a change necessary.

- List the managerial functions that will be necessary as you tackle this process and select at least one tool that will be used in each function. Be sure to justify the selection of the tool.

References

Swenson, D. X. 2016. Managing and Leading During Organizational Change. Chapter 22 in *Health Information Management: Concepts, Principles, and Practice*, 5th ed. Oachs, P. and A. Watters, eds. Chicago: AHIMA.

6.43

Project: contract management

Subdomain VI.I.2
Recommend clinical, administrative, and specialty service applications

Subdomain VI.J.2
Develop negotiation skills in the process of system selection

1. As HIM director, you are in charge of the purchase process of an encoder for your 20 coders. You have pulled out the criteria that you will use to make the determination and put it in the grid below. Based on this information from the requests for proposal choose an encoder vendor and justify your choice.

2. The IT department, who was not part of the selection process, has found out that you are closing the deal on the new encoder. They ask about the interfaces between the EHR and the encoder. You realize that this is a key area that you forgot to address and learn that it is an additional cost of $2,500.00. Design a negotiation strategy to attempt to reduce or eliminate this cost.

Type of Encoder	Vendor 1 Knowledge-based	Vendor 2 Logic-based	Vendor 3 Knowledge-based
Grouping and Pricing:			
DRG	X	X	X
APC	X	X	X
ASC	X	X	
Integrated coding references	X	X	X
Built in code edits	X	X	X
Productivity reports	X	X	
Platform	Installed	Either	Web-based
Support:			
Technical	X	X	X six months free, $500 per month after first six months
Coding		X	
Cost	$25,000 initial cost, additional $1,000 per user over 10	32,000 initial cost, additional $500.00 per user over 10	$17,500 initial cost, additional $500 per user over 10
Annual Maintenance	$5,000.00 annually	10% of total cost annually	$2,500.00 annually

References

Oachs, P. 2016. Work Design and Process Improvement. Chapter 25 in *Health Information Management: Concepts, Principles, and Practice*, 5th ed. Oachs, P. and A. Watters, eds. Chicago: AHIMA.

Olson, B. D. 2016. Project Management. Chapter 27 in *Health Information Management: Concepts, Principles, and Practice*, 5th ed. Oachs, P. and A. Watters, eds. Chicago: AHIMA.

6.44

Vendor contracts

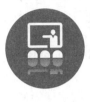

Subdomain VI.J.1
Evaluate vendor contracts

You are the coding manager for Pine Valley Regional Hospital and are in negotiations to outsource some of your coding. The vendor has drawn up a contract for your approval.

1. Review the remote coding contract that follows and determine the one significant area that has not been addressed.

2. Recommend language to insert into the contract to correct the omission.

AGREEMENT FOR REMOTE CODING SERVICES

THIS AGREEMENT made on the date and year indicated below, between **DAWSON & ASSOCIATES, LLC** (hereinafter referred to as "Contractor") and **Pine Valley Regional Hospital (PVRH)** ("Client");

WHEREAS, Client desires the services of remote coding of its Medicare, Medicaid, and commercial payor assigned charts that are scanned or made available to coders; and WHEREAS, Contractor desires to provide the service of remote coding; NOW, THEREFORE, in consideration of the mutual promises made herein and for other good and valuable consideration, it is hereby agreed by and between the parties as follows:

1. Contractor shall provide remote coding services.

   a) The Contractor understands and agrees to provide all information necessary to set up a Contract coder in the OVMC systems. This may include personal information about the contract coder including DOB, last four digits of their social security number, phone number and address in order for remote access to be added.

   b) Contract coders with 3M Coding and Reimbursement encoder and Meditech software will be sought.

   c) Contract coders will abide by the Official Coding and Reporting Guidelines, coding advice published in Coding Clinic for ICD-10-CM, CPT Assistant, except in the instance of unique payor requirements. Contract coders will also abide by PVRH coding policies and procedures.

   d) Company must provide proof of current coding credentials – RHIT and or CCS or CCA required with at least 1 year experience in acute care setting in either inpatient or ambulatory surgery coding.

2. In consideration of the above service, Client shall pay to Contractor the sum of FIFTY DOLLARS PER HOUR ($50):

3. Contractor will review any new contract coder provided to an PVRH facility. Contractor shall provide bi-annual quality reviews on remote coding staff at no charge to Client. At least twenty (20) records will be reviewed for each staff member per bi-annual audit.

e) Contractor will review the first fifty (50) records of any new contract coder that is assigned to PVRH at no charge to the Client. The review results will be shared with PVRH.

f) Results of bi-annual review will be shared with Client by November 1 of every year.

g) Results of 95% for DRG assignment or less than 95% for ICD-10-CM Coding or CPT Coding a performance improvement action plan will be initiated consisting of 5% random reviews every week until quality goals are met.

4. Contractor agrees to lock in pricing with minimal increases (less than 3% increase per hourly rate) for the next 3 years.

5. Client agrees to pay Contractor the full amount of the invoice with thirty (30) days of receipt of the invoice. A service charge of one and one-half percent (1.5%) per month shall be charged for any invoices not paid within thirty (30) days of delivery of said invoice.

6. Client shall make available to Contractor at Client's expense, the means by which the Contractor can access the Client's records and Clients computer network including. (Delete - any and all hardware and software necessary including a secure ID card for Contractor to access any of Client's records and access to Client's computer network.)

    a) Contractor will be required to support their staff set up for remote access. In addition the company must provide:

       i) Adequate equipment for their contracting staff that can support remote coding

       ii) Connectivity to internet

7. Contractor is at all times acting and performing as an independent contractor and is not and shall not be deemed to be an employee of Client for any purpose whatsoever. Contractor has the full power over the determination of the hours to be worked and method of completing Contractor's responsibilities hereunder. As an independent contractor, Contractor will not receive workers' compensation, unemployment compensation, or any other fringe benefit which normally accrue to employees of Client and is responsible for providing Contractor's own benefits and paying all income withholding taxes, including FICA.

8. Upon termination of this Agreement, each party shall promptly return to the other all data, materials, and other property of the other held by it.

9. Client agrees that any and all intellectual property including copies thereof used by Contractor to perform its services are and shall remain the exclusive property of Contractor and may not be used by Client for any purpose not specifically authorized by Contractor. Intellectual property shall include, but is not limited to, processes, computer software, and educational materials.

10. Both parties will indemnify and hold the other party harmless against any liabilities, damages, and expenses including reasonable attorney fees resulting from any third-party claim or suit arising from Contractor's performance under this Agreement.

11. All notices and communications in connection with this Agreement shall be in writing and shall be considered given when delivered personally to the recipient's address as stated in this Agreement or when sent by fax to the last fax number of the recipient known to the person giving notice.

12. Either party may terminate this Agreement at any time by giving the other written notice of termination. Such notice of termination shall be effective thirty (30) days after notice is delivered. Contractor shall be responsible for carrying out all duties that have been scheduled within that thirty (30)-day termination period and Client

shall be responsible for full payment of all services scheduled and performed prior to the actual date of termination.

13. This Agreement shall be governed by the laws of the State of Ohio.

14. This is the entire agreement between the parties with respect to this matter.

15. This Agreement may not be changed except in writing and signed by authorized representatives of both parties.

CLIENT: **Pine Valley Regional Hospital**

By: _____

_____

[Type or print name]

Address: _____

_____

Its: _____

Date: _____

CONTRACTOR: **DAWSON & ASSOCIATES, LLC**

By: _____

_____

[Type or print name]

Address: _____

_____

Its: _____

Date: _____

Source of contract Dee Mandley and Associates. Adapted and reprinted with permission.

References

Oachs, P. 2016. Work Design and Process Improvement. Chapter 25 in *Health Information Management: Concepts, Principles, and Practice*, 5th ed. Oachs, P. and A. Watters, eds. Chicago: AHIMA.

6.45

IG plan

Subdomain VI.K.1
Manage information as a key strategic resource and mission tool

1. Defend the position that information is an organizational strategic asset.

2. Explain the importance of having an information governance plan in place to manage an organization's information assets.

References

American Health Information Management Association. 2016. Information governance basics: Why IG for healthcare? http://www.ahima.org/topics/infogovernance/igbasics.

6.46

Project management—Gantt chart

Subdomain VI.I.3
Apply project management techniques to ensure efficient workflow and appropriate outcomes

Subdomain VI.I.4
Facilitate project management by integrating work efforts

As coding manager, you are in charge of a new encoder purchase. This is your first attempt at project management and you want to manage it effectively. You create a Gantt chart to illustrate the project from vendor selection to go live.

1. Determine the baseline duration of the critical path of the project.
2. Determine the variance that causes a week's delay.
3. Determine the variance that puts the project back on track.
4. Give an opinion on whether this was a successful project implementation or not and support your position.
5. Evaluate the impact of the document completion task on the overall project.

Task Name	Baseline Duration	Baseline Start	Baseline Finish	Actual Duration	Actual Start	Actual Finish
Purchase and Installation of Encoder		**Mon 2/15/16**	**Fri 7/15/16**		**Mon 2/15/16**	**Mon 7/18/16**
Select Vendor	**55 days**	**Mon 2/15/16**	**Fri 4/29/16**	**62 days**	**Mon 2/15/16**	**Tue 5/10/16**
Create List of Vendors	10 days	Mon 2/15/16	Fri 2/26/16	10 days	Mon 2/15/16	Fri 2/26/16
Send Out Request for Proposal (RFP)	20 days	Mon 2/29/16	Fri 3/25/16	20 days	Mon 2/29/16	Fri 3/25/16
Select Vendor	20 days	Mon 3/28/16	Fri 4/22/16	20 days	Mon 3/28/16	Fri 4/22/16
Finalize Contract	**5 days**	**Mon 4/25/16**	**Fri 4/29/16**	**12 days**	**Mon 4/25/16**	**Tue 5/10/16**
Department Head Signature	2 days	Mon 4/25/16	Tue 4/26/16	2 days	Mon 4/25/16	Tue 4/26/16
CEO Signature	3 days	Wed 4/27/16	Fri 4/29/16	10 days	Wed 4/27/16	Tue 5/10/16
Complete Document Requests	**5 days**	**Mon 5/2/16**	**Fri 5/6/16**	**5 days**	**Wed 5/11/16**	**Tue 5/17/16**
List of Payers	5 days	Mon 5/2/16	Fri 5/6/16	5 days	Wed 5/11/16	Tue 5/17/16
List of Discharge Dispositions	5 days	Mon 5/2/16	Fri 5/6/16	5 days	Wed 5/11/16	Tue 5/17/16
List of Reimbursement Amounts by Payer	5 days	Mon 5/2/16	Fri 5/6/16	5 days	Wed 5/11/16	Tue 5/17/16
Build Interfaces	40 days	Mon 5/9/16	Fri 7/1/16	30 days	Wed 5/18/16	Tue 6/28/16
Installation	1 day	Mon 7/4/16	Mon 7/4/16	1 day	Wed 6/29/16	Wed 6/29/16
Testing	5 days	Tue 7/5/16	Mon 7/11/16	10 days	Thu 6/30/16	Wed 7/13/16
Training	3 days	Tue 7/12/16	Thu 7/14/16	2 days	Thu 7/14/16	Fri 7/15/16
Go Live	1 day	Fri 7/15/16	Fri 7/15/16	1 day	Mon 7/18/16	Mon 7/18/16

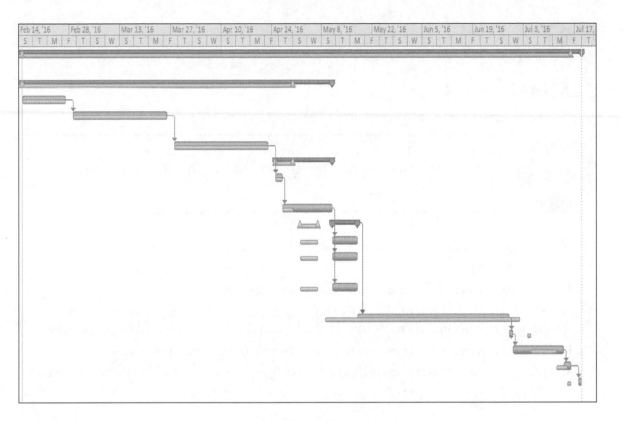

GANTT chart created by M.J. Foley. Reprinted with permission.

References

Olson, B. D. 2016. Project Management. Chapter 27 in *Health Information Management: Concepts, Principles, and Practice*, 5th ed. Oachs, P. and A. Watters, eds. Chicago: AHIMA.

6.47

Sentinel events

Subdomain VI.C.2
Identify cost-saving and efficient means of achieving work processes and goals

Apply The Joint Commission's definition of sentinel event to determine if the following are sentinel events or not.

1. Baby boy Brown is discharged to the Carmichael family
2. Mrs. Richards has extensive cardiac damage from several myocardial infarctions, along with multiple co-morbid conditions and dies during cardiac bypass surgery
3. Patient Smith leaves the emergency department against medical advice
4. Patient Thomas leaves the emergency department against medical advice and two days later commits suicide

References

Joint Commission. 2016. Sentinel events. http://www.jointcommission.org/assets/1/6/CAMH_24_SE_all_CURRENT.pdf.

6.48

PI tools

Subdomain VI.C.1
Utilize tools and techniques to monitor, report, and improve processes

Select the most appropriate performance improvement (PI) tool or technique for each scenario below.

1. A HIM performance improvement committee wants to determine the priorities in addressing the project at hand.

2. Administration has requested a chart showing the processes changes that have been achieved from January to June.

3. A revenue cycle PI team wants to illustrate the percent of denials that are a result of a registration error.

4. A PI team wants to display data that will show if there are uncommon variations in the process.

References

Shaw, P. L. and D. Carter. 2015. *Quality and Performance Improvement in Healthcare: A Tool for Programmed Learning*, 6th ed. Chicago: AHIMA.

6.49

Data collection methods

Subdomain VI.F.1
Summarize a collection methodology for data to guide strategic and organizational management

You have just been hired as a coding supervisor at a local hospital. The coding department has many issues including a two-week backlog of coding, a DNFB of over $7.5 million dollars, and over 50 unanswered physician queries. Describe how you can use the three different data collection tools (interview, survey tools, and direct observation) to capture data that can help you improve the coding process.

References

Shaw, P. L. and D. Carter. 2015. *Quality and Performance Improvement in Healthcare: A Tool for Programmed Learning*, 6th ed. Chicago: AHIMA.

Further Student Reading

Forrestal, E. 2016. Research methods. Chapter 19 in *Health Information Management: Concepts, Principles, and Practice*, 5th ed. Oachs, P. and A. Watters, eds. Chicago: AHIMA.

6.50

Discipline

Subdomain VI.D.3
Adhere to work plans, policies, procedures, and resource requisitions in relation to job functions

A random audit showed that one of the scanner techs was not following the proper procedure for entering late records. You discussed this with him and gave him a verbal warning. Per protocol you monitored that scanner's handling of late records for a month and found several more instances of them being processed incorrectly. This time the scanner received a written warning. How will you handle a third occurrence of this issue?

References

LeBlanc, M. M. 2016. Human Resources Management. Chapter 23 in *Health Information Management: Concepts, Principles, and Practice*, 5th ed. Oachs, P. and A. Watters, eds. Chicago: AHIMA.

6.51

Budgets

Subdomain VI.G.1
Plan budgets

Consider that you are going to be the HIM director for a large physician group that is just organizing the practice. They are planning to utilize fully electronic records. The electronic health record system and computers will be coming from a separate IT budget. However, you need to plan a departmental and capital budget for the first year of business. What items should you list under each budget? Keep in mind that the group has decided that anything more than $500 should be on the capital budget, except payroll expenses.

References

Revoir, R. and N. Davis. 2016. Financial Management. Chapter 26 in *Health Information Management: Concepts, Principles, and Practice*, 5th ed. Oachs, P. and A Watters, eds. Chicago: AHIMA.

6.52

Data dictionary

Subdomain VI.K.1
Apply knowledge of database architecture and design

1. A data dictionary for patient address and phone number is shown below. Margaret, a registration clerk, is trying to enter the patient's state of Arizona. Every time she starts typing it, Arkansas pops up. Identify the issue preventing the correct state from being entered.

2. Margaret begins to enter the patient's telephone number of 616-256-6767 and only gets as far as 616-256-67 and the field won't accept any more characters.

References

Sharp, M. and C. Madlock-Brown. 2016. Data Management. Chapter 6 in *Health Information Management: Concepts, Principles, and Practice*, 5th ed. Oachs, P. and A. Watters, eds. Chicago: AHIMA.

6.53

Managed care versus accountable care

Subdomain VI.F.3
Describe the differing types of organizations, services, and personnel and their interrelationships across the health care delivery system

1. Identify the characteristics of managed care.
2. Identify the characteristics of an accountable care organization (ACO).
3. Summarize the significant difference between managed care and ACOs.

References

Casto, A. B. and E. Forrestal. 2015. *Principles of Healthcare Reimbursement,* 5th ed. Chicago: AHIMA.

6.54

Data stewardship

Subdomain VI.F.4
Apply information and data strategies in support of information governance initiatives

1. Jim has just been hired as a cancer registrar at a large tertiary care facility. He will be one of four abstractors for the registry. After two days of job training spent going over the registry's data dictionary definitions, Jim is frustrated. He wants to dig in and start abstracting actual cases. Educate Jim on the importance of the data dictionary and the correct application of its definitions for the registry.

2. Apply the concept of data stewardship to this process.

References

Sharp, M. 2016. Secondary data sources. Chapter 7 in *Health Information Management Technology: An Applied Approach*, 5th ed. Sayles, N. B. and L. Gordon, eds. Chicago: AHIMA.

6.55

Data quality management

Subdomain VI.F.5
Utilize enterprise-wide information assets in support of organizational strategies and objectives

A new EHR is going to be purchased for the physician practice you manage. Use three of the characteristics of data quality from AHIMA's Data Quality Management Model, and illustrate how incorporating those characteristics into the EHR will support patient care decisions.

References

AHIMA. 2016. A new view of HIM: introducing the Core Model. http://library.ahima.org/xpedio/groups/public/documents/ahima/bok1_049283.pdf

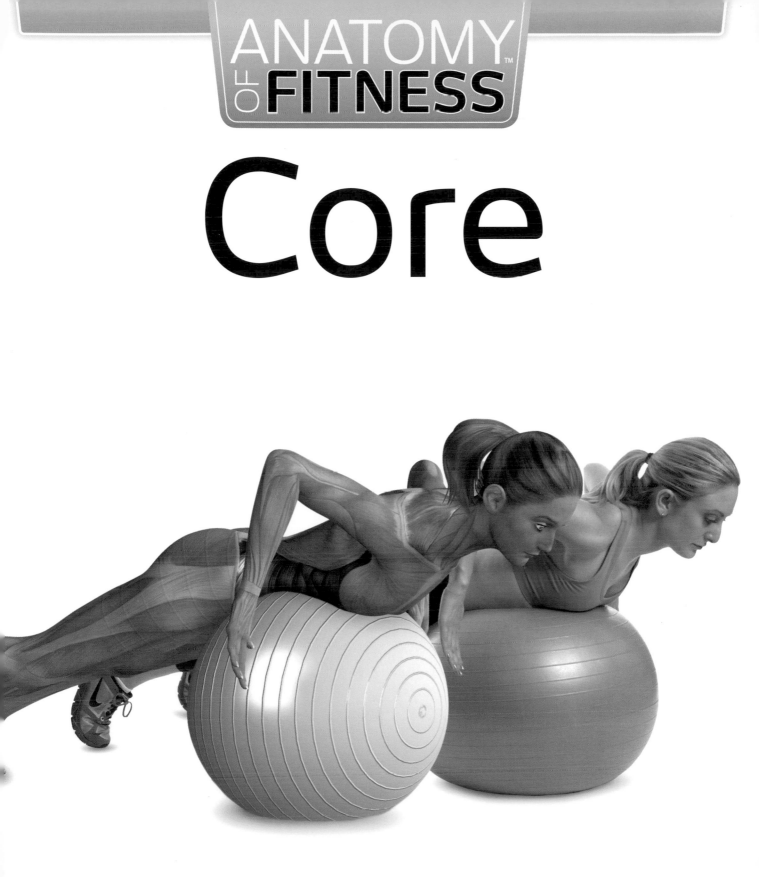

ANATOMY of FITNESS™

Core

Hollis Lance Liebman

Published by Hinkler Books Pty Ltd 2016
45–55 Fairchild Street
Heatherton Victoria 3202 Australia
www.hinkler.com.au

hinkler

Copyright © Hinkler Books Pty Ltd 2013, 2016

Created by Moseley Road Inc.
Editorial Director: Lisa Purcell
Art Director: Brian MacMullen
Photographer: Jonathan Conklin Photography, Inc.
Editor: Erica Gordon-Mallin
Cover design: Sam Grimmer
Designers: Danielle Scaramuzzo, Patrick Johnson
Author: Hollis Lance Liebman
Model: Cori D. Cohen
Illustrator: Hector Aiza/3D Labz Animation India
Prepress: Graphic Print Group

All rights reserved. No part of this publication may be reproduced, stored
in a retrieval system, or transmitted in any way or by any means, electronic,
mechanical, photocopying, recording or otherwise, without the prior written
permission of Hinkler Books Pty Ltd.

ISBN: 978 1 7436 7729 2

Printed and bound in China

Always do the warm-up exercises before attempting any individual exercises. It is recommended that you check with
your doctor or healthcare professional before commencing any exercise regime. While every care has been taken in
the preparation of this material, the publishers and their respective employees or agents will not accept responsibility
for injury or damage occasioned to any person as a result of participation in the activities described in this book.

Contents

CORE STRENGTHENERS

Your core

In the last decade, working the core has become all the rage. But core consciousness is no mere fad—awareness of the importance of a strong, stable core is the key to a stronger self.

These days, fitness enthusiasts invoke the word *core* so often that it can be hard to tell what it really means. Everyone from the new mother wanting to firm her midsection to the weekend tennis warrior seeking more power and accuracy in his backhand swing to the sedentary executive just looking to get through the day without lower-back pain seems to be talking about the core. And for anyone who wants improved posture, or simply to look slimmer and fitter, the idea of "working the core" holds great currency.

What is the core?

The core comprises a system of muscles in the lower-trunk area including the lower back, abdomen, and hips. These muscles work together to provide support and mobility, and it is through them that all bodily movement, in every conceivable direction, originates.

The major core muscles include the spinal flexors, spinal extensors, hip flexors, and hip extensors. The spinal flexors are also known as the anterior abdominals—the muscle group usually referred to as simply the abdominals or the "abs." The abdominal group consists of the rectus abdominis, transversus abdominis, and internal and external obliques. The rectus abdominis, commonly called the "six-pack," is responsible for maintaining spinal stability as well as shortening the distance between your torso and hips. The transversus abdominis provides thoracic and pelvic stability. Both the internal and external obliques are responsible for your ability to bend from side to side and rotate your torso.

The spinal extensors, also known as the posterior abdominals, include the erector spinae, quadratus lumborum, and multifidus spinae. The Christmas tree-shaped erector spinae is actually a group of muscles and tendons that stretches from the lumbar to the cervical spine. The erector spinae is responsible for stabilization as well as movement of your spine.

The hip flexors are the iliopsoas, rectus femoris, sartorius, tensor fasciae latae, pectineus, adductor longus, adductor brevis, and gracilis. The hip extensors include the gluteus maximus and the hamstrings, which are made up of the biceps femoris, semitendinosus, and semimembranosus. The hip flexors and extensors act as the basement of this muscular powerhouse, supporting movement and allowing you to flex and extend your hips.

A strong core is paramount to keeping your body functionally sound and operational. Many quick-fix diets, pieces of exercise equipment, and even surgeries promise a sleeker, better-looking abdominal area, but it is through core training that focuses on the strength and flexibility of these muscle groups—coupled with a healthful diet—that you can achieve real, long-lasting results.

A stronger core = a stronger body

Aside from the obvious aesthetic benefits of maintaining a lean and tight core, there are important functional pluses as well. Imagine easing back pain, improving your balance, standing straighter (and in the process, looking taller), and lifting heavy objects without stress or strain. A strong core allows you to execute everyday movements with ease, even as you age. Core training is an insurance policy for keeping the body performing at peak levels.

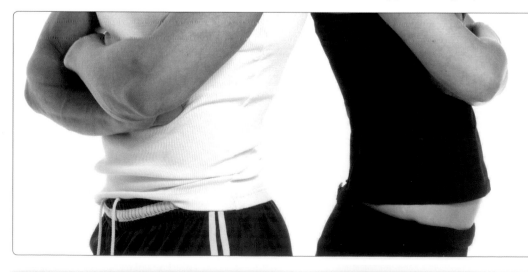

Good things in small packages

The core is the only muscle system in the body that we train for compactness—rather than for volume, as we tend to do for other muscle groups, such as those of the chest or arms. As you train your core, the ultimate goal is not only to have a sleek, toned midsection, but also to attain a functionally sound core that can rotate, contract, and support you whichever way you move.

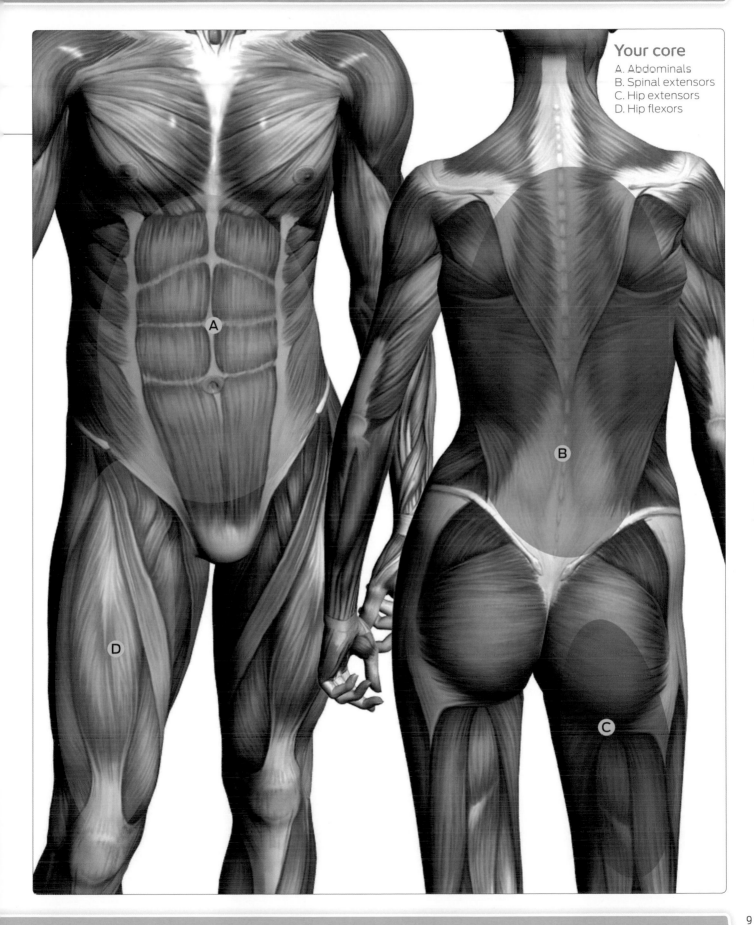

Your core
A. Abdominals
B. Spinal extensors
C. Hip extensors
D. Hip flexors

Maintaining a strong core will also lend optimal support to ancillary (assisting) muscles. In fact, the core is so central to your body's movement that it is called upon whenever any muscle in the body is used. Have you ever exercised your upper arms and discovered later that your midsection was quite sore? That was your core at work.

Your body's central power station

The core is constantly assisting other muscle groups as they function, acting as the fulcrum for all motion. When you squat down to pick up something from the floor, your core muscles work to maintain the integrity of vertical movement. And when you lift an object overhead you mainly recruit your deltoids and triceps, but your core muscles are also working to both support and balance you, keeping your torso steady as you lift. If your core muscles were not engaging, proper trunk alignment would be nearly impossible. That kind of motion, unassisted by the core, would be both much more difficult and potentially dangerous due to spinal compression.

The core acts as the central power station from which all muscular movement originates. Your ability to squat down

to retrieve an object comes from the simultaneous firing of the quadriceps and gluteal muscles, with the core assisting by contracting and keeping the body in line. Whether you are working out or just carrying out your everyday tasks, attempting muscular contraction without aid from the core is like turning on the television without plugging it in.

Core-training basics

Core training is about treating the body as a unified whole. You may feel the effects of some of the exercises in this book in one region of your body more strongly than in others, but these workouts are designed to improve muscular function, strengthening, and stabilization throughout your entire body.

You draw upon your core muscles every day. Although rarely in daily life will you find yourself contracting your biceps or extending your arms to full lockout from your chest as if you're doing a bench press, it's not uncommon to lift an object off the ground and rotate your trunk in order to put it down. This movement is accomplished through reliance on not one isolated muscle, but rather on a group of muscles, including the core, working together.

Put it in neutral

Neutral position, also known as neutral spine and neutral posture, is a key element of core training. You need to understand it before commencing a core-training regimen.

Neutral position is one of the most efficient positions from which to begin movement; it ensures that you properly target and strengthen your core muscles. While in neutral, your spine is in the proper alignment between postural extremes. In its natural alignment, your spine isn't straight—it curves at the neck, upper back, and lower back. These curves act as protection against spinal stress and strain.

Adjusting the tilt of your pelvis will also adjust the alignment of your spine. If you rotate your pelvis backward, you'll notice that the curve of your lower back increases; rotating it forward diminishes that curve.

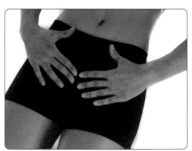

To find your neutral position while lying on your back, place your thumbs on your hip bones and your fingers over your pubic bone (the bone between your legs), to create a triangle. In neutral position, all of the bones will line up on the same plane—neither tipping back nor shifting to one side.

To find neutral position while lying on your stomach, press your pubic bone into your exercise mat until you feel your back flatten slightly or your stomach lightly lift. Tuck your chin so that your forehead rests against your mat.

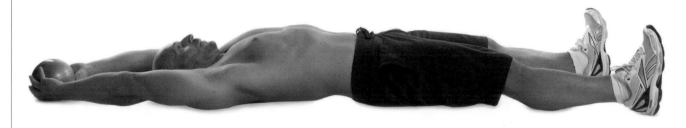

Challenge your core

Our widespread dependence on artificial support, such as chair backs that shoulder for us the work of sitting up straight, has left many of us with weak spines and soft middles. Imagine all of those hours spent slouching, without challenging your core, so that upon rising your back feels strained to the point of pain. If you have a sedentary job, you are likely to benefit greatly from challenging your core through exercise. You can also augment your fitness regimen with a simple addition to your work environment.

If you spend hours behind a desk, try replacing your office chair with a fitness ball. To maintain your balance while sitting on an unstable ball, you must make constant minute postural adjustments, which strongly engages your core. Some manufacturers are now producing specialized balance ball chairs.

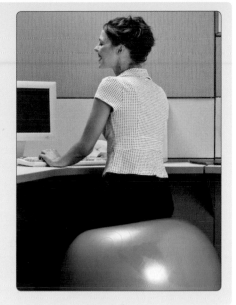

The three keys to core fitness

The keys to successfully executing a core workout are breathing, form, and speed. With a firm command of these three elements, you can develop your core muscles efficiently and effectively. Endless repetitions are neither necessary nor advisable; you need only carry out a few calculated sets to achieve a deep muscular burn.

Breathing

Keep your breathing pace natural and steady. Couple a deep inhale with the negative, or stretching, of the muscle. Think of the inhalation as pulling back the arrow on an archer's bow before launch, and follow it with a deep exhale on the positive, or extended, portion of the movement as if you were releasing the arrow. Aim for a slow or controlled negative followed by an explosive positive and a slight hold at the peak contraction or finished position.

Form

Form is critical to effective core training. Every exercise has its proper starting position, movement path, and action. As you read through the steps to a new exercise, think about those three things, and take the time to properly execute each step with control and precision. Maintain that control through every repetition; controlled exercising develops strength, stamina, flexibility, and ease of movement.

Speed

Neither rush through your reps nor greatly slow them; instead, adopt a natural pace that you can sustain throughout the set while keeping proper form. It is human nature to avoid pain, which is why so many gym-goers perform excessive sets at a lowered intensity or with a limited range of motion. But a few focused and well-executed sets that focus on the muscle's full range and a peak contraction at the top will always be far more effective than too many go-through-the-motions sets.

Give your all during each and every rep performed. That guy at the gym who claims that he can do a thousand sit-ups would in reality be lucky to complete a hundred that truly work his core, because the neck and lower back—not to mention speed and momentum—usually do all the work when so many repetitions are involved. For best results, less is more: aim to lengthen the muscle, then contract and squeeze. Place the tension on the core muscles at hand without calling in recruits.

From warm-up to cool-down

Cold muscles are susceptible to strains, pulls, and tears, so before you begin any workout session, it's best to "thaw out" your muscles. Your body performs optimally when it is warmed and primed for performance. Just 5 to 10 minutes of moderate cardiovascular work, such as pedaling a stationary bicycle or walking on a treadmill, followed by 5 minutes of stretching, warms up your body, preparing it for the rigorous demands you'll place upon it, and protecting it from injury.

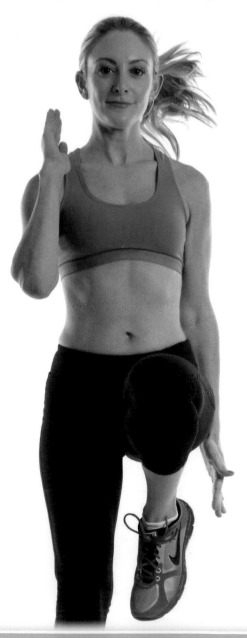

Stretching improves the flexibility in a given muscle and increases its range of motion, which promotes the development of lean muscle tissue. It also improves the rate and quality of your body's processing of nutrients.

Just as you should warm up before you begin your core-training workout, you should cool down after it. Exercise elevates your heart rate and loosens your muscles. A few minutes of stretching and cardio activity will effectively lower your heart rate and help to rid your body of lactic acid and other toxins created as by-products of your workout. Proper warm-ups and cool-downs help ensure long-term performance in and out of the gym.

Core stability and core strength

This book focuses on both core strength and core stability. Stability exercises work the muscles that support your core during motion. To stabilize is to both secure your spine and work your visible abdominal muscles. During the execution of a core-stabilizing exercise, your spine should remain in a neutral position without any movement. Stability exercises focus on improving your core functionality over defining your abdominal musculature.

Core-strengthening exercises work the core directly, building strength and endurance as well as muscles. These are the moves that can give you the "six-pack" abs look, in which each segment of the rectus abdominis is highly defined. Core-strengthening exercises generally target the rectus abdominis, the transversus abdominis, and the obliques. In the process, the muscles of your midsection become more compact, taking inches from your waistline.

How to use this book

The step-by-step chapters of this book include a few warm-up stretches followed by both core-stabilizing and core-strengthening exercises, as well as cool-downs. For each exercise, you'll find a short overview of the move, photos with step-by-step instructions demonstrating how to do it, some tips on how to perform it, and an anatomical illustration annotating key muscles. Some exercises have accompanying variations, shown in the modification box.

Alongside each exercise is a quick-read panel that features at-a-glance illustrations that highlight the targeted areas, an estimate of the level of difficulty, and the average amount of time you'll need to complete the exercise. The last category is a caution list: if you have one of the issues listed, it is best to avoid that exercise.

Core and cardio

Core training isn't just about flat abs—a core-training regimen can also offer you a full body workout that improves cardiovascular fitness.

Before you begin your exercise session, try a few High Knees to raise your heart rate. To perform this fat-burning move, begin running in place, raising your knees to waist height and staying on the balls of your feet. Be sure to keep your core engaged, and really pump your arms for extra aerobic benefit.

Exercises such as Mountain Climber (see pages 56–57) combine the best of core and cardio.

Working out at home

A clear plan and the will to improve are all you need to begin an at-home core-training regimen that is just as effective as working with a personal trainer at an exclusive gym.

You don't need a multilevel health club with all the latest equipment and extras in order to cultivate an attention-grabbing physique. In truth, some of the fittest bodies have been sculpted in low-tech gyms and even at home with some basic equipment—the only extras you'll need are the desire to improve and a targeted plan. In fact, a targeted fitness plan performed at home can prove superior to a schedule at a commercial health club that includes a daunting array of high-tech machinery and filled-up classes. At home, you can focus without distractions and work at your own pace, experimenting as you see fit in order to keep your exercise sessions interesting.

Home-gym equipment

Effective at-home core training calls for very few pieces of specialized equipment—your own body weight is your best asset, providing resistance. To add variety to your fitness regimen, take advantage of objects around the house: use a chair as a prop for dips and push-ups or take advantage of steps for lunges. Broomsticks come in handy for balancing

exercises and twisting movements. A large, thick towel or carpet will provide light cushioning and prevent you from sliding on the floor if you don't have a mat.

There are also plenty of relatively inexpensive pieces of equipment that change up your home workout. Hand weights or dumbbells add resistance, and they take up very little space. To keep clutter to a minimum, purchase adjustable dumbbells that allow you to easily vary the weight levels. Look for a set with a solid-locking mechanism that makes adding and subtracting weight disks a breeze.

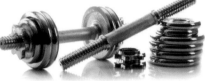

You can also augment your workout with elastic resistance bands; anchoring one of these under your feet or attaching it to a sturdy object allows you to easily switch exercise angles and increase intensity. These bands, which come in several

A core-training corner

Even in the smallest of homes, you can create a fully functional core-training area. Basically, your space need not be much larger than an exercise mat.

Lay out your mat away from the clutter of daily life, if possible. The fewer distractions you face, the more you can concentrate on your breathing, form, and speed. It's also convenient to have a closet or shelf nearby, so that you can store your fitness equipment, such as balls and weights, and set it up without fuss.

Devise a schedule for yourself, designating regular workout times to spend in your core-training corner. You want your training to become a habit.

Creating an inviting and invigorating corner will further your effort to make working out a habit. If simplicity appeals to you, keep your space spare and serene, but don't be afraid to bring in objects that inspire you. A large mirror or anatomical posters of the human skeleton and the major muscles of the back and front might make interesting additions to your space. Although not strictly necessary, these extra visuals can help keep you focused while also providing information that can enhance your exercise experience. The more the space appeals to you, the more you will want to go there.

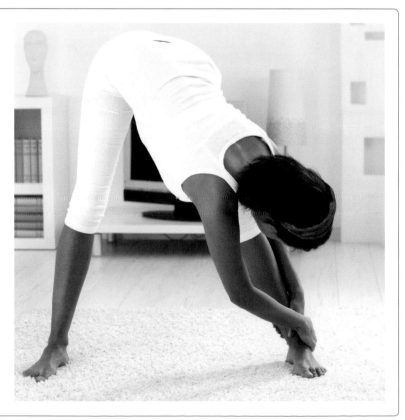

Fitness balls

A low-tech extra like the antiburst fitness ball shown adds another dimension to your at-home routine. This heavy-duty inflatable ball—known by many names, including Swiss ball, exercise ball, body ball, and balance ball—was originally developed for use by physical therapy patients, but it is now standard equipment in commercial and home gyms everywhere. Working on a fitness ball, which ranges in diameter from 15 to 33 inches (35–85 cm), calls for you to constantly adjust your balance, which forces the engagement of many more muscles, especially those of your core. You can perform both core-stabilizing and core-strengthening exercises on a fitness ball.

progressive resistance levels, add another layer of variety to your routine. Weighing next-to-nothing and taking up almost no space, they are the perfect pieces of equipment for travelers who want to keep up their fitness regimens even while away from home.

Balls have many uses in a core-training program. A weighted medicine ball can take the place of hand weights or dumbbells. A fitness ball, shown in many of the following exercises, is a large, heavy-duty inflatable ball that helps you improve your balance and flexibility.

Your workout wardrobe

Think comfort, utility, and, yes, style when deciding what to wear for your workout. Dress for breathability, insulation, and functional comfort, choosing garments that allow you to move freely. This doesn't mean that you should throw on a shapeless T-shirt or baggy sweatpants; form-fitting shorts and tops move with your natural musculature rather than restricting it. Even if you're working out at home, a great outfit can inspire you. Try exercising in front of a mirror—at the start of your workout plan, you may not like how you look in body-hugging garments, but as you stick to your plan, you'll see the changes to your shape even more clearly. Now that's motivation.

Invest in shoes with good cushioning and support; your feet are your foundation. You'll find core training–specific athletic shoes on the market, but a sturdy cross-trainer will serve your needs very well, too.

A time and place for fitness

Effective exercise begins with setting aside time and a place. This is your chance to give back to your body and maintain the machine that is you. Pick a distraction-free location that allows you to clearly focus on your fitness goals. Such elements as music, room temperature, and lighting all have effects on ensuring the best possible workout. A great thing about working out at home is that you can keep these elements personalized to your own taste.

Make sure that your workout surface is comfortable. If you are exercising on a mat, roll it out properly, making sure

that it lies flat with no loose ends curling upward. Leave plenty of space around it. It is important that you be able to freely elongate your muscles; incomplete extensions can lead to incomplete muscular development. A full range of motion is vital to your progress.

Now that you are set to begin your workout, it is important that you be "present." This may seem like a no-brainer at first, but in today's ultra-fast-paced world, it is easy to become distracted by what you think you may be missing while working out. Try to leave all of your concerns outside of your workout space. Turn off the pads, pods, and various other electronic distractions—the world will still exist in all its complexity once your session is over.

For many, making time and space to take care of the body is the highest hurdle; simply getting ready to exercise, whether this involves driving to the gym or setting up a mat at home, takes discipline, time management, and commitment. But we all share the same 24 hours in a day; from the stay-at-home dad to the corporate executive, we lead busy lives. You absolutely can and must make the commitment to take care of your body, whether you slot in that 15 minutes before work, 20 minutes during lunchtime, or 30 minutes after dinner. Make the most of your 24 hours by bettering yourself.

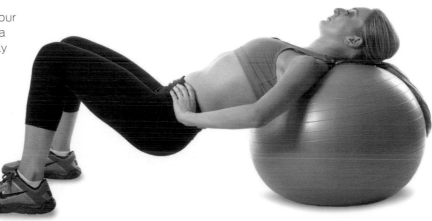

Nourishing your core

Consistent exercise is only part of the successful core-training equation: you must combine targeted training with healthy nutrition to achieve a strong and healthy body.

When you train your core, you are aiming for a physique that is both low in visible body fat and high in lean muscle tissue—a physique most definitely attainable. You can maintain a fit core over the long term by carrying out a solid day-to-day plan that combines stretching, strengthening and cardiovascular exercise with sound food choices.

Food as fuel
For best results, it is vital to fuel properly. The old adage that you are what you eat applies quite literally to the physique. Almost anyone can get thin or even skinny—just severely limit food intake. Relying on drastic reductions of calories, though, often comes at the expense of precious muscle tissue. And a starvation diet usually results in a rebound effect, with the overzealous dieter soon gaining back all the lost weight and then some.

When it comes to fat loss, the most common mistake lies in overtraining and, in the process, breaking the body down to the point of lethargy and exhaustion, while also failing to eat enough to power the body. In this scenario, the body reacts to the lack of food as if it were facing true famine and will burn muscle tissue while holding on to fat stores it can reserve for future use. Your scale may display a lower number, but you still have the same amount of body fat as ever. Rid yourself of any fixation on low weight—replace a "skinny" mentality with a "lean" consciousness.

Too many of us skip breakfast or depend on a last-minute stimulant like coffee, which may fuel us through a few hours—but burnout is inevitable. For optimal results, consume small, frequent meals throughout the day in order to keep your body energized, sparing muscle and instead utilizing stored fat as fuel.

Balancing your diet
The food that makes up your diet can be divided into three groups, or macronutrients: proteins, which help to build muscle mass; fats, which are good for joint lubrication, maintaining body temperature, and promoting healthy cell function in your hair and skin; and carbohydrates, which provide energy.

Look not at calories but rather at macronutrients. Proteins, carbohydrates, and fats are the numbers with which successful "dieters" concern themselves. If you know how many grams of each you consume daily, your can calculate your total caloric intake by adding the three macronutrients.

Carbs: friend or foe?
Carbohydrates can be simple, complex, or fibrous. Simple carbs, such as fruit, are broken down quickly by the body and provide short bursts of energy, while complex carbs, such as oatmeal, are slower to break down and provide sustained energy for longer periods. Fibrous carbs like broccoli and asparagus aid digestion and provide fiber, which assists in the removal of waste from the body.

Many different theories surround the role of carbohydrates in the diet. To some they are the enemy, while others tout them as absolutely necessary parts of every meal. The truth is that they should have a place in the diet of anyone seeking to get fit and look great.

All too often, when you want to lose weight, you begin your day with a carb-free breakfast, eat a midday meal like salad that is high in fibrous carbs, and then arrive home from work ravenous and proceed to consume an excess of complex and simple carbs. Starting out without carbs limits the energy you can draw upon throughout the day. A lunchtime salad,

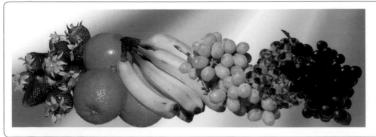

A rainbow diet
Eating the colors of the rainbow may sound like an elementary school lesson plan, but its underlying message is important for adults and children alike. Choose from a varied palette of fruits and vegetables from red berries to green spinach to violet plums—and all the shades in between. Splashing your plate with different-colored fruits and vegetables is an easy and smart way to ensure that you are getting the vitamins and minerals you need.

with lots of fibrous carbs but few if any complex ones, may leave you struggling to get through the next few hours. And consuming an overabundance of complex and simple carbs in the evening, when your body does not need this energy, is likely to result in stored fat. Following this eating pattern means that you are likely to wake up the next day noticeably softer—and liable to begin the process of carb restriction and then introduction all over again.

Instead, for optimal fueling and fat loss, eat breakfast like a king, lunch like a prince, and dinner like a pauper. Generally speaking, a ratio of 40 percent protein to 40 percent carbohydrates and 20 percent fats should compose your nutritional intake. Additionally, tapering your carb intake, starting with the largest portion early in the day before switching to more fibrous or low-caloric choices, will help to keep your fat furnace burning.

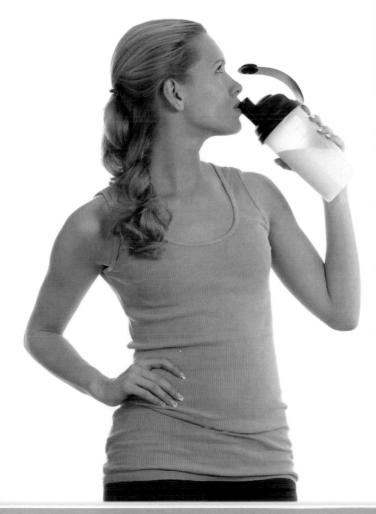

Eating to lose

A day of healthy eating doesn't mean 24 hours of depriving yourself. To lose fat and raise energy, think of your meals as regular refueling: consume 5 to 6 small meals every 3 hours or so. The key is to maintain a positive nitrogen balance and peak blood sugar levels, which you can accomplish by including some protein with every meal and ample carbs for optimal fueling throughout the day.

When planning your daily menu, include 3 whole meals, with 2 supplemental high-energy snacks, such as ready-to-drink protein shakes. The following is just a sample menu of a healthy day of eating.

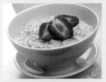

Breakfast: An omelet made from two egg whites and one yolk, with a small bowl of oatmeal topped with strawberries

Morning snack: A protein shake and a handful of raw nuts

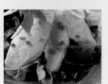

Lunch: Chicken-breast salad topped with kidney beans

Afternoon snack: A protein shake and a piece of fruit

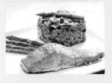

Dinner: Baked fish, poached asparagus, and brown rice

If you are used to the typical deprivation-style weight-loss diet, you may at first feel as if you are eating too much, but you're really eating the same amount—just parceled into smaller packages. Your body will soon adjust to your new meal schedule; with the increased activity levels of your core training, it will come to expect to be fed every few hours or so. Remember: one must eat to lose.

A recipe for fueling

Consume at least one gram of protein per pound of your body weight from lean sources (think lean beef, white-meat poultry, fish, eggs, low-fat cottage cheese, and Greek yogurt) in order to preserve and/or gain lean muscle mass. "Good" fats such as monounsaturated fats (found in olives and avocados, for instance), polyunsaturated fats (found in nuts and seeds), and omega-3s (found in walnuts, flax seeds, and coldwater oily fish such as salmon, sardines, and anchovies) will provide a feeling of satiety, help to lubricate your joints, moisturize your skin, and assist in protecting your heart.

Hydrate, hydrate

Consuming adequate fluid is another key factor in maximizing exercise performance and preventing injury. Proper hydration maintains optimal organ function and helps you feel your best during and after your core workout. It is healthy to work up a sweat while exercising; sweating is your body's way of protecting you from overheating during periods of physical exertion. Failure to replace fluids lost through perspiration, can produce serious effects. Early signs of dehydration include thirst, flushed skin, premature fatigue, accelerated pulse and breathing rates, and decreased exercise capacity.

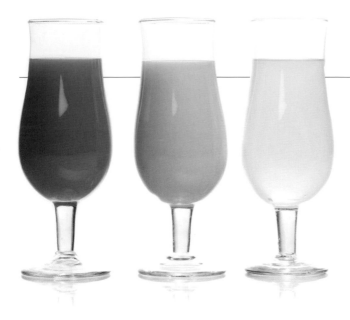

after low- to moderate-intensity exercise that lasts up to an hour. Anyone exercising for more than an hour at a higher intensity should consume beverages that contain a combination of carbohydrates and electrolytes. A smart choice is 100-percent pure coconut water, which contains fewer calories and less sugar and sodium than many popular sports drinks. Another healthy way to replace fluids and electrolytes lost during exercise is to eat a serving of fruit or vegetables after your workout.

Trimming the fat

The healthy range for real, long-lasting fat loss is one to two pounds per week. You can best achieve this goal through a combination of good nutrition (to fuel the body), proper weight training (to harden the body), and ample cardiovascular activity (to burn stored fat). When these three elements are all strong, your body will support you time and time again—and you'll see real improvement, as well.

These symptoms can give way to dizziness and severe weakness if dehydration is allowed to persist. Most nutrition authorities recommend drinking water before, during, and

The Glycemic Index

The Glycemic Index (GI), which some have found to be the nutritional key to long-term fat loss, measures the rate at which carbohydrates affect our blood sugar levels. A lower-GI food is likely to be digested at a relatively slow rate, impose a lower insulin demand on the body, and ultimately lead to less fat storage.

According to the Glycemic Index, foods with a high GI score of 70 and above include white bread, white rice, extruded breakfast cereals, and glucose. Those foods with a medium range of 56 to 69 include whole-wheat products, and sucrose (found in brown sugar and maple syrup, for instance). Foods considered to have a low GI score of 55 or below include most vegetables, legumes, whole grains, nuts, and fructose (found in colas and honey); for a lean physique, these low-GI foods should constitute the majority of carbohydrates consumed.

GI values of some common foods

Low GI
55 and below

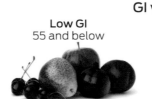

- apples
- beets
- berries
- cherries
- chickpeas
- citrus fruits
- jams & marmalades
- kidney beans
- lentils
- lettuce
- milk (skim)
- nuts
- pasta
- peaches
- peppers
- plums
- snow peas
- spinach
- tomatoes
- wheat kernels
- yogurt (low-fat)

Medium GI
56–69

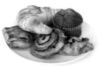

- angel food cake
- apricots
- barley
- brown rice
- brown sugar
- cranberry juice
- croissants
- Danish pastries
- maple syrup
- muesli
- muffins
- oat bran
- pineapples
- pita bread
- pizza
- popcorn
- pumpernickel bread
- raisins
- rye bread
- shortbread
- shredded wheat

High GI
70 and above

- alcoholic drinks
- bacon
- baked beans
- broad beans
- butter
- corn flakes
- doughnuts
- eggs
- French fries
- ice cream
- jelly beans
- parsnips
- potato chips
- pretzels
- puffed wheat
- sausages
- waffles
- watermelons
- white bread
- white potatoes
- white rice

Vitamins and supplements

It is always best to obtain nutrients from whole foods. If you find certain nutrient-rich foods unpalatable or they aren't readily available where you live, however, then it is crucial to take a multivitamin that contains at least 100 percent of the recommended daily value (DV) for the nutrients you need. This information can be found on the supplement package.

Sticking to the plan

If you're like so many of us these days, trying to fit as much as possible into a hectic schedule, you often skip meals and snack on highly processed sugar-laden foods during lunchtime, only to come home later at night and gorge on anything and everything in sight. The result is a constant yo-yo game of weight gain and weight loss.

A better plan: follow a "grazing" system of several small meals consumed throughout the day. This system keeps energy levels up and encourages the body to use fat as it fuel source.

Of course, life isn't a never-ending sprint toward optimum condition, but rather a steady jog to a healthy and consistent baseline. Every once in while you may peak for an athletic event (a race or marathon, for instance) or a special occasion (like a wedding or reunion), but aim for healthy eating and effective exercise as a consistent lifestyle. You'll look great, and will function well, too.

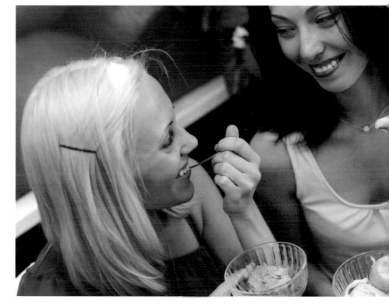

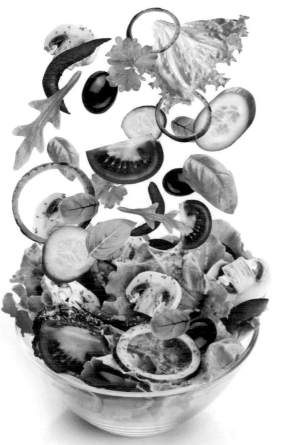

A healthy lifestyle means enjoying your life, so even as you begin your any diet, factor in the occasional indulgence or "cheat" meal. Rather than sabotaging your efforts, a treat can offset the mental fatigue that often accompanies strenuous dieting. Have your cheat meal when needed (once or twice per week), and then return to your diet.

Eating out and eating healthy

All you need is a bit of planning to make sure that you eat healthy whether dining at home, at work, or at a restaurant. With a little effort the night before, you can prepare a nutritious lunch for the next workday. Grilling some chicken breast or microwaving some yams and vegetables yields a balanced lunch. A small bag of raw nuts and a couple of pieces of fruit makes the perfect midafternoon snack. The fewer processed foods (breads, cereals, sauces) you consume, the more efficiently your body will run.

Feel free to join your friends for an evening out sharing a meal—just choose the most healthful menu options. At a Chinese restaurant, order steamed chicken, vegetables, and brown rice with sauce on the side. At a Mexican restaurant indulge in the grilled chicken or shrimp over a salad and black beans topped with salsa. At an Italian restaurant, look for grilled chicken or fish over whole-wheat pasta and a light tomato sauce; at a Mediterranean restaurant, opt for the hummus over a salad with a whole-wheat pita. No matter what the cuisine, you always have a healthy choice.

Full-body anatomy

Front View

Annotation Key
* indicates deep muscles

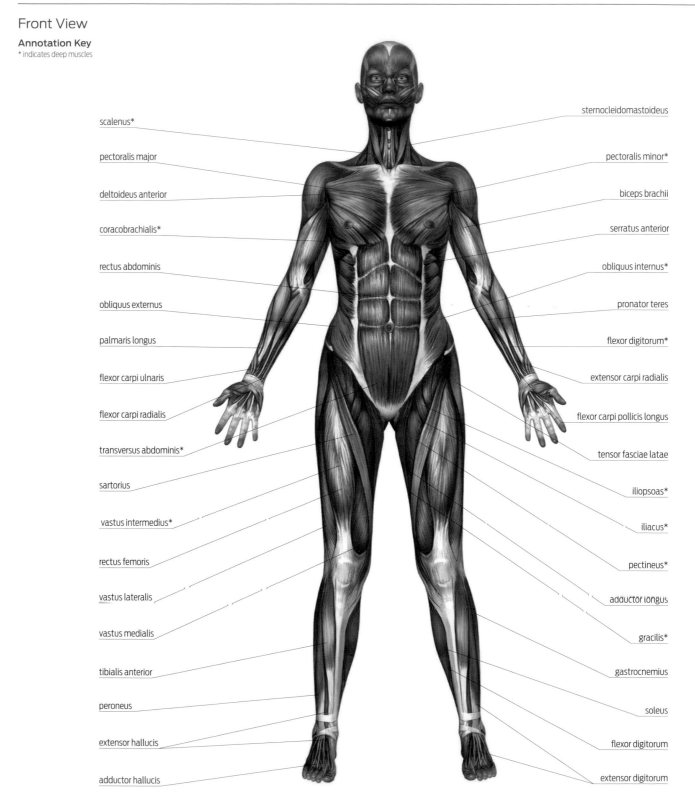

scalenus*

pectoralis major

deltoideus anterior

coracobrachialis*

rectus abdominis

obliquus externus

palmaris longus

flexor carpi ulnaris

flexor carpi radialis

transversus abdominis*

sartorius

vastus intermedius*

rectus femoris

vastus lateralis

vastus medialis

tibialis anterior

peroneus

extensor hallucis

adductor hallucis

sternocleidomastoideus

pectoralis minor*

biceps brachii

serratus anterior

obliquus internus*

pronator teres

flexor digitorum*

extensor carpi radialis

flexor carpi pollicis longus

tensor fasciae latae

iliopsoas*

iliacus*

pectineus*

adductor longus

gracilis*

gastrocnemius

soleus

flexor digitorum

extensor digitorum

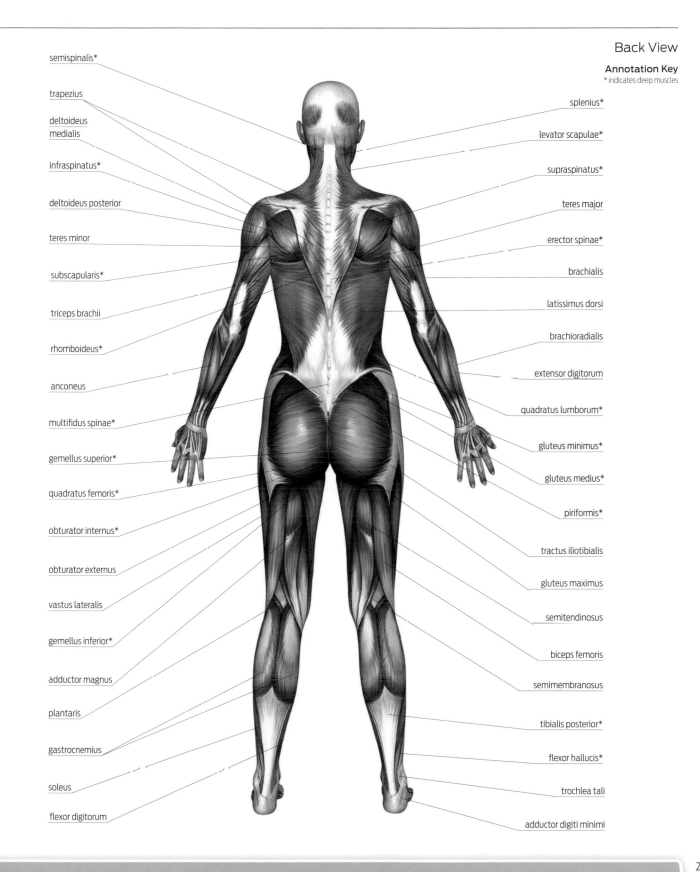

Back View

Annotation Key
* indicates deep muscles

semispinalis*

trapezius

deltoideus medialis

infraspinatus*

deltoideus posterior

teres minor

subscapularis*

triceps brachii

rhomboideus*

anconeus

multifidus spinae*

gemellus superior*

quadratus femoris*

obturator internus*

obturator externus

vastus lateralis

gemellus inferior*

adductor magnus

plantaris

gastrocnemius

soleus

flexor digitorum

splenius*

levator scapulae*

supraspinatus*

teres major

erector spinae*

brachialis

latissimus dorsi

brachioradialis

extensor digitorum

quadratus lumborum*

gluteus minimus*

gluteus medius*

piriformis*

tractus iliotibialis

gluteus maximus

semitendinosus

biceps femoris

semimembranosus

tibialis posterior*

flexor hallucis*

trochlea tali

adductor digiti minimi

Contents

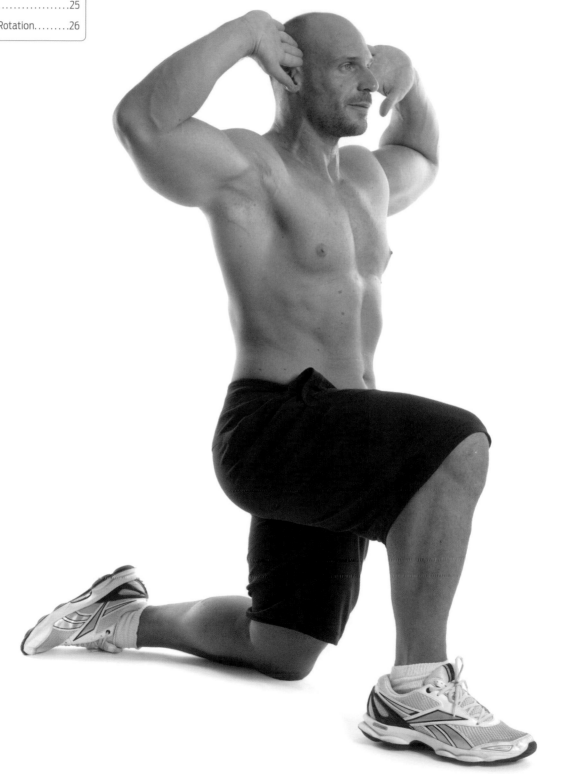

Are you ready to really work your core, pushing yourself to the limit? The following sample of warm-up exercises will prepare your muscles for the core-training regimen to come. Warming up properly reduces your risk of injury, so make warming up a ritual that you complete at the start of every core-training workout, and include a few cardio exercises, such as running in place or jumping jacks, that get your heart pumping and your spirit energized. Your core muscles will thank you.

Warm-Ups

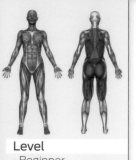

Level
· Beginner

Duration
· 2–3 minutes

Benefits
· Stretches lower-back and gluteal muscles

Caution
· Severe back issues

Back & Side Stretches

Supine Lower-Back Stretch

Supine Lower-Back Stretch is an excellent warm-up that stretches your lower-back and gluteal muscles, preparing them for the workout ahead.

1 Lie on your back, with legs bent and hands clasped around your knees.

2 Slowly pull your knees toward your chest until you feel a stretch in your lower back.

3 Hold for 30 seconds, relax, and repeat for an additional 30 seconds.

Annotation Key
Bold text indicates target muscles
Black text indicates other working muscles
* indicates deep muscles

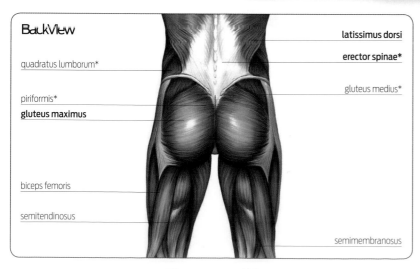

Back View

quadratus lumborum*

piriformis*

gluteus maximus

biceps femoris

semitendinosus

latissimus dorsi

erector spinae*

gluteus medius*

semimembranosus

Correct form
· Keep your knees and feet together.

Avoid
· Raising your head off the floor.

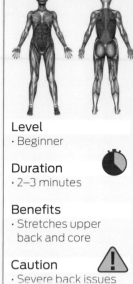

Side Stretch

When performing Side Stretch, you should feel a good stretch along the sides of your body. Focus on keeping the lower part of your body strongly rooted and stable, like a tree with branches leaning over in the wind.

1 Stand with one hand on your hip and the other arm over your head and leaning toward the opposite side.

2 Reach up and over, and lean your torso to the side.

3 Hold for 30 seconds, relax, and repeat for an additional 30 seconds.

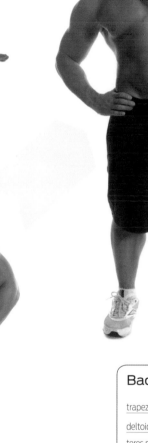

Level
· Beginner

Duration
· 2–3 minutes

Benefits
· Stretches upper back and core

Caution
· Severe back issues

Annotation Key
Bold text indicates target muscles
Black text indicates other working muscles
* indicates deep muscles

Front View

intercostales externi

intercostales interni*

serratus anterior

obliquus internus*

obliquus externus

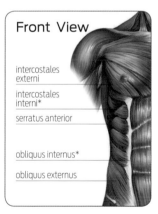

Back View

trapezius

deltoideus posterior

teres minor

teres major

latissimus dorsi

erector spinae*

multifidus spinae*

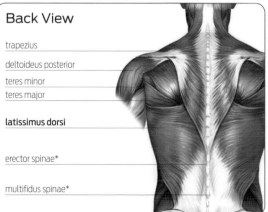

Correct form
· Be sure to keep your torso straight on.

.Avoid
· Bending forward or backward at the trunk.

Half-Kneeling Rotation

Half-Kneeling Rotation is a warm-up stretch that increases your spinal mobility, improves your posture, and enhances your core rotation. Concentrate on engaging your core muscles, making sure that your stomach does not bulge outward as your upper body rotates from one side to the other.

1 Kneel on one leg with your right leg bent at 90 degrees in front of you, foot on the floor. Your hands should be beside your head and your elbows should be flared outward.

2 Keeping your back straight, rotate your left shoulder toward your right knee.

3 Hold for 10 seconds, and then repeat on the other side. Work up to 10 repetitions on each side.

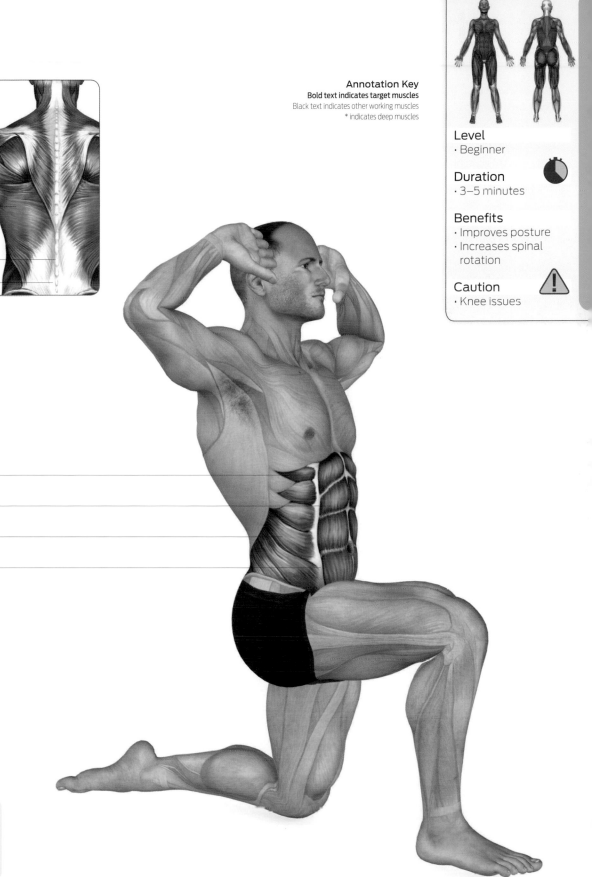

Back View

deltoideus posterior

latissimus dorsi

erector spinae*

multifidus spinae*

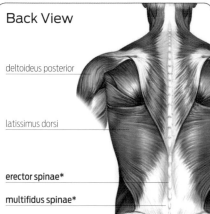

Annotation Key
Bold text indicates target muscles
Black text indicates other working muscles
* indicates deep muscles

Level
· Beginner

Duration
· 3–5 minutes

Benefits
· Improves posture
· Increases spinal
  rotation

Caution
· Knee issues

serratus anterior

rectus abdominis

obliquus externus

obliquus internus*

Correct form
· Keep your back straight.

Avoid
· Overextension.

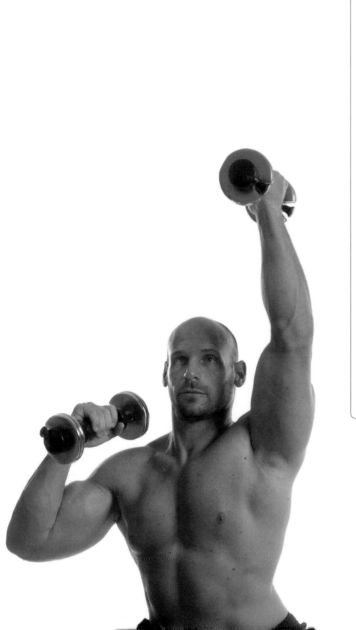

Contents

Your abdominals, obliques, glutes, hip adductors, hip flexors, and spinal column work together to support you each and every day. It's only right, then, that you should put some effort into supporting them.

The following exercises make for a more stable core, which will augment your performance as you move through a spectrum of daily activities. Whether you are reaching for the high shelf at the supermarket, running for the bus, or swinging a baseball bat, performing these exercises will build a more balanced, centered, and powerful body. So try holding that Side Plank 10 seconds longer than usual, or making T-Stabilization a morning ritual.

Core Stabilizers

Plank

Plank is an isometric, or contracted, core-stabilizing exercise, designed to work your entire core. It is performed everywhere from yoga and Pilates studios to hard-core gyms for a good reason: it is a reliable way to build endurance in your abs and back, as well as in the stabilizer muscles.

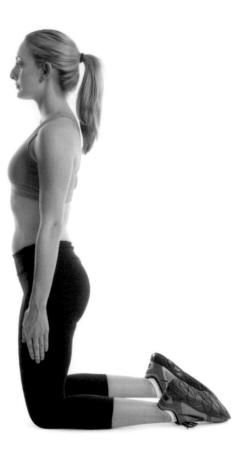

1 Kneel on an exercise mat, and then place your hands on the floor to come into onto all-fours.

2 Plant your forearms on the floor, parallel to each other.

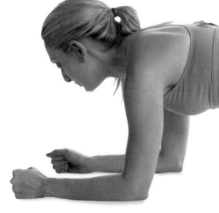

Correct form
· Keep your abdominal muscles tight.
· Keep your body in a straight line.

Avoid
· Bridging too high, which can take stress off working muscles.

3 Raise your knees off the floor and lengthen your legs until they are in line with your arms. Remain suspended in Plank for 30 seconds, building up to 2 minutes.

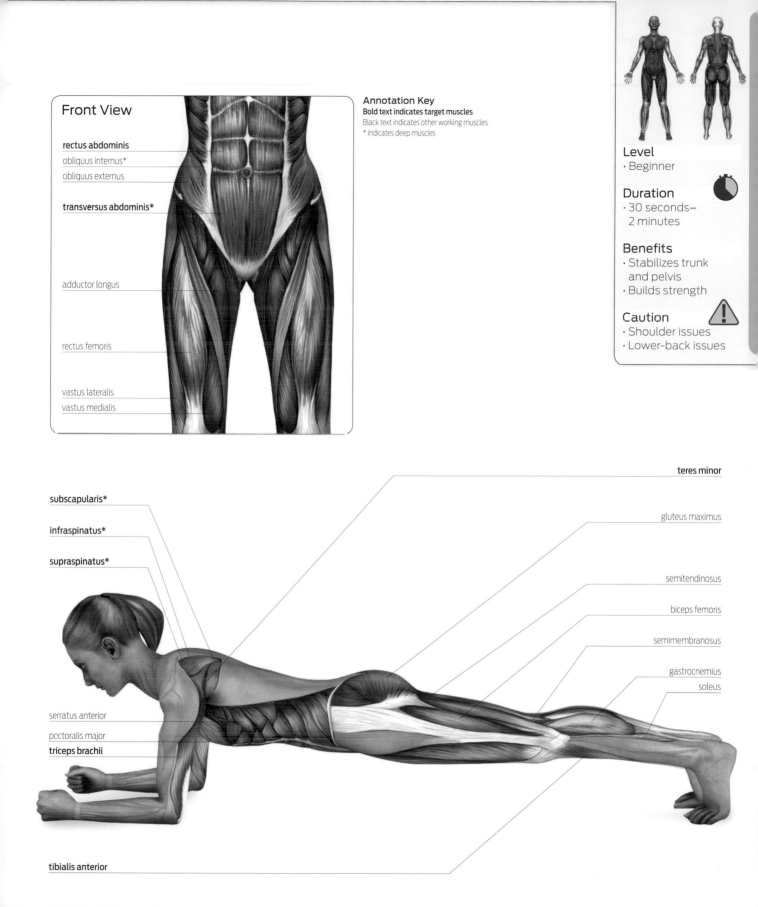

Front View

rectus abdominis

obliquus internus*

obliquus externus

transversus abdominis*

adductor longus

rectus femoris

vastus lateralis

vastus medialis

Annotation Key
Bold text indicates target muscles
Black text indicates other working muscles
* indicates deep muscles

Level
· Beginner

Duration
· 30 seconds–
  2 minutes

Benefits
· Stabilizes trunk
  and pelvis
· Builds strength

Caution
· Shoulder issues
· Lower-back issues

teres minor

subscapularis*

infraspinatus*

supraspinatus*

gluteus maximus

semitendinosus

biceps femoris

semimembranosus

gastrocnemius

soleus

serratus anterior

pectoralis major

triceps brachii

tibialis anterior

Plank-Up

Plank-Up is an advanced core-stabilizing exercise that expands upon the basic Plank exercise. Try to maintain a steady rhythm as you move from one arm to the other.

1 Begin on your hands and knees in a facedown position. Plant your forearms on the floor parallel to each other.

2 Raise your knees off the floor and lengthen your legs until they are in line with your arms.

3 Lift up with your right arm until it is fully extended, and then straighten your left arm until you are balanced on both arms in a completed push-up position.

Correct form
· Plant each hand, rather than using momentum, which places too much stress on the joints.
· Keep your abs tucked tightly during the movement.

Avoid
· Crashing down suddenly; instead, use a steady 4-count motion: 2 up for both arms, then 2 down.

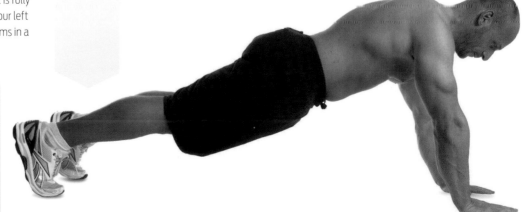

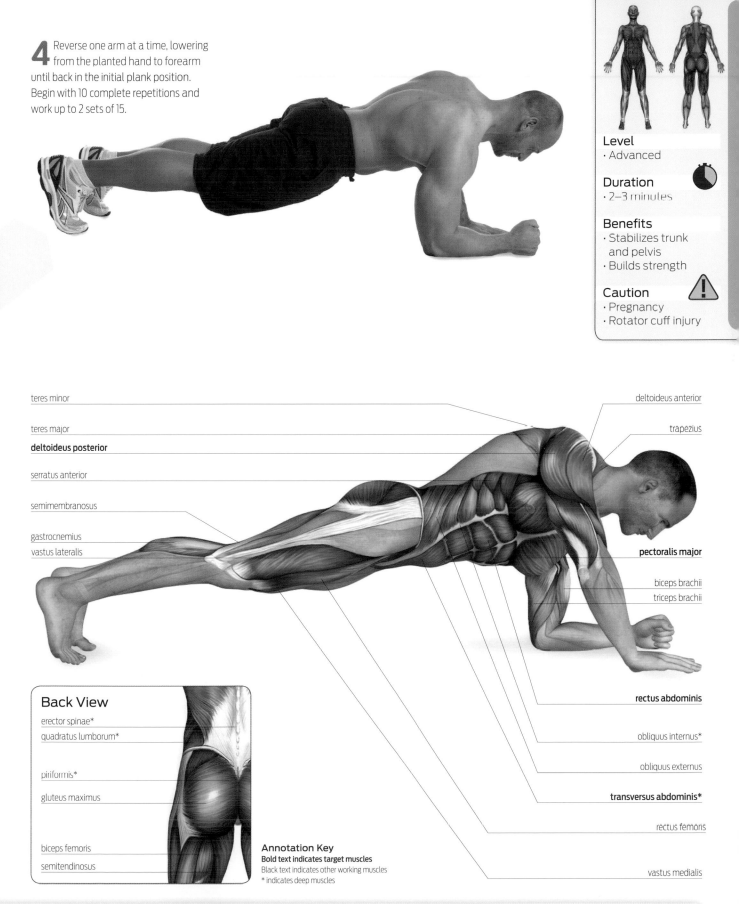

4 Reverse one arm at a time, lowering from the planted hand to forearm until back in the initial plank position. Begin with 10 complete repetitions and work up to 2 sets of 15.

Level
• Advanced

Duration
• 2–3 minutes

Benefits
• Stabilizes trunk and pelvis
• Builds strength

Caution
• Pregnancy
• Rotator cuff injury

teres minor

teres major

deltoideus posterior

serratus anterior

semimembranosus

gastrocnemius

vastus lateralis

deltoideus anterior

trapezius

pectoralis major

biceps brachii

triceps brachii

rectus abdominis

obliquus internus*

obliquus externus

transversus abdominis*

rectus femoris

vastus medialis

Back View

erector spinae*

quadratus lumborum*

piriformis*

gluteus maximus

biceps femoris

semitendinosus

Annotation Key
Bold text indicates target muscles
Black text indicates other working muscles
* indicates deep muscles

Side Plank

Side Plank stabilizes your spine, but it is also great for strengthening your abdominals, lower back, and shoulders. Contracting your abdominals in Side Plank is a great way to whittle down your waistline. For best results, try holding for a few seconds longer than you initially think you can.

Correct form
· Push evenly from both your forearm and hips.

Avoid
· Placing too much strain on your shoulders; they should neither sink into their sockets nor lift toward your ears.

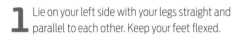

1 Lie on your left side with your legs straight and parallel to each other. Keep your feet flexed.

2 Bend your left arm to form a 90-degree angle with the knuckles of your hand facing forward. Place your right hand on your waist or extend your arm along your side.

3 Pressing your forearm down into the floor, raise your hips until your body is in a long, straight line. Hold for 30 seconds, working up to 1 minute. Release, and repeat on the other side.

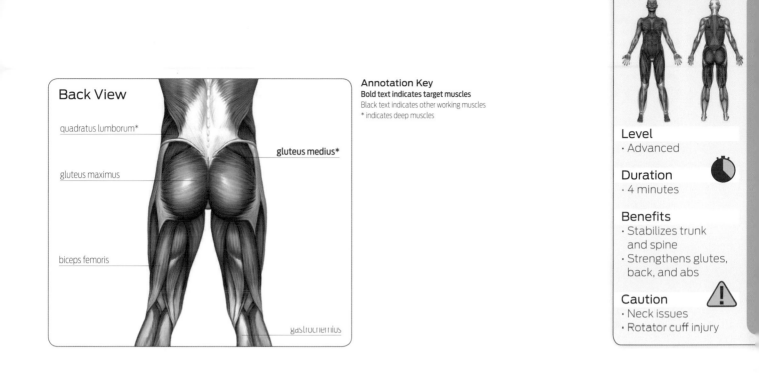

Back View

quadratus lumborum*

gluteus medius*

gluteus maximus

biceps femoris

gastrocnemius

Annotation Key
Bold text indicates target muscles
Black text indicates other working muscles
* indicates deep muscles

Level
· Advanced

Duration
· 4 minutes

Benefits
· Stabilizes trunk
  and spine
· Strengthens glutes,
  back, and abs

Caution
· Neck issues
· Rotator cuff injury

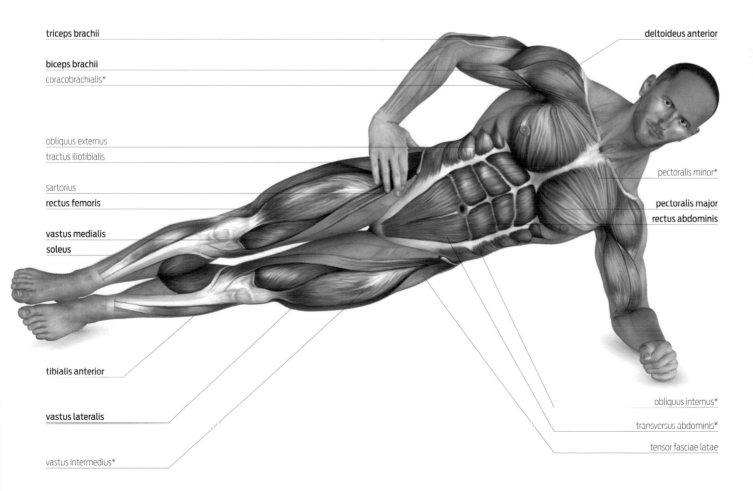

triceps brachii

biceps brachii

coracobrachialis*

obliquus externus

tractus iliotibialis

sartorius

rectus femoris

vastus medialis

soleus

tibialis anterior

vastus lateralis

vastus intermedius*

deltoideus anterior

pectoralis minor*

pectoralis major

rectus abdominis

obliquus internus*

transversus abdominis*

tensor fasciae latae

Side Plank with Reach-Under

In Side Plank with Reach-Under, strength lies in stillness rather than in motion. As you maintain the static position of your torso and legs while moving one of your arms, you are effectively strengthening your abs, lower back, and shoulders.

1 Lie on your left side with your legs straight and parallel to each other. Keep your feet flexed.

2 Bend your left arm to form a 90-degree angle, with the knuckles of your hand facing forward. Place your right hand on your waist or extend your arm along your side.

3 Pressing your left forearm into the floor, raise your hips off the floor until your body forms a long, straight line.

4 Twist your upper torso toward the floor as you reach your right arm under your chest as far as you can stretch.

5 Twist your upper torso back to front as you extend your right arm toward the ceiling.

6 Complete 4 repetitions, and then switch sides and repeat. Work up to performing 2 sets of 15 on each side.

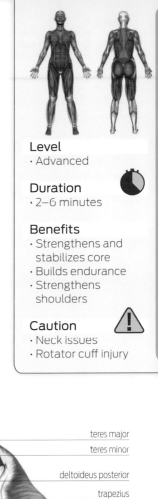

Correct form

· Both your forearm and your hips should drive the raising motion.
· Allow your head and neck to follow the movement of your torso, so that you are looking toward the floor during the reach-under and straight ahead in the finished position with your top arm extended.
· Keep your feet flexed and stacked.

Avoid

· Placing too much strain on your shoulders.
· Losing your alignment when your top arm is extended.

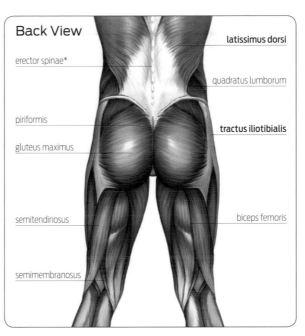

Back View

erector spinae*

piriformis

gluteus maximus

semitendinosus

semimembranosus

latissimus dorsi

quadratus lumborum

tractus iliotibialis

biceps femoris

Level
· Advanced

Duration
· 2–6 minutes

Benefits
· Strengthens and stabilizes core
· Builds endurance
· Strengthens shoulders

Caution
· Neck issues
· Rotator cuff injury

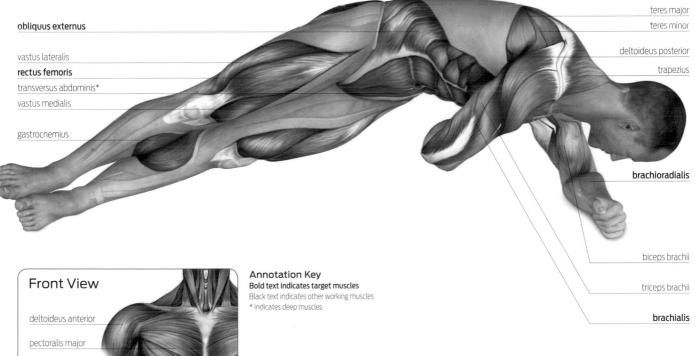

obliquus externus

vastus lateralis

rectus femoris

transversus abdominis*

vastus medialis

gastrocnemius

teres major

teres minor

deltoideus posterior

trapezius

brachioradialis

biceps brachii

triceps brachii

brachialis

Front View

deltoideus anterior

pectoralis major

serratus anterior

rectus abdominis

obliquus internus*

Annotation Key
Bold text indicates target muscles
Black text indicates other working muscles
* indicates deep muscles

Side Plank with Band Row

Side Plank with Band Row is an effective strengthener for your abdominal muscles, as well as the muscles in your upper and lower back and shoulders. As you pull the band and then release it, concentrate on moving your top arm smoothly and with control as the rest of your body stays still.

1 Attach one end of the exercise band to a nearby stabilized object. Lie on your left side, with your legs straight, stacked one on top of the other.

2 Bend your left arm so that if forms a 90-degree angle, with the knuckles of your hand facing forward.

Correct form
· Both your forearm and your hips should drive the raising motion.
· Make sure the band is pulled taut in the contracted position.
· Keep your legs stable throughout the exercise.
· Pull the band all the way to your chest.

Avoid
· Tensing either of your shoulders.
· Losing alignment in your body.

3 With your right arm, grasp one end of the exercise band. Extend your top arm in front of you, holding the band parallel to the floor.

4 Push off your forearm while raising your hips off the floor until your body forms one straight line.

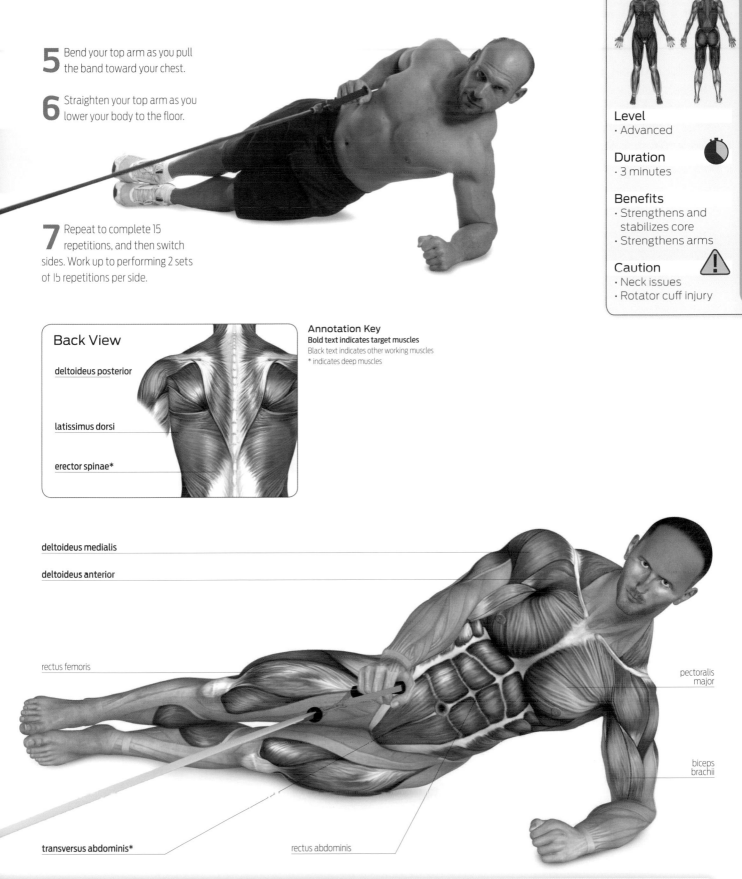

5 Bend your top arm as you pull the band toward your chest.

6 Straighten your top arm as you lower your body to the floor.

7 Repeat to complete 15 repetitions, and then switch sides. Work up to performing 2 sets of 15 repetitions per side.

Level
· Advanced

Duration
· 3 minutes

Benefits
· Strengthens and stabilizes core
· Strengthens arms

Caution
· Neck issues
· Rotator cuff injury

Back View

deltoideus posterior

latissimus dorsi

erector spinae*

Annotation Key
Bold text indicates target muscles
Black text indicates other working muscles
* indicates deep muscles

deltoideus medialis

deltoideus anterior

rectus femoris

pectoralis major

biceps brachii

transversus abdominis*

rectus abdominis

Fire-Hydrant In-Out

Fire Hydrant In-Out is a hard-working core-stabilizing exercise, as well as a great abdominal strengthener. It targets your inner thighs, hamstrings, and glutes, with assistance from your abdominal muscles.

Correct form
· Press your hands into the floor to keep your shoulders from sinking.
· Squeeze your glutes with your leg fully extended.

Avoid
· Lifting your hip as you lift your bent leg to the side.
· Rushing through the exercise; make sure that you feel each portion of the repetition.

1 Begin on your hands and knees, with your palms on the floor and spaced shoulder-width apart. Your spine should be in a neutral position.

2 Keeping your right leg bent at a 90-degree angle, raise it laterally, or to the side.

Level
· Beginner

Duration
· 3 minutes

Benefits
· Stabilizes pelvis
· Strengthens glutes

Caution
· Wrist pain
· Knee issues

3 Straighten your right leg until it is fully extended behind you so that it is in line with your torso.

4 Bend your right knee and bring your leg back into its 90-degree position, and then lower it to meet your left leg. Work up to 15 repetitions. Repeat on the other side.

Annotation Key
Bold text indicates target muscles
Black text indicates other working muscles
* indicates deep muscles

Front View

rectus abdominis

obliquus externus

obliquus internus*

transversus abdominis*

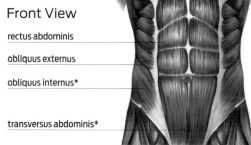

tensor fasciae latae

gluteus maximus

gluteus medius*

vastus lateralis

tractus iliotibialis

adductor magnus

adductor longus

sartorius

vastus medialis

T-Stabilization

T-Stabilization, another advanced variation on the traditional Plank, is a proven exercise for targeting your abs, hips, lower back, and obliques.

1 Assume the finished push-up position with your arms extended to full lockout, your fingers facing forward, your legs outstretched, and your body weight supported on your toes.

2 Turn your hips to one side, stacking one foot on top of the other and raising your top arm across your body until you are pointing toward the ceiling.

3 Hold for 30 seconds, lower, and then repeat on the other side. Work your way up to holding for 1 minute on each side.

Correct form
· Keep your body in one straight line.

Avoid
· Arching or bridging your back.

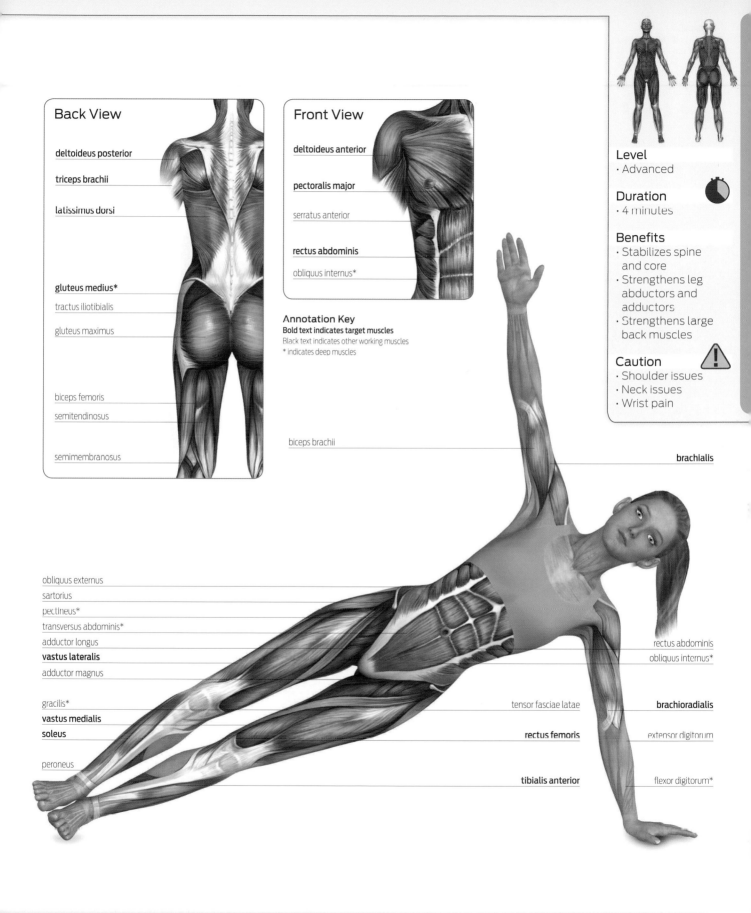

Back View

deltoideus posterior

triceps brachii

latissimus dorsi

gluteus medius*

tractus iliotibialis

gluteus maximus

biceps femoris

semitendinosus

semimembranosus

Front View

deltoideus anterior

pectoralis major

serratus anterior

rectus abdominis

obliquus internus*

Annotation Key
Bold text indicates target muscles
Black text indicates other working muscles
* indicates deep muscles

Level
• Advanced

Duration
• 4 minutes

Benefits
• Stabilizes spine and core
• Strengthens leg abductors and adductors
• Strengthens large back muscles

Caution
• Shoulder issues
• Neck issues
• Wrist pain

biceps brachii

brachialis

obliquus externus

sartorius

pectineus*

transversus abdominis*

adductor longus

vastus lateralis

adductor magnus

gracilis*

vastus medialis

soleus

peroneus

rectus abdominis

obliquus internus*

tensor fasciae latae

brachioradialis

rectus femoris

extensor digitorum

tibialis anterior

flexor digitorum*

Fitness Ball Atomic Push-Up

Performing the Fitness Ball Atomic Push-Up causes many major muscle groups to fire at once. When executed properly, this exercise tones your upper body, engages your core, and works your hip flexors.

1 Begin on your hands and knees with your fingers facing forward and a fitness ball placed behind you. Rest your shins on the ball, and straighten your legs so that your body forms a straight line.

2 While keeping your back flat, bend your knees to draw the fitness ball into your core.

Correct form
· Keep your hips level with your torso.

Avoid
· Piking or bridging your body.

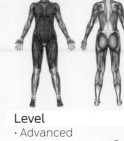

3 Straighten your legs, moving the ball farther behind you, and then perform a push-up. Start with 5 repetitions, working your way up to 2 sets of 12 to 15.

Level
· Advanced

Duration
· 2 minutes

Benefits
· Stabilizes spine and core

Caution
· Lower-back pain
· Wrist pain
· Shoulder issues

Front View

tensor fasciae latae

iliopsoas*

pectineus*

sartorius

adductor brevis

adductor longus

gracilis*

Annotation Key
Bold text indicates target muscles
Black text indicates other working muscles
* indicates deep muscles

obliquus internus*

rectus abdominis

deltoideus posterior

deltoideus anterior

obliquus externus

transversus abdominis*

brachialis

biceps brachii

triceps brachii

rectus femoris

tibialis anterior

vastus lateralis

Fitness Ball Pike

Fitness Ball Pike targets your hip flexors and external obliques, as well as your rectus abdominis and spinal erectors. In starting position, your sense of balance comes into play, and as you raise your hips your core muscles are greatly challenged. For best results, concentrate on keeping your movement smooth.

Correct form
· Raise your hips evenly.
· Move as slowly as possible.
· Keep both hands anchored to the floor.
· Keep your gaze directed toward the floor.

Avoid
· Rounding your back.
· Tilting your hips to either side.
· Straining your neck by trying to look forward.

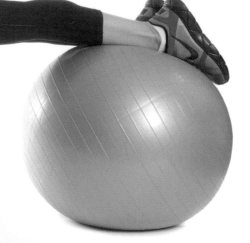

1 Assume a push-up position with your arms shoulder-width apart and your shins resting on a fitness ball.

2 While keeping your legs straight, roll the ball toward your body while raising your hips as high as you are able.

3 Lower and repeat, performing 20 repetitions. Rest if desired, and then complete another set of 20.

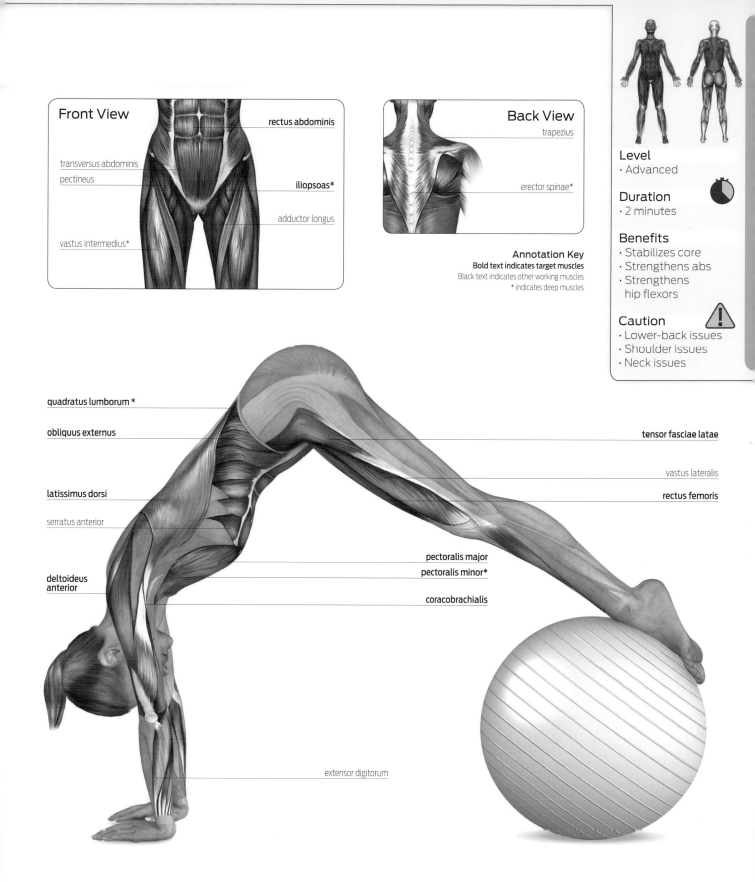

Front View

rectus abdominis

transversus abdominis

pectineus

iliopsoas*

adductor longus

vastus intermedius*

Back View

trapezius

erector spinae*

Annotation Key
Bold text indicates target muscles
Black text indicates other working muscles
* indicates deep muscles

Level
· Advanced

Duration
· 2 minutes

Benefits
· Stabilizes core
· Strengthens abs
· Strengthens
  hip flexors

Caution
· Lower-back issues
· Shoulder issues
· Neck issues

quadratus lumborum *

obliquus externus

latissimus dorsi

serratus anterior

deltoideus
anterior

tensor fasciae latae

vastus lateralis

rectus femoris

pectoralis major

pectoralis minor*

coracobrachialis

extensor digitorum

Fitness Ball Jackknife

Fitness Ball Jackknifes does an excellent job of working your hip flexors. It also targets both the front and back core muscles—especially your rectus abdominis and spinal erectors respectively.

Correct form
· Brace your core.
· Keep both hands anchored to the floor.
· Keep your gaze directed toward the floor.

Avoid
· Rounding your back.
· Straining your neck by trying to look forward.

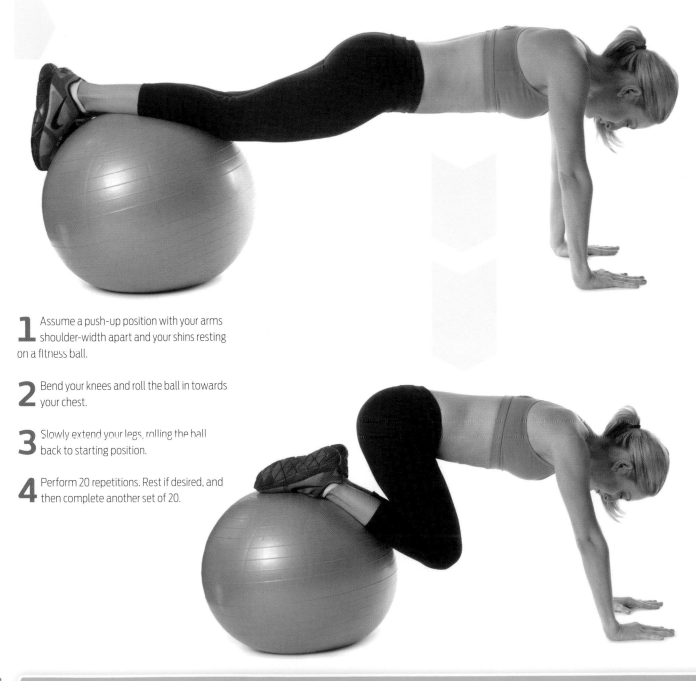

1 Assume a push-up position with your arms shoulder-width apart and your shins resting on a fitness ball.

2 Bend your knees and roll the ball in towards your chest.

3 Slowly extend your legs, rolling the ball back to starting position.

4 Perform 20 repetitions. Rest if desired, and then complete another set of 20.

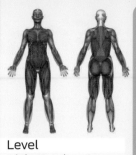

Level
· Advanced

Duration
· 2 minutes

Benefits
· Stabilizes core
· Strengthens abs
· Strengthens
  hip flexors

Caution
· Lower-back issues
· Shoulder issues
· Neck issues

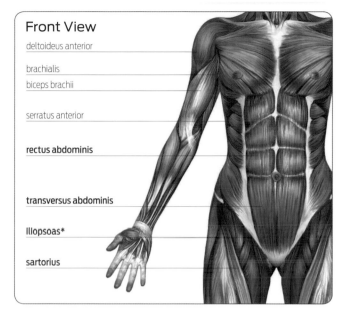

Front View
deltoideus anterior

brachialis

biceps brachii

serratus anterior

rectus abdominis

transversus abdominis

Iliopsoas*

sartorius

Back View
subscapularis*

rhomboideus

erector spinae*

Annotation Key
Bold text indicates target muscles
Black text indicates other working muscles
* indicates deep muscles

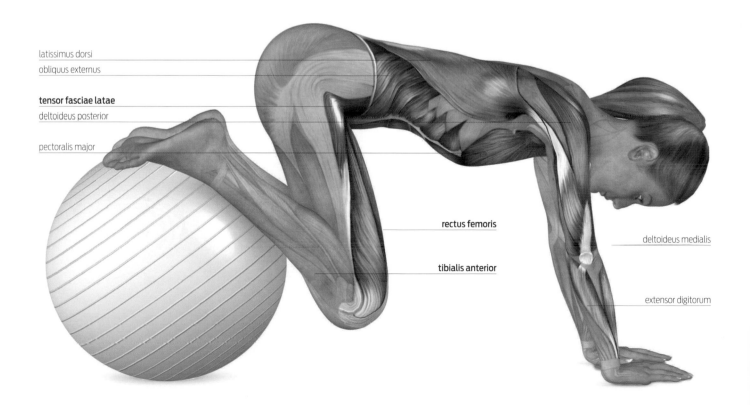

latissimus dorsi

obliquus externus

tensor fasciae latae

deltoideus posterior

pectoralis major

rectus femoris

tibialis anterior

deltoideus medialis

extensor digitorum

Fitness Ball Lateral Roll

Fitness Ball Lateral Roll offers a unique,
dynamic way to build core stability. It calls
for you to fully engage your core and rely
on your balance and stability to drive the
subtle movement.

1 Lie face-up on a fitness ball, with
your upper back firmly supported.
Plant your feet shoulder-width apart or
a little wider. Your hips and thighs should
be parallel to your torso; if necessary, raise
your hips to achieve this alignment.

2 Extend your arms out to the sides.

3 Take "baby steps" as you move
toward the side of the ball.

4 Take equally small steps back to
the center of the ball.

5 Repeat on the other side.
Complete 3 sets of 10 per side.

Annotation Key
Bold text indicates target muscles
Black text indicates other working muscles
* indicates deep muscles

Level
· Intermediate

Duration
· 4 minutes

Benefits
· Stabilizes core
· Strengthens abs
  and quadriceps

Caution
· Lower-back issues
· Neck issues

triceps brachii

rectus abdominis
iliopsoas*
adductor longus
adductor magnus
vastus intermedius*

obliquus internus*
transversus abdominis
obliquus externus
sartorius

adductor brevis

tensor fasciae latae

rectus femoris

vastus medialis

Correct form
· Keep your core braced.
· Keep your hips raised.
· Keep both arms extended.

Avoid
· Dropping your hips.
· Moving to the side too quickly.

Fitness Ball Rollout

Fitness Ball Rollout is a fun and challenging exercise for effectively stabilizing your core. Aim for controlled, steady movement throughout.

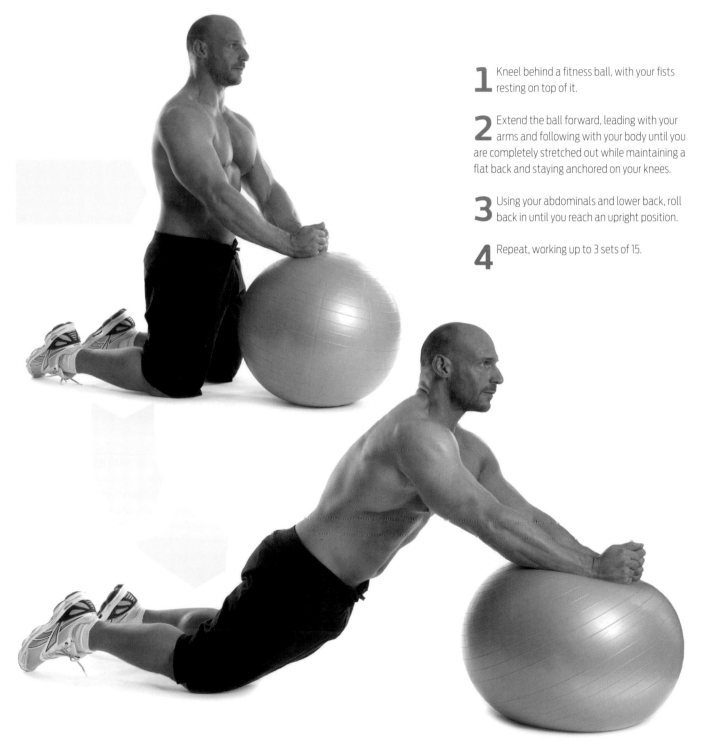

1 Kneel behind a fitness ball, with your fists resting on top of it.

2 Extend the ball forward, leading with your arms and following with your body until you are completely stretched out while maintaining a flat back and staying anchored on your knees.

3 Using your abdominals and lower back, roll back in until you reach an upright position.

4 Repeat, working up to 3 sets of 15.

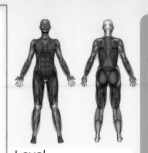

Back View

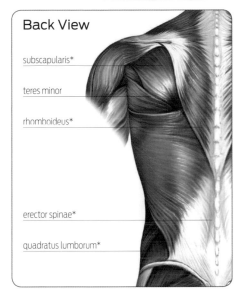

subscapularis*

teres minor

rhomboideus*

erector spinae*

quadratus lumborum*

Correct form
· Keep your body elongated.

Avoid
· Bridging your back and
  allowing your hips to sag.

Level
· Intermediate

Duration
· 3 minutes

Benefits
· Builds strength
  and dexterity

Caution
· Pregnancy
· Lower-back issues

Annotation Key
Bold text indicates target muscles
Black text indicates other working muscles
* indicates deep muscles

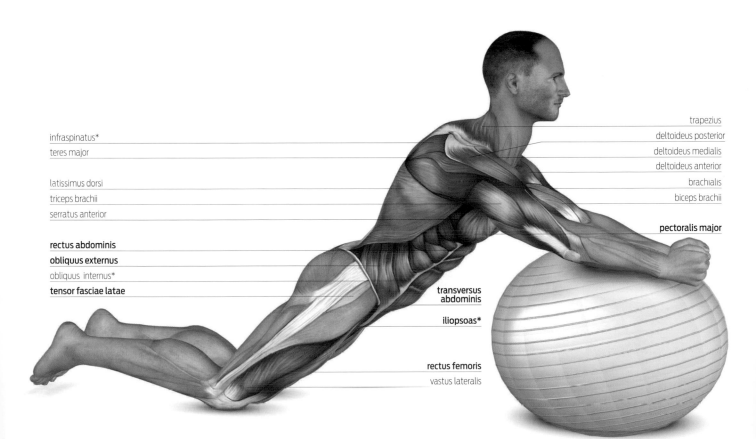

infraspinatus*

teres major

latissimus dorsi

triceps brachii

serratus anterior

rectus abdominis

obliquus externus

obliquus internus*

tensor fasciae latae

transversus
abdominis

iliopsoas*

rectus femoris

vastus lateralis

trapezius

deltoideus posterior

deltoideus medialis

deltoideus anterior

brachialis

biceps brachii

pectoralis major

Fitness Ball
Hyperextension

Fitness Ball Hyperextension, executed on the large fitness ball, is a safe and effective alternative to traditional hyperextension machines. Performing this exercise is a great way to work your lower-back muscles.

1 Begin in a facedown position on top of a fitness ball, with your abdominals covering most of the ball, your legs spread with toes on the floor, and your arms behind your head. Push your toes into the floor for stability.

2 Raise your torso so that it forms a line with the lower half of your body.

3 Squeeze your glutes as you lower your upper body, and then raise it back to the starting position.

4 Continue lowering and raising, working up to 3 sets of 15 to 20.

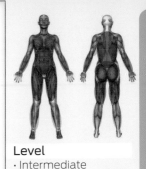

Front View

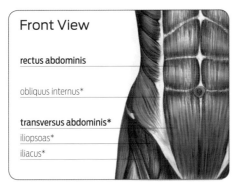

rectus abdominis

obliquus internus*

transversus abdominis*

iliopsoas*

iliacus*

Back View

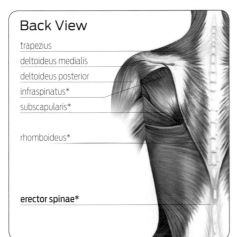

trapezius

deltoideus medialis

deltoideus posterior

infraspinatus*

subscapularis*

rhomboideus*

erector spinae*

Correct form
· Complete the full range of motion in both the negative (downward stretch) and positive (upward motion) of the exercise.

Avoid
· Overcontracting or hyperextending your back at the top of the movement.

Level
· Intermediate

Duration
· 5 minutes

Benefits
· Strengthens gluteal and lower-back muscles

Caution
· Lower-back issues
· Neck issues

extensor digitorum

deltoideus anterior

brachialis

triceps brachii

latissimus dorsi

serratus anterior

pectoralis major

obliquus externus

gluteus maximus

tensor fasciae latae

rectus femoris

tibialis anterior

Annotation Key
Bold text indicates target muscles
Black text indicates other working muscles
* indicates deep muscles

Mountain Climber

Mountain Climber is a core-stabilizing, timed distance exercise. This high-intensity move gets your heart rate going, improving your cardiovascular fitness, while it challenges your legs and core. This all-around exercise also helps to develop muscular endurance in your arms.

1 Begin in a completed push-up position with your body forming a straight line.

2 Bend one knee, and bring it as close to your chest as possible.

3 Return to the starting position and repeat with your other leg. Continue to alternate for 30 seconds, working up to 2 minutes.

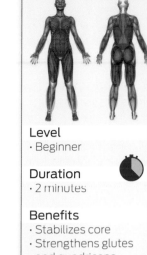

Modifications

Harder: Instead of jumping one foot straight forward, jump the foot diagonally forward so that it crosses under your torso. Then, jump the foot back to starting position. Repeat, alternating sides, to give your oblique muscles a challenging workout.

Annotation Key
Bold text indicates target muscles
Black text indicates other working muscles
* indicates deep muscles

Level
· Beginner

Duration
· 2 minutes

Benefits
· Stabilizes core
· Strengthens glutes and quadriceps
· Improves coordination

Caution
· Pregnancy
· Lower-back issues

deltoideus posterior

serratus anterior

rectus abdominis

gluteus maximus
obliquus externus

obliquus internus*
transversus abdominis*
tensor fasciae latae
biceps femoris

deltoideus anterior
brachialis
triceps brachii
biceps brachii
sartorius
adductor longus

rectus femoris
gastrocnemius

Correct form
· Keep the movement steady, but do not race through it.

Avoid
· Excessive back-bridging.

tibialis anterior

Body-Weight Squat

Body-Weight Squat is a full-body exercise. Completing it correctly means using your core properly. It may look like an easy move, but there is more to it: as well as engaging your leg muscles, it engages nearly every muscle in your lower body. Perfecting this exercise is a great way to combat the weakness that often develops from a sedentary lifestyle.

1 Stand upright, with your feet shoulder-width apart and your arms outstretched in front of you.

2 Bend your legs and lower your body until your thighs are parallel to the floor, pushing your buttocks out slightly and maintaining a flat back.

3 Push through your heels back into an upright position

4 Repeat, working up to 3 sets of 15.

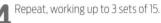

Correct form
· Keep your head up and your chest out so that your body forms a straight line.

Avoid
· Allowing your knees to hyperextend past your feet.

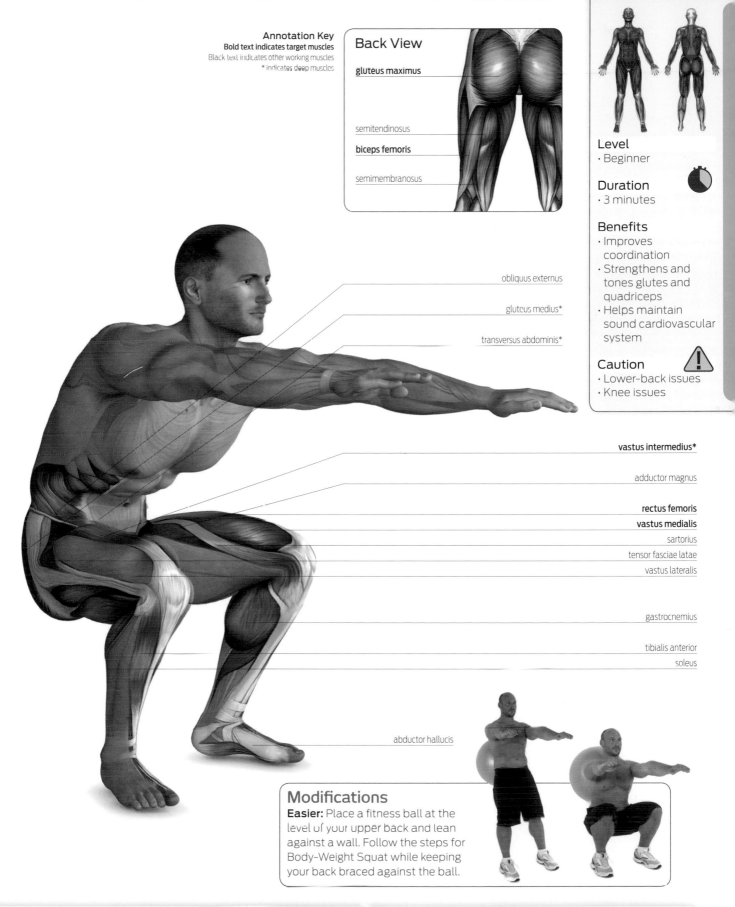

Annotation Key
Bold text indicates target muscles
Black text indicates other working muscles
* indicates deep muscles

Back View
gluteus maximus

semitendinosus

biceps femoris

semimembranosus

Level
· Beginner

Duration
· 3 minutes

Benefits
· Improves coordination
· Strengthens and tones glutes and quadriceps
· Helps maintain sound cardiovascular system

Caution
· Lower-back issues
· Knee issues

obliquus externus

gluteus medius*

transversus abdominis*

vastus intermedius*

adductor magnus

rectus femoris
vastus medialis
sartorius
tensor fasciae latae
vastus lateralis

gastrocnemius

tibialis anterior
soleus

abductor hallucis

Modifications
Easier: Place a fitness ball at the level of your upper back and lean against a wall. Follow the steps for Body-Weight Squat while keeping your back braced against the ball.

Medicine Ball Squat to Press

Medicine Ball Squat to Press works your entire body. A multifunctional exercise, it calls upon a spectrum of different muscles to engage at the same time.

1 Stand upright, holding the medicine ball in front of your chest. Plant your feet shoulder-width apart, and stick your buttocks slightly outward.

2 Lower toward the floor until your thighs are parallel to the floor.

Correct form
· Keep your head up and your chest out so your body forms a straight line.

Avoid
· Allowing your knees to hyperextend past your feet.

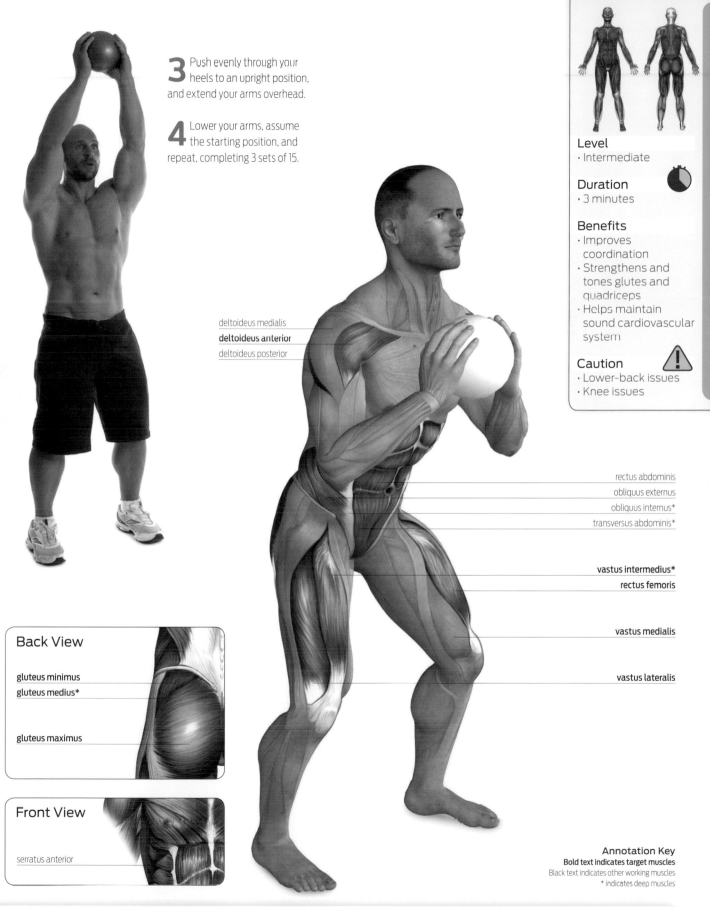

3 Push evenly through your heels to an upright position, and extend your arms overhead.

4 Lower your arms, assume the starting position, and repeat, completing 3 sets of 15.

Level
· Intermediate

Duration
· 3 minutes

Benefits
· Improves coordination
· Strengthens and tones glutes and quadriceps
· Helps maintain sound cardiovascular system

Caution
· Lower-back issues
· Knee issues

deltoideus medialis
deltoideus anterior
deltoideus posterior

rectus abdominis
obliquus externus
obliquus internus*
transversus abdominis*

vastus intermedius*
rectus femoris

vastus medialis

vastus lateralis

Back View

gluteus minimus
gluteus medius*

gluteus maximus

Front View

serratus anterior

Annotation Key
Bold text indicates target muscles
Black text indicates other working muscles
* indicates deep muscles

Balance Push-Up

Balance Push-Up is an advanced upper-body exercise. To complete it correctly demands proper stabilization of your core.

1 Assume a push-up position with your hands balanced on a fitness ball, shoulder-width apart.

2 Keeping your body in one straight line, bend your arms and lower your chest until it is nearly touching the fitness ball.

3 Straighten your arms, pushing to full extension.

4 Repeat, aiming for 3 sets of 10.

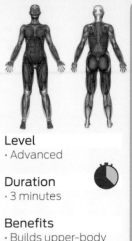

Correct form
· Keep your hands planted on the ball.
· Try to keep the ball as still as possible.
· Keep your heels lifted so that you are balancing on your toes.

Avoid
· Arching your back.
· Rushing through the movement.

Annotation Key
Bold text indicates target muscles
Black text indicates other working muscles
* indicates deep muscles

Front View

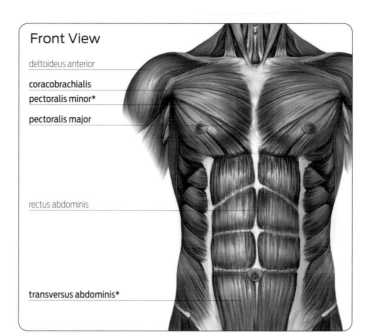

deltoideus anterior
coracobrachialis
pectoralis minor*
pectoralis major

rectus abdominis

transversus abdominis*

Level
· Advanced

Duration
· 3 minutes

Benefits
· Builds upper-body strength and stability
· Stabilizes spine and core

Caution
· Lower-back pain
· Wrist pain
· Shoulder issues

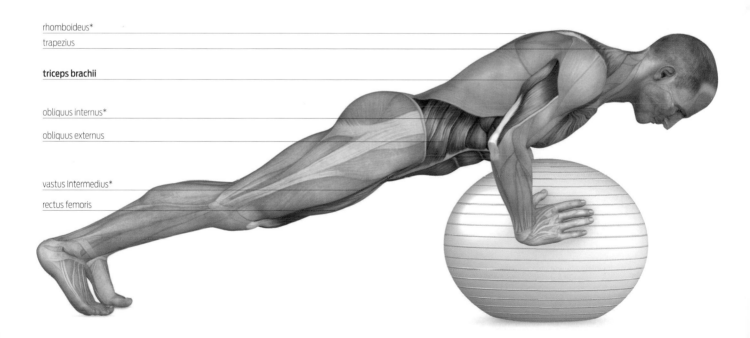

rhomboideus*
trapezius

triceps brachii

obliquus internus*
obliquus externus

vastus Intermedius*
rectus femoris

Kneel on Ball

Kneel on Ball really challenges your core stability. Before attempting this advanced exercise solo, it is best tryout with a fitness partner guiding you while you find your balance. Once balanced, fully engage your core and concentrate on keeping the ball as still as possible while your partner spots you.

1 Stand upright with a fitness ball in front of you.

2 Place one knee on top of the ball, and then slowly place the other one on the ball as well. Ask a partner to hold your torso in place while you find your balance.

3 Remain balanced for 15 seconds, stretching your arms out to your sides. Release.

4 Repeat, working up to 3 sets of 30-second balances.

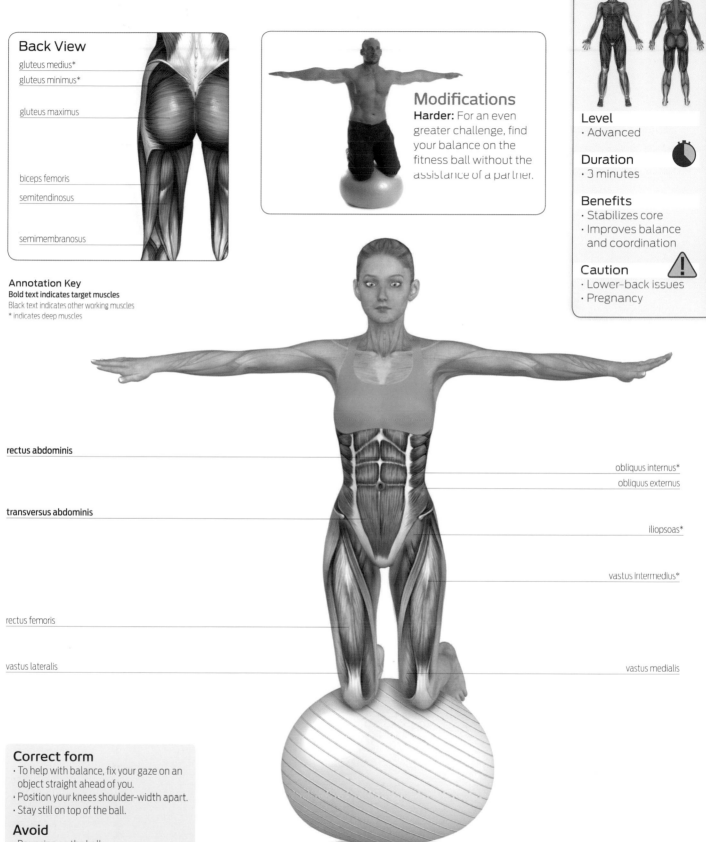

Back View

gluteus medius*
gluteus minimus*
gluteus maximus

biceps femoris
semitendinosus

semimembranosus

Annotation Key
Bold text indicates target muscles
Black text indicates other working muscles
* indicates deep muscles

Modifications
Harder: For an even greater challenge, find your balance on the fitness ball without the assistance of a partner.

Level
· Advanced

Duration
· 3 minutes

Benefits
· Stabilizes core
· Improves balance and coordination

Caution
· Lower-back issues
· Pregnancy

rectus abdominis

transversus abdominis

rectus femoris

vastus lateralis

obliquus internus*
obliquus externus

iliopsoas*

vastus intermedius*

vastus medialis

Correct form
· To help with balance, fix your gaze on an object straight ahead of you.
· Position your knees shoulder-width apart.
· Stay still on top of the ball.

Avoid
· Bouncing on the ball.

Medicine Ball Over-the-Shoulder Throw

As simple as it may look, Medicine Ball Over-the-Shoulder Throw trains multiple muscles at once. It is a multipurpose exercise that helps you develop coordination, balance, and power while working on core stability and strength.

1 Stand upright, with a medicine ball in your hands, held low with your arms extended. Rotate your core, moving your extended arms slightly upward and to the side so that the medicine ball follows your body's twist.

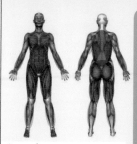

Correct form
· Follow through with your swing.
· Bend your legs slightly as you twist.
· Follow the ball with your gaze.

Avoid
· Rushing through the movement.

2 Twist your torso in the other direction as you raise your arms in an arc. At the top of the arc, with your torso twisted, release the ball to your partner.

3 Lower your arms and return your torso to center.

4 Repeat. Perform 15 repetitions, and then switch sides, working up to 3 sets of 15 repetitions per side.

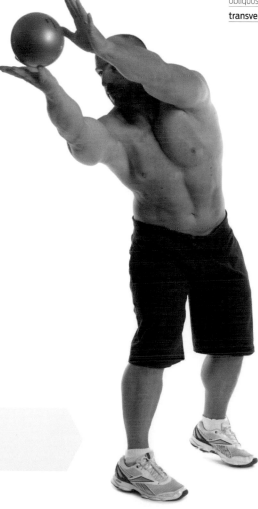

Annotation Key
Bold text indicates target muscles
Black text indicates other working muscles
indicates deep muscles

serratus anterior
intercostales externi
intercostales interni*
obliquus externus

rectus abdominis
obliquus internus*
transversus abdominis

Level
· Beginner

Duration
· 3 minutes

Benefits
· Stabilizes core
· Improves balance and coordination
· Strengthens shoulders and upper back

Caution
· Lower-back issues
· Rotator cuff injury

Back View
infraspinatus*
teres minor
subscapularis*
supraspinatus*
latissimus dorsi

Fitness Ball Split Squat

Fitness Ball Split Squat is an advanced leg exercise. But it doesn't just involve your legs: to perform it correctly requires drawing upon a sound core so that your whole body gets a workout.

1 Stand with a fitness ball behind you. Place your hands on your hips.

2 Bend one leg to rest your ankle and the top of your foot on the ball.

3 Bend the knee of your front leg until the thigh is nearly parallel to the floor while simultaneously bending your back leg.

4 Straighten both legs to return to a standing position. Repeat to perform 15 repetitions. Switch legs and repeat, building up to 3 sets of 15 per leg.

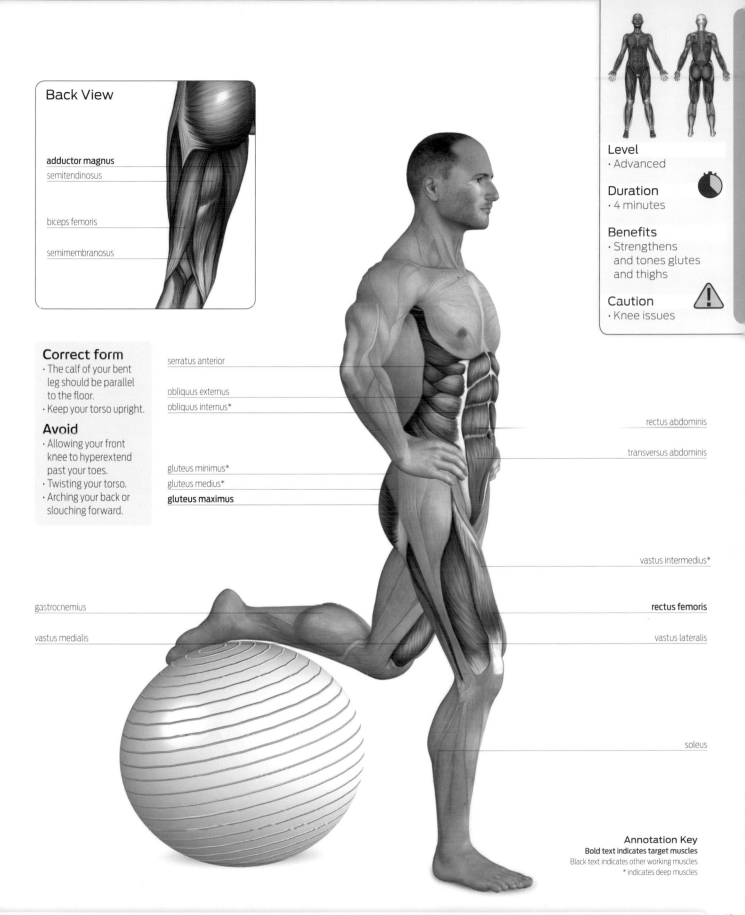

Back View

adductor magnus
semitendinosus

biceps femoris

semimembranosus

Level
· Advanced

Duration
· 4 minutes

Benefits
· Strengthens
  and tones glutes
  and thighs

Caution
· Knee issues

Correct form
· The calf of your bent
  leg should be parallel
  to the floor.
· Keep your torso upright.

Avoid
· Allowing your front
  knee to hyperextend
  past your toes.
· Twisting your torso.
· Arching your back or
  slouching forward.

serratus anterior

obliquus externus
obliquus internus*

gluteus minimus*
gluteus medius*
gluteus maximus

rectus abdominis

transversus abdominis

vastus intermedius*

rectus femoris

vastus lateralis

gastrocnemius

vastus medialis

soleus

Annotation Key
Bold text indicates target muscles
Black text indicates other working muscles
* indicates deep muscles

Fitness Ball Prone Row to External Rotation

Fitness Ball Prone Row to External Rotation is an advanced exercise that challenges your rotator cuffs and upper back. It also effectively works your core. This exercise is best preceded by a thorough warm-up to loosen your shoulder girdle.

1 Begin facedown on top of a fitness ball, with your torso supported. Balance on your toes, with your legs separated for stability.

2 Bend your arms to form 90-degree angles, with your upper arms parallel to the floor.

3 Pull your arms back as high as possible into a rowing position.

4 Rotate your forearms until they are parallel to the floor.

5 Reverse the movement until your fingers are nearly touching the floor.

6 Repeat to perform 3 sets of 15.

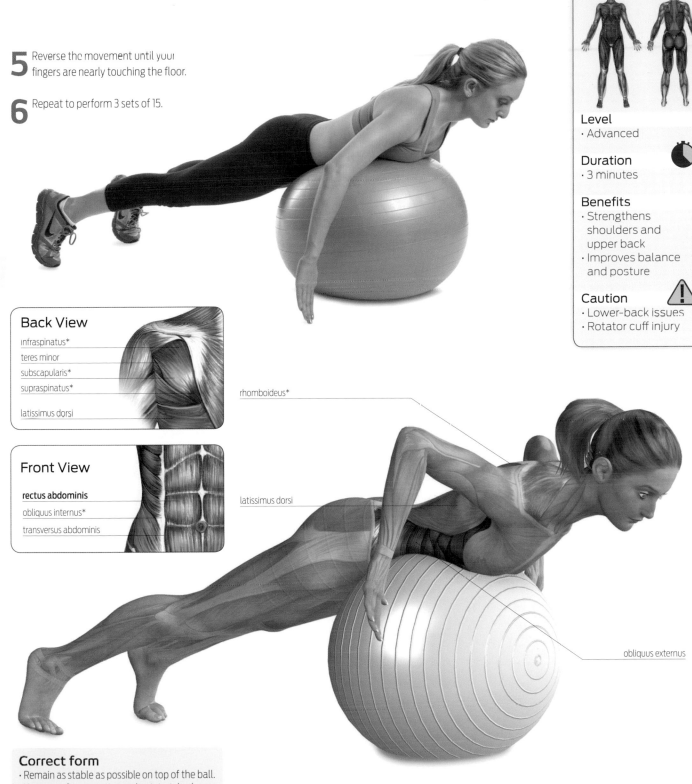

Level
· Advanced

Duration
· 3 minutes

Benefits
· Strengthens shoulders and upper back
· Improves balance and posture

Caution
· Lower-back issues
· Rotator cuff injury

Back View
infraspinatus*
teres minor
subscapularis*
supraspinatus*
latissimus dorsi

Front View
rectus abdominis
obliquus internus*
transversus abdominis

rhomboideus*

latissimus dorsi

obliquus externus

Correct form
· Remain as stable as possible on top of the ball.
· Keep your fingers active and outstretched.

Avoid
· Hyperextending your back.
· Allowing one or both feet to lift off the floor.
· Straining your neck by trying to look up.

Annotation Key
Bold text indicates target muscles
Black text indicates other working muscles
* indicates deep muscles

Fitness Ball Seated External Rotation

Fitness Ball Seated External Rotation targets your upper back and shoulders, particularly your rotator cuff muscles, in addition to the muscles of your core.

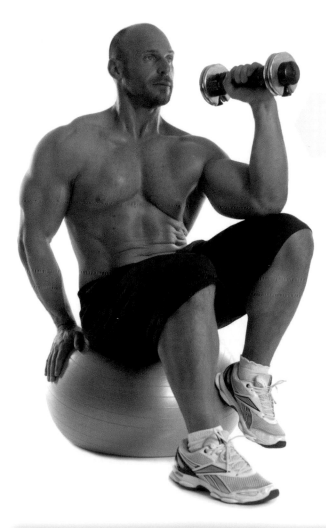

1 Sit on top of the fitness ball, with one foot firmly planted on the floor and the other slightly raised.

2 In your left hand, grasp a light dumbbell, and then rest your elbow on your raised knee. Position your left arm to hold the dumbbell against your chest, forearm level with the floor.

3 Rotate your left arm until your fist is pointing toward the ceiling.

4 Lower your left arm, and repeat to complete 15 repetitions.

5 Switch sides and repeat. Work up to performing 2 sets of 15.

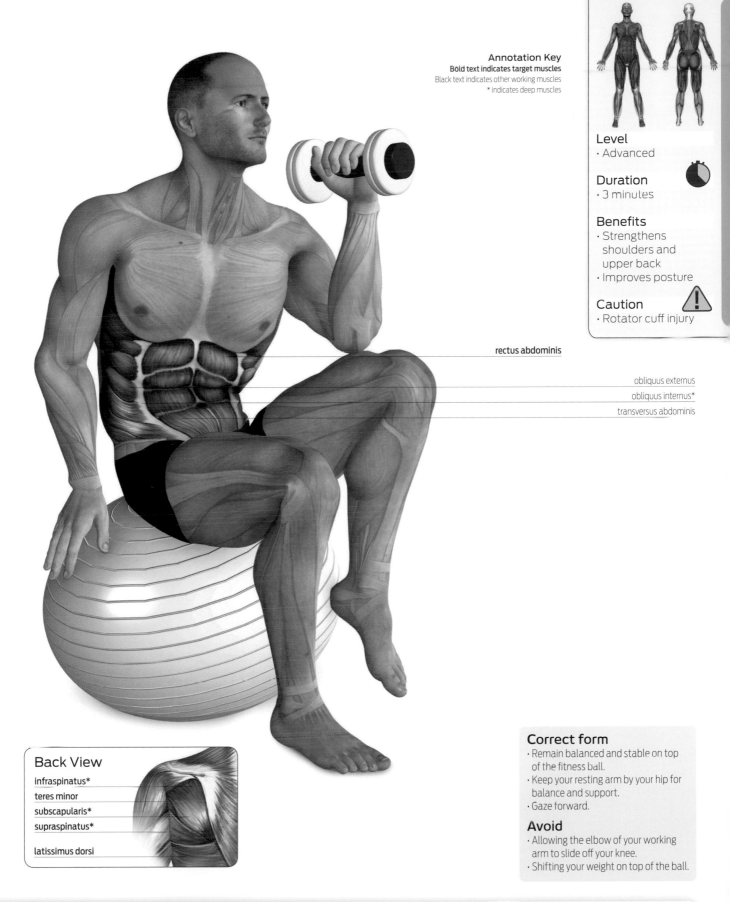

Annotation Key
Bold text indicates target muscles
Black text indicates other working muscles
* indicates deep muscles

Level
· Advanced

Duration
· 3 minutes

Benefits
· Strengthens shoulders and upper back
· Improves posture

Caution
· Rotator cuff injury

rectus abdominis

obliquus externus
obliquus internus*
transversus abdominis

Back View
infraspinatus*
teres minor
subscapularis*
supraspinatus*

latissimus dorsi

Correct form
· Remain balanced and stable on top of the fitness ball.
· Keep your resting arm by your hip for balance and support.
· Gaze forward.

Avoid
· Allowing the elbow of your working arm to slide off your knee.
· Shifting your weight on top of the ball.

Medicine Ball Walkover

Medicine Ball Walkover calls upon the major muscles of your upper body, challenging them to stay active and engaged as you carry out the movement.

1 Assume a push-up position, with your arms wider than shoulder-distance apart and the medicine ball under one hand.

2 Slowly bend both arms, lowering yourself toward the floor as if you were beginning a normal push-up.

3 Begin to straighten your arms as you raise your body toward starting position. Quickly pass the ball from one hand to the other.

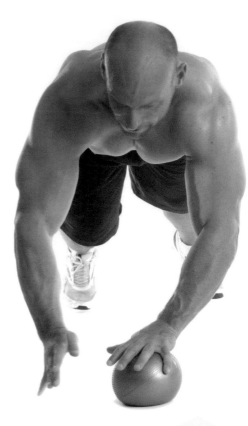

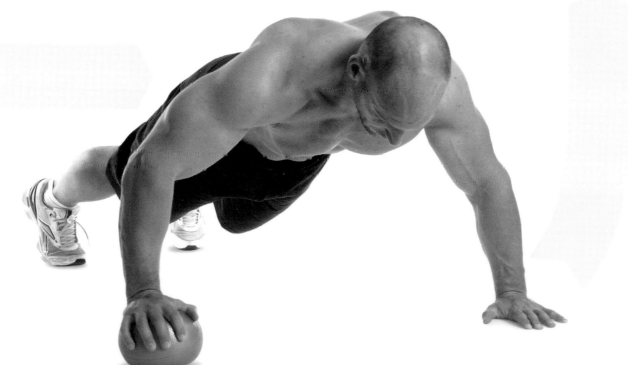

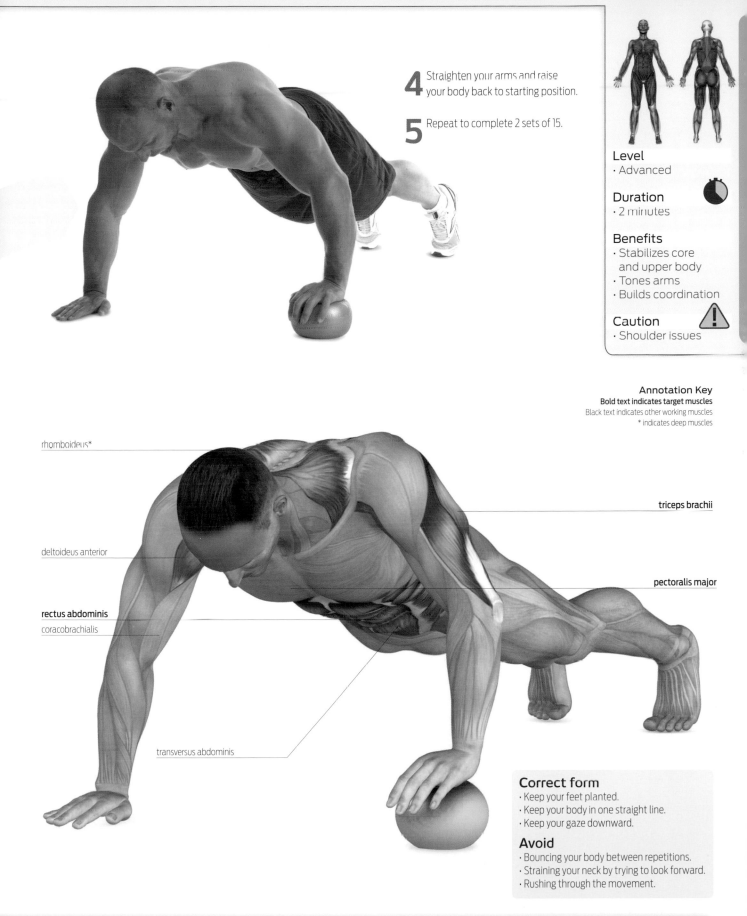

4 Straighten your arms and raise your body back to starting position.

5 Repeat to complete 2 sets of 15.

Level
· Advanced

Duration
· 2 minutes

Benefits
· Stabilizes core and upper body
· Tones arms
· Builds coordination

Caution
· Shoulder issues

Annotation Key
Bold text indicates target muscles
Black text indicates other working muscles
* indicates deep muscles

rhomboideus*

triceps brachii

deltoideus anterior

pectoralis major

rectus abdominis

coracobrachialis

transversus abdominis

Correct form
· Keep your feet planted.
· Keep your body in one straight line.
· Keep your gaze downward.

Avoid
· Bouncing your body between repetitions.
· Straining your neck by trying to look forward.
· Rushing through the movement.

Fitness Ball Band Fly

Fitness Ball Band Fly is an excellent exercise for working your chest. Of course, this movement will also call your core into play.

1 Run an exercise band under your fitness ball. Lie back, with your upper back supported by the ball. With your arms extended out to your sides, hold one handle of the band in each hand.

2 Bend your arms slightly as you begin to contract your chest in a hugging motion.

3 Lengthen your arms to full extension until your chest is fully contracted.

4 Return to starting position and repeat, working up to 3 sets of 15.

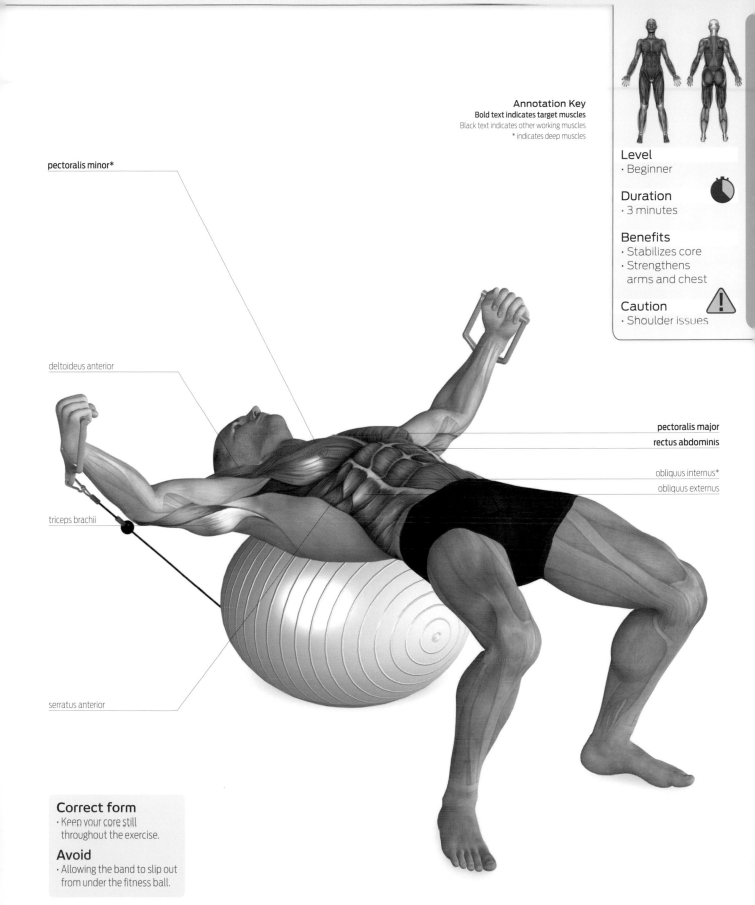

pectoralis minor*

Annotation Key
Bold text indicates target muscles
Black text indicates other working muscles
* indicates deep muscles

Level
· Beginner

Duration
· 3 minutes

Benefits
· Stabilizes core
· Strengthens
  arms and chest

Caution
· Shoulder issues

deltoideus anterior

pectoralis major

rectus abdominis

obliquus internus*

obliquus externus

triceps brachii

serratus anterior

Correct form
· Keep your core still
  throughout the exercise.

Avoid
· Allowing the band to slip out
  from under the fitness ball.

Fitness Ball Walk-Around

Fitness Ball Walk-Around offers a great challenge for your core stability. It also works your arms and sharpens your sense of balance.

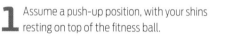

1 Assume a push-up position, with your shins resting on top of the fitness ball.

2 One at a time, "walk" your hands to the side and turn your body so that it rotates in a half circle.

3 Walk your hands in the reverse direction, returning your body to starting position.

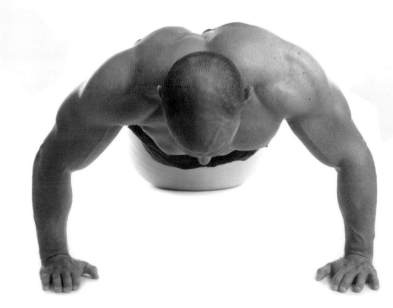

Correct form
· Keep the fitness ball as still and stable as possible.
· Keep your legs, torso, and neck in a straight line.
· Keep your gaze downward.
· Keep your hands' "steps" small enough that you can control the movement.

Avoid
· Twisting your body.
· Straining your neck by trying to look forward.
· Rushing through the movement.

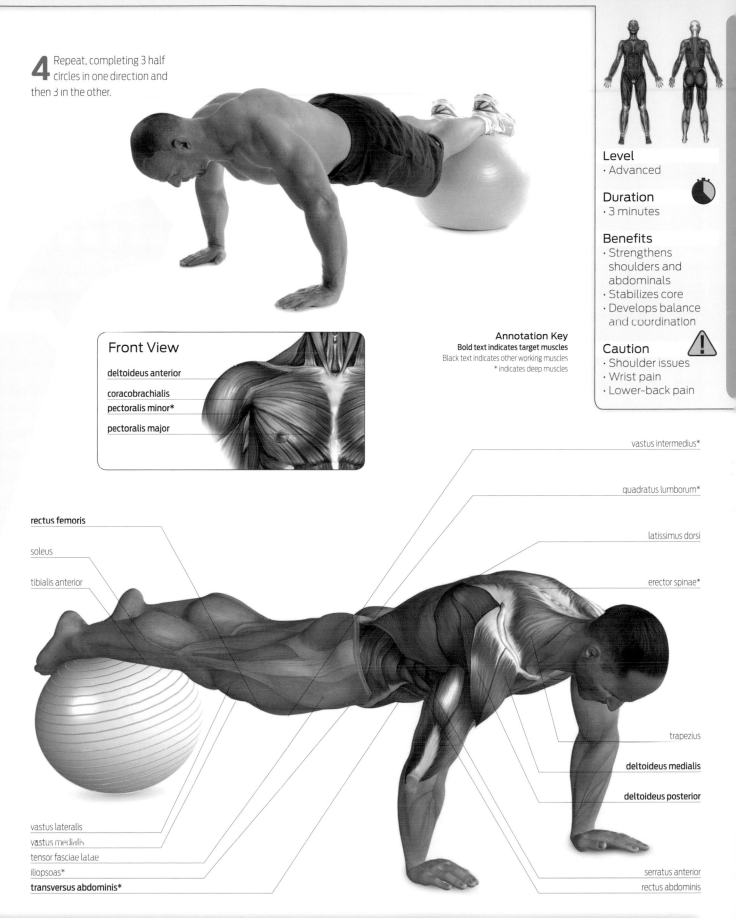

4 Repeat, completing 3 half circles in one direction and then 3 in the other.

Level
· Advanced

Duration
· 3 minutes

Benefits
· Strengthens shoulders and abdominals
· Stabilizes core
· Develops balance and coordination

Caution
· Shoulder issues
· Wrist pain
· Lower-back pain

Front View

deltoideus anterior

coracobrachialis

pectoralis minor*

pectoralis major

Annotation Key
Bold text indicates target muscles
Black text indicates other working muscles
* indicates deep muscles

vastus intermedius*

quadratus lumborum*

latissimus dorsi

erector spinae*

trapezius

deltoideus medialis

deltoideus posterior

serratus anterior

rectus abdominis

rectus femoris

soleus

tibialis anterior

vastus lateralis

vastus medialis

tensor fasciae latae

iliopsoas*

transversus abdominis*

Medicine Ball Pullover on Fitness Ball

Medicine Ball Pullover on Fitness Ball is great for working the latissimus dorsi. The latissimus dorsi, often just called the "lats," is the largest of the back muscles and engages any time you pull something, such as when you open a door.

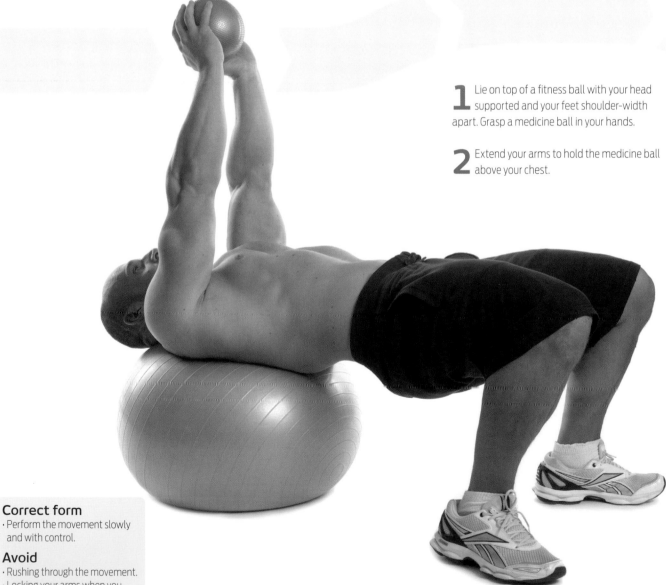

1 Lie on top of a fitness ball with your head supported and your feet shoulder-width apart. Grasp a medicine ball in your hands.

2 Extend your arms to hold the medicine ball above your chest.

Correct form
· Perform the movement slowly and with control.

Avoid
· Rushing through the movement.
· Locking your arms when you bring the ball behind your head.

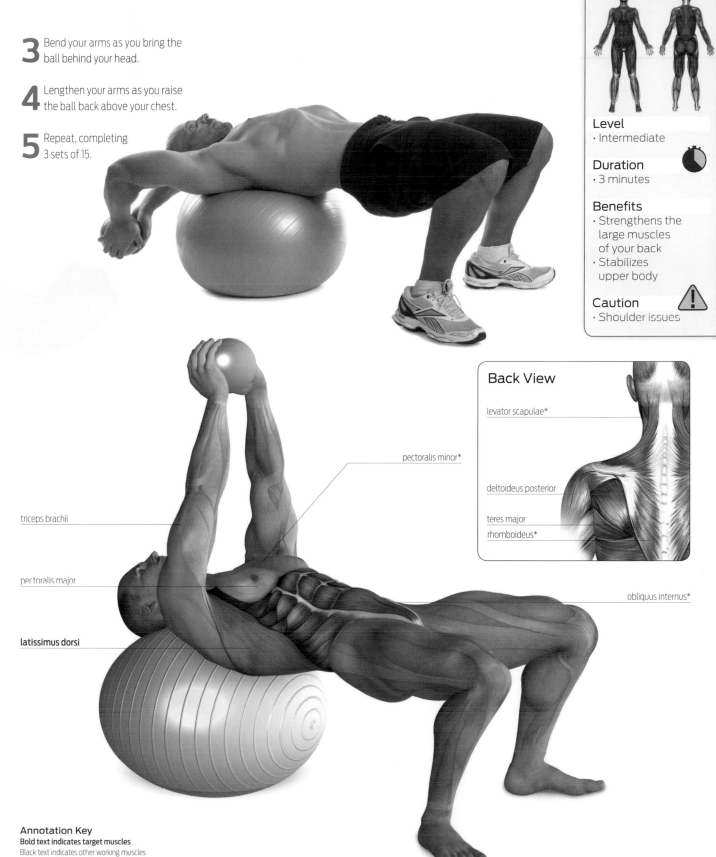

3 Bend your arms as you bring the ball behind your head.

4 Lengthen your arms as you raise the ball back above your chest.

5 Repeat, completing 3 sets of 15.

Level
· Intermediate

Duration
· 3 minutes

Benefits
· Strengthens the large muscles of your back
· Stabilizes upper body

Caution
· Shoulder issues

Back View

levator scapulae*

deltoideus posterior

teres major

rhomboideus*

pectoralis minor*

triceps brachii

pectoralis major

latissimus dorsi

obliquus internus*

Annotation Key
Bold text indicates target muscles
Black text indicates other working muscles
* indicates deep muscles

Side Lunge and Press

Side Lunge and Press is a combo exercise that works both your upper and lower body. The lunge to the side develops the often-neglected adductors and abductors, as well as your core, and the press works out your shoulders.

Correct form
· Ease into the lunge.
· Keep your torso stable and upright.

Avoid
· Rushing through the movement.

1 Stand upright, holding a dumbbell in each hand.

2 Raise both dumbbells over your head, arms straight.

3 Bend your right leg as you lunge to the right side. At the same time, bend your right arm to lower the dumbbell to just above shoulder height.

4 Raise the arm, and return your bent leg to center. Repeat on the other side, working up 3 sets of 15 repetitions per side.

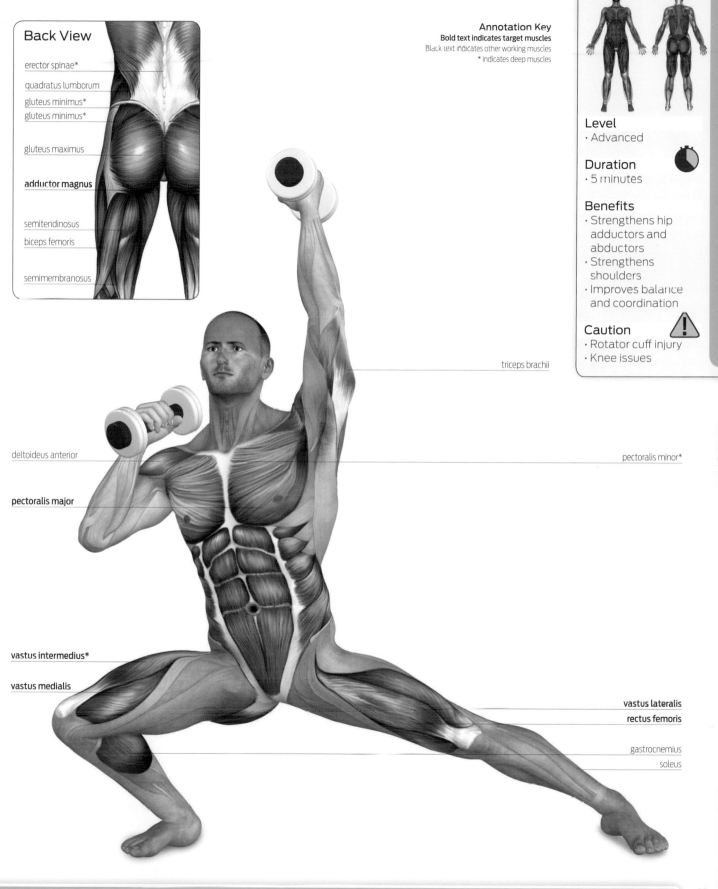

Back View

erector spinae*

quadratus lumborum

gluteus minimus*

gluteus minimus*

gluteus maximus

adductor magnus

semitendinosus

biceps femoris

semimembranosus

Annotation Key
Bold text indicates target muscles
Black text indicates other working muscles
* indicates deep muscles

triceps brachii

pectoralis minor*

deltoideus anterior

pectoralis major

vastus intermedius*

vastus medialis

vastus lateralis

rectus femoris

gastrocnemius

soleus

Level
· Advanced

Duration
· 5 minutes

Benefits
· Strengthens hip adductors and abductors
· Strengthens shoulders
· Improves balance and coordination

Caution
· Rotator cuff injury
· Knee issues

Hip Crossover

Hip Crossover effectively targets your lower-back and oblique muscles. As with many core exercises, when executing Hip Crossover, aim for controlled movements. You want your muscles—not momentum—to move you.

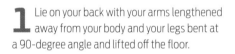

1 Lie on your back with your arms lengthened away from your body and your legs bent at a 90-degree angle and lifted off the floor.

2 Brace your abs, and lower your knees to the side, dropping them as close to the floor as possible without lifting your shoulders off the floor.

3 Return to the starting position, hold for a moment, and then repeat on the other side. Work up to 15 repetitions per side.

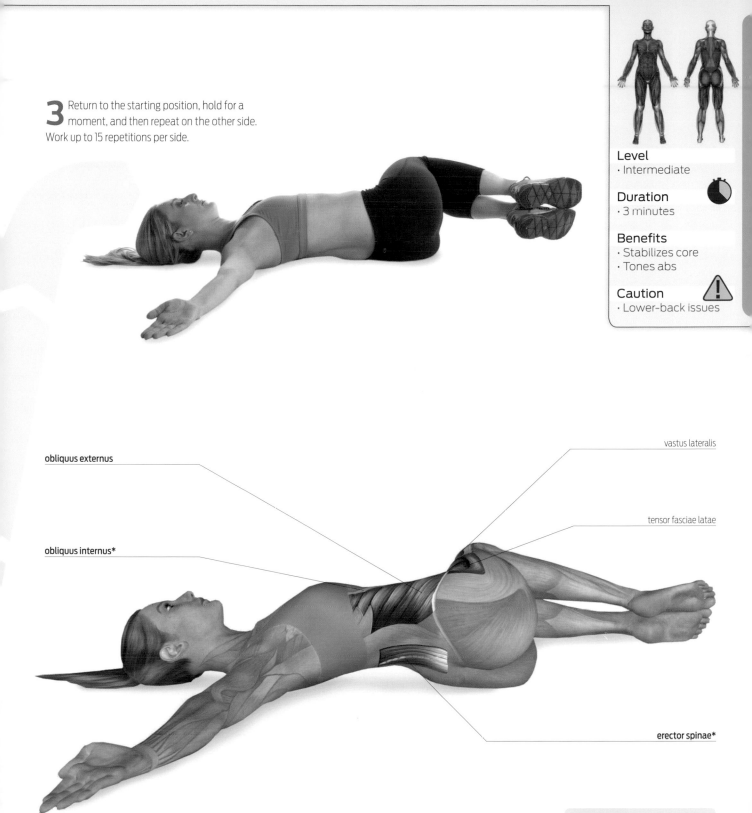

Level
· Intermediate

Duration
· 3 minutes

Benefits
· Stabilizes core
· Tones abs

Caution
· Lower-back issues

obliquus externus

obliquus internus*

vastus lateralis

tensor fasciae latae

erector spinae*

Correct form
· Keep your core centered.
· Move carefully and with control.

Avoid
· Excessively swinging your legs.

Annotation Key
Bold text indicates target muscles
Black text indicates other working muscles
* indicates deep muscles

Hip Raise

Adding movement to the traditional shoulder bridge, Hip Raise really challenges your core strength. It is not only an abdominal and lower-back exercise, but it targets your gluteal and hamstring muscles, too.

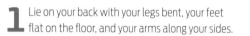

1 Lie on your back with your legs bent, your feet flat on the floor, and your arms along your sides.

2 Push through your heels while raising your pelvis until your torso is aligned with your thighs.

3 Lower and then repeat, working up to 3 sets of 15.

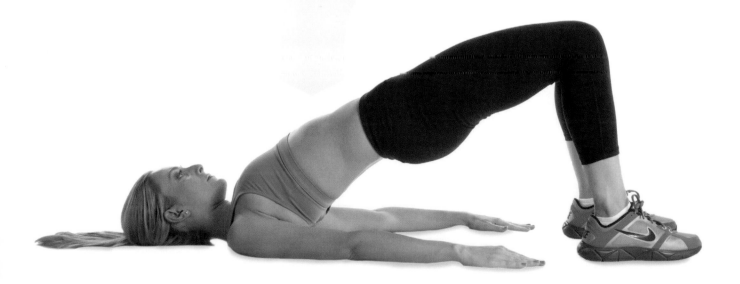

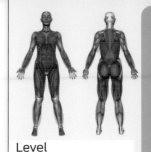

Back View

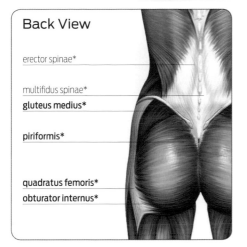

erector spinae*

multifidus spinae*
gluteus medius*

piriformis*

quadratus femoris*
obturator internus*

Correct form
· Push through your heels, not your toes.
· Roll your shoulders under once you are
  in the raised position.
· Tighten your thighs and buttocks.

Avoid
· Tucking you chin toward your chest.
· Overextending your abdominals past
  your thighs in the raised position.

Annotation Key
Bold text indicates target muscles
Black text indicates other working muscles
* indicates deep muscles

Level
· Beginner

Duration
· 3 minutes

Benefits
· Strengthens glutes
  and hamstrings
· Stretches chest
  and spine

Caution
· Lower-back issues
· Neck Issues
· Shoulder issues

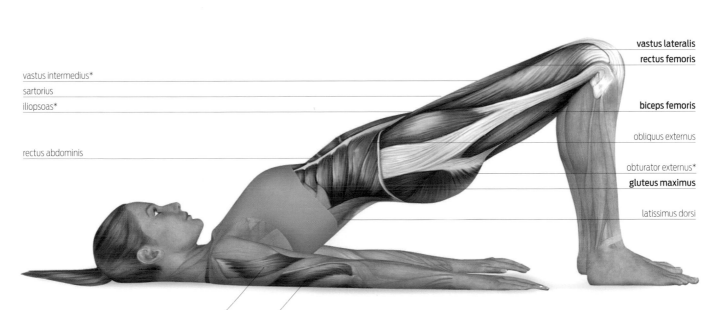

vastus lateralis
rectus femoris

biceps femoris

obliquus externus

obturator externus*
gluteus maximus

latissimus dorsi

vastus intermedius*
sartorius
iliopsoas*

rectus abdominis

deltoideus medialis

triceps brachii

Fitness Ball Hip Raise

Fitness Ball Hip Raise targets your core muscles, particularly the glutes. Along the way, your hamstrings get a great workout, too.

Correct form
· Place your feet flat on the fitness ball in the starting position.
· Push through your heels rather than your toes.
· Keep the fitness ball as stable as possible.

Avoid
· Pushing the ball away as you raise or lower your body.

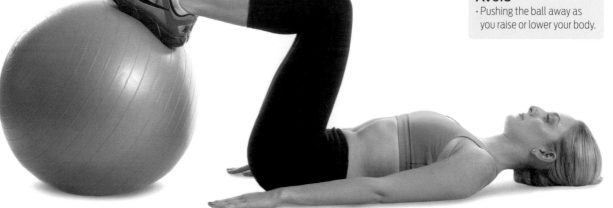

1 Lie on your back with your arms along your sides. Bend your knees, and rest your feet on the fitness ball.

2 Push through your heels while raising your pelvis until your torso is aligned with your thighs.

3 Lower and repeat, building up to for 3 sets of 15.

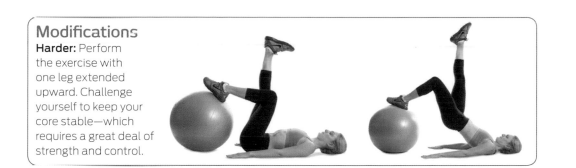

Modifications

Harder: Perform the exercise with one leg extended upward. Challenge yourself to keep your core stable—which requires a great deal of strength and control.

Front View

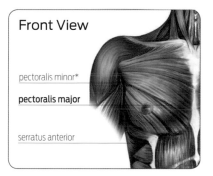

pectoralis minor*

pectoralis major

serratus anterior

Annotation Key
Bold text indicates target muscles
Black text indicates other working muscles
* indicates deep muscles

Level
· Intermediate

Duration
· 3 minutes

Benefits
· Strengthens glutes and hamstrings
· Stretches chest and spine

Caution
· Lower-back issues
· Neck issues
· Shoulder issues

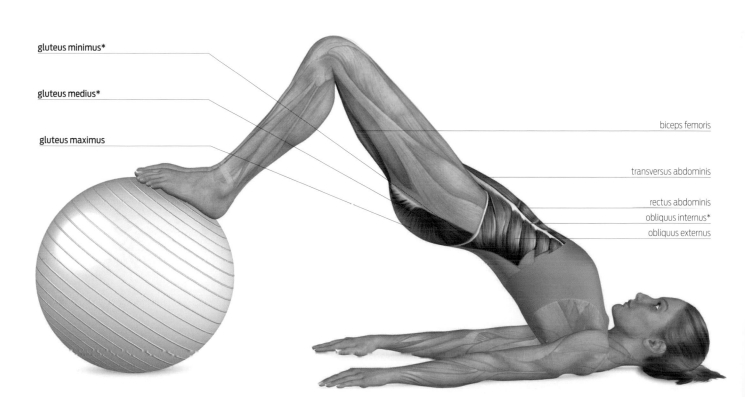

gluteus minimus*

gluteus medius*

gluteus maximus

biceps femoris

transversus abdominis

rectus abdominis

obliquus internus*

obliquus externus

Fitness Ball Bridge

Bridging exercises are great for toning the legs and buttocks. Fitness Ball Bridge adds another layer of challenge to this classic—working on an unstable ball means that you must keep your entire core fully engaged so that you maintain your balance.

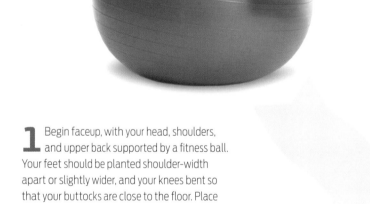

1 Begin faceup, with your head, shoulders, and upper back supported by a fitness ball. Your feet should be planted shoulder-width apart or slightly wider, and your knees bent so that your buttocks are close to the floor. Place your hands on your hips.

2 Pushing through your heels, raise your torso until your upper body is parallel to the floor.

3 Lower to starting position. Repeat, aiming for 3 sets of 15.

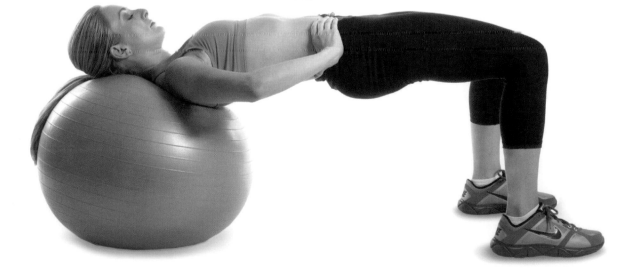

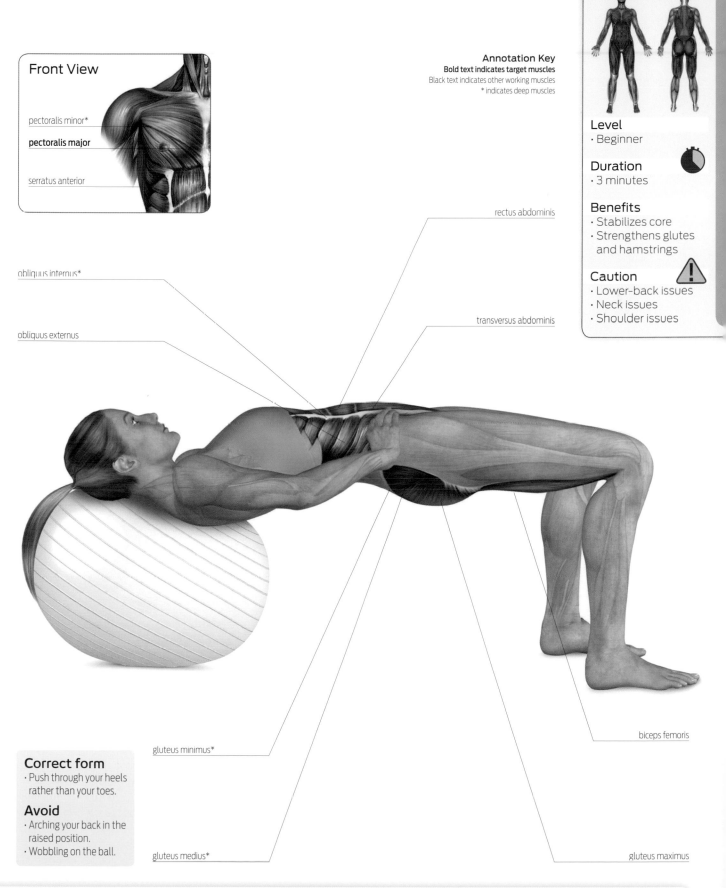

Front View

pectoralis minor*

pectoralis major

serratus anterior

Annotation Key
Bold text indicates target muscles
Black text indicates other working muscles
* indicates deep muscles

Level
· Beginner

Duration
· 3 minutes

Benefits
· Stabilizes core
· Strengthens glutes
and hamstrings

Caution
· Lower-back issues
· Neck issues
· Shoulder issues

rectus abdominis

transversus abdominis

obliquus internus*

obliquus externus

gluteus minimus*

biceps femoris

Correct form
· Push through your heels
rather than your toes.

Avoid
· Arching your back in the
raised position.
· Wobbling on the ball.

gluteus medius*

gluteus maximus

Stiff-Legged Deadlift

Stiff-Legged Deadlift is a standard among body-builders who want to work their hamstrings. Add this exercise to your regimen, and you'll also target your glutes and the erector muscles in your back.

1 Hold a pair of dumbbells in front of your thighs, with your knees bent and your buttocks pushed out slightly.

2 Keeping your back flat, lower your dumbbells toward the floor.

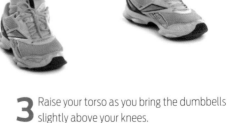

3 Raise your torso as you bring the dumbbells slightly above your knees.

4 Repeat, building up to 3 sets of 15.

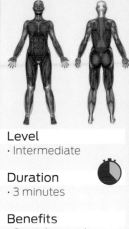

Correct form
· Keep your back flat throughout the exercise.
· Gaze forward.

Avoid
· Arching or rounding your back.
· Avoid standing completely up at the top to keep the tension on the hamstrings and glutes.

Level
· Intermediate

Duration
· 3 minutes

Benefits
· Stretches and strengthens hamstrings, glutes and back muscles
· Improves lower-body flexibility

Caution
· Lower-back issues

Annotation Key
Bold text indicates target muscles
Black text indicates other working muscles
* indicates deep muscles

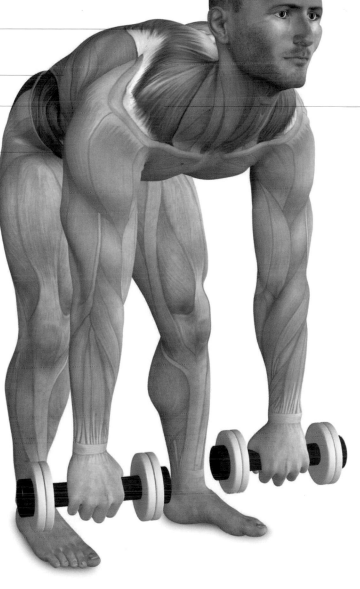

rhomboideus*

latissimus dorsi

obliquus externus

rectus abdominis

trapezius

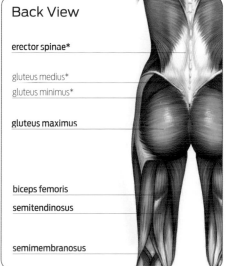

Back View

erector spinae*

gluteus medius*

gluteus minimus*

gluteus maximus

biceps femoris

semitendinosus

semimembranosus

Standing One-Legged Row

Standing One-Legged Row will greatly challenge the stabilization of your core, testing your balance and the functionality of your entire upper body. This exercise works your lats and arms, as well as your legs. Although it may seem difficult at first, with regular practice it will become easier as your core stability improves.

1 Stand upright, holding a dumbbell in your right hand.

2 Extend your right leg behind you. At the same time, lean forward, extending your left arm in front of you for balance and bending your left leg slightly.

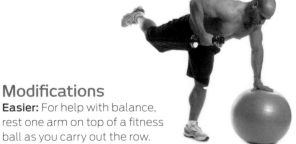

Modifications
Easier: For help with balance, rest one arm on top of a fitness ball as you carry out the row.

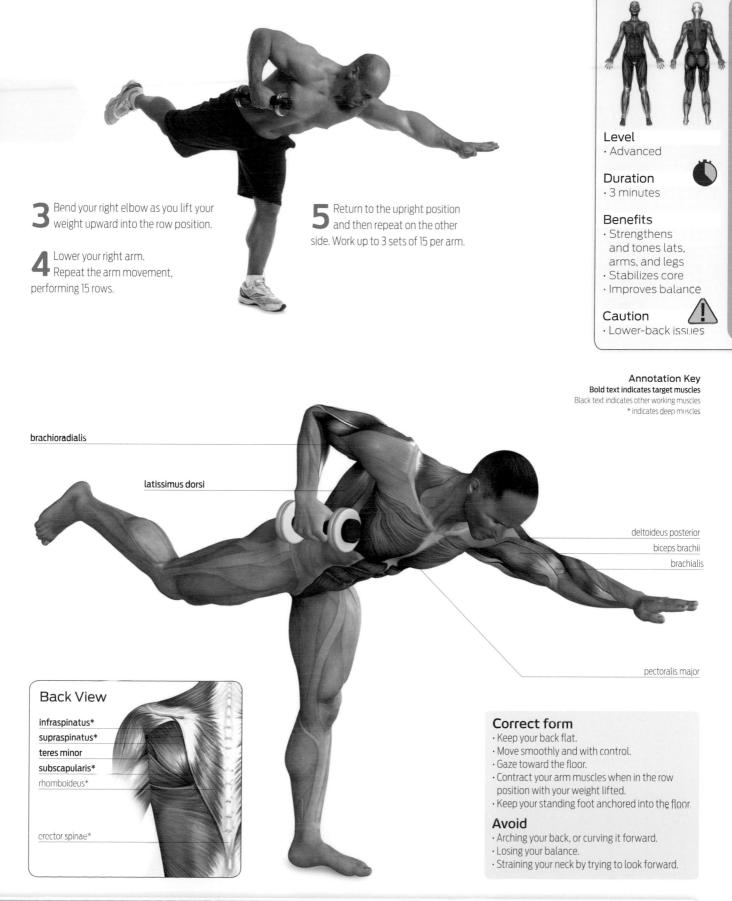

3 Bend your right elbow as you lift your weight upward into the row position.

4 Lower your right arm. Repeat the arm movement, performing 15 rows.

5 Return to the upright position and then repeat on the other side. Work up to 3 sets of 15 per arm.

Level
· Advanced

Duration
· 3 minutes

Benefits
· Strengthens and tones lats, arms, and legs
· Stabilizes core
· Improves balance

Caution
· Lower-back issues

Annotation Key
Bold text indicates target muscles
Black text indicates other working muscles
* indicates deep muscles

brachioradialis

latissimus dorsi

deltoideus posterior
biceps brachii
brachialis

pectoralis major

Back View

infraspinatus*
supraspinatus*
teres minor
subscapularis*
rhomboideus*

erector spinae*

Correct form
· Keep your back flat.
· Move smoothly and with control.
· Gaze toward the floor.
· Contract your arm muscles when in the row position with your weight lifted.
· Keep your standing foot anchored into the floor.

Avoid
· Arching your back, or curving it forward.
· Losing your balance.
· Straining your neck by trying to look forward.

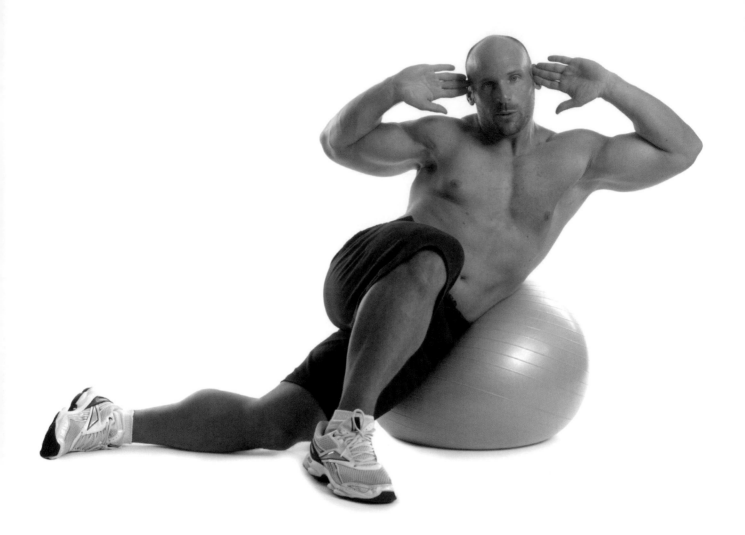

Contents

et's be honest: many of us work out because we want to look better, whether this means fitting into a smaller jeans size, unveiling visibly defined abs at the beach, or "just" sporting that much-coveted toned appearance.

Strengthening the core, that muscular power station at the center of the body, is a remarkably effective way to do just that. Along the way, you will also feel better: slimmer, stronger, and more powerful. Mix and match from the following exercises to suit your fitness goals. For instance, Fitness Ball Side Crunch, performed regularly, will help you achieve to-die-for obliques, while the simple Sit-Up, performed correctly, will really tone those abdominals.

Core Strengtheners

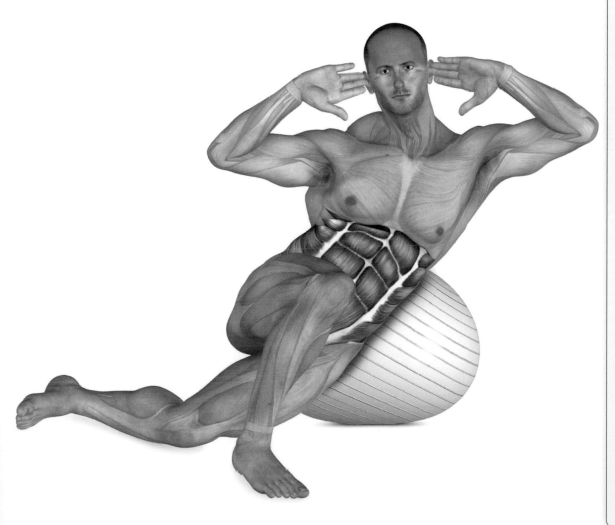

Sit-Up

No core-training regimen would be complete without the Sit-Up. This workout staple is effective for both strengthening and defining the abdominal muscles, and it works your hip flexors, too. Form is crucial—to avoid stressing your spine and/or the muscles in your head and neck, make sure that your abdominals are driving the movement.

1 Lie on your back, with your legs bent and your feet planted on the floor. Bend your arms, and place your hands behind your head so that your elbows flare outward.

2 Engage your abdominals as you raise your shoulders and torso.

3 With control, lower your shoulders and torso back to starting position.

4 Repeat. Work up to 3 sets of 20.

Correct form
· Lead with your abdominals, not with your neck.
· Keep your feet planted on the floor.
· Keep the movement slow and controlled.

Avoid
· Relying on momentum to move up or down.
· Using your neck or lower back to drive the movement.
· Twisting your necks, torso, or hips.

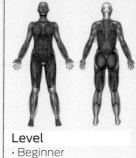

Annotation Key
Bold text indicates target muscles
Black text indicates other working muscles
* indicates deep muscles

Level
· Beginner

Duration
· 3 minutes

Benefits
· Strengthens abs
· Stabilizes core

Caution
· Lower-back issues
· Neck issues

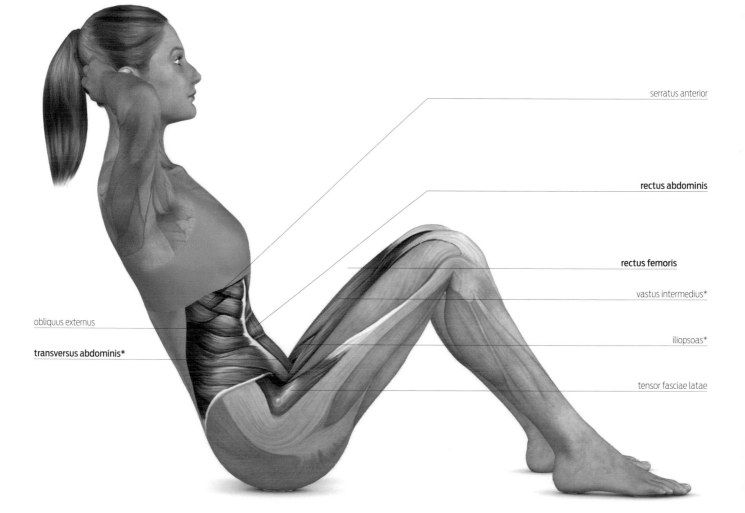

serratus anterior

rectus abdominis

rectus femoris

vastus intermedius*

obliquus externus

iliopsoas*

transversus abdominis*

tensor fasciae latae

Rise and Reach

Rise and Reach is a simple exercise, yet it is highly effective for both strengthening and defining your abdominal muscles while also working your hip flexors. Practicing proper form will protect your spine, as well as the muscles in your head and neck, from any stress or strain.

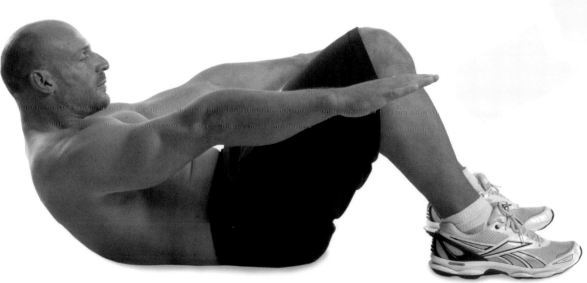

1 Lie on your back with your legs bent and your feet firmly planted on the floor. Extend your arms straight along your sides.

2 Lift your shoulders, head, and neck slightly off the floor.

3 Using your abdominal muscles to drive the movement, raise your upper torso off the floor toward your legs.

4 Lower and repeat, working up to 3 sets of 20.

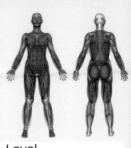

Correct form
· Lead with your abdominals, not with your neck.
· Keep your feet planted on the floor.

Avoid
· Using excessive momentum.
· Overusing your lower back.

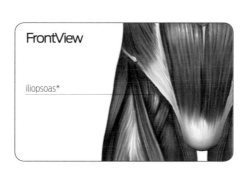

FrontView

iliopsoas*

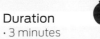

Level
· Beginner

Duration
· 3 minutes

Benefits
· Strengthens abs
· Stabilizes core

Caution
· Lower-back issues
· Neck issues

Annotation Key
Bold text indicates target muscles
Black text indicates other working muscles
* indicates deep muscles

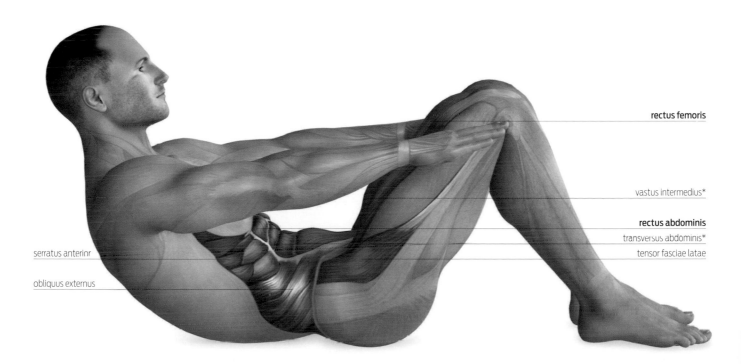

rectus femoris

vastus intermedius*

rectus abdominis

transversus abdominis*

tensor fasciae latae

serratus anterior

obliquus externus

One-Armed Sit-Up

One-Armed Sit-Up is a challenging twist on the traditional Sit-Up, engaging the obliques and the latissimus dorsi, as well as the rectus abdominis.

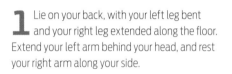

1 Lie on your back, with your left leg bent and your right leg extended along the floor. Extend your left arm behind your head, and rest your right arm along your side.

2 Pushing through your left heel, raise your shoulders and torso off the floor until you are sitting nearly upright and your left arm is directly over your head.

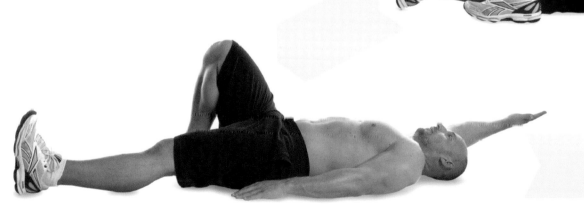

3 Gradually lower to the floor.

Correct form
· Anchor the foot of your bent leg into the floor.
· Draw upon your core muscles to drive the movement.
· Keep your extended arm as straight as possible.

Avoid
· Relying on momentum to sit up or down.
· Using your neck or lower back to drive the movement.
· Twisting your neck, torso, or hips.

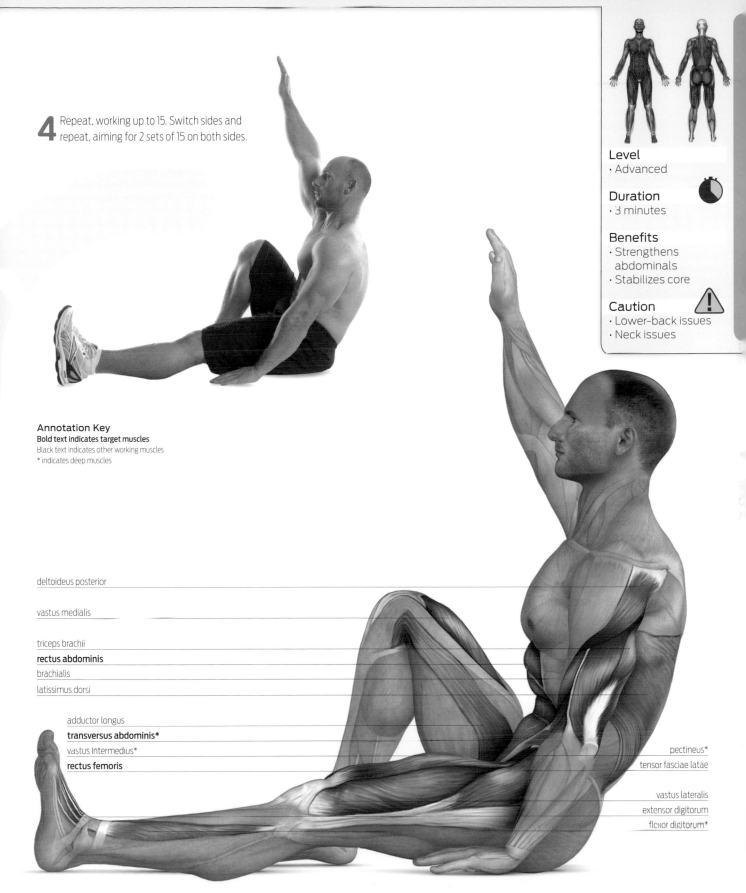

4 Repeat, working up to 15. Switch sides and repeat, aiming for 2 sets of 15 on both sides.

Level
· Advanced

Duration
· 3 minutes

Benefits
· Strengthens abdominals
· Stabilizes core

Caution
· Lower-back issues
· Neck issues

Annotation Key
Bold text indicates target muscles
Black text indicates other working muscles
* indicates deep muscles

deltoideus posterior

vastus medialis

triceps brachii

rectus abdominis

brachialis

latissimus dorsi

adductor longus

transversus abdominis*

vastus intermedius*

rectus femoris

pectineus*

tensor fasciae latae

vastus lateralis

extensor digitorum

flexor digitorum*

Medicine Ball Sit-Up

Medicine Ball Sit-Up takes a basic exercise one step further. By grasping the medicine ball throughout the exercise, your arms are unable to propel you upward. As a result, your abdominals have to work extra hard—reaping greater benefits in the process.

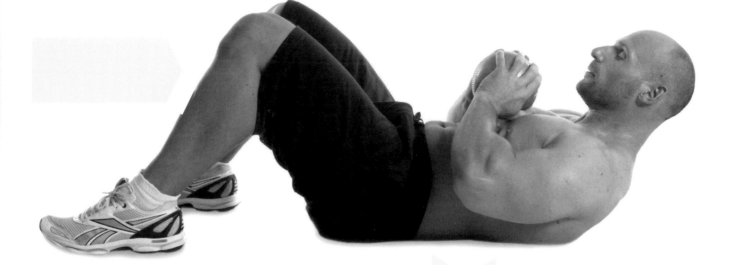

1 Lie on your back with your legs bent and your feet firmly planted on the floor. Grasp a medicine ball between your hands and hold it just in front of your chest.

2 Raise your shoulders and torso off the floor toward your legs.

3 Lower and repeat, working up to 3 sets of 20.

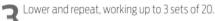

Correct form
· Lead with your abdominals, not with your neck.
· Keep your feet planted on the floor.
· Keep the medicine ball in front of your chest throughout all stages of the exercise.

Avoid
· Using excessive momentum.
· Overusing your lower back.

Annotation Key
Bold text indicates target muscles
Black text indicates other working muscles
* indicates deep muscles

Level
· Intermediate

Duration
· 3 minutes

Benefits
· Strengthens abs
· Stabilizes core

Caution
· Lower-back issues
· Neck issues

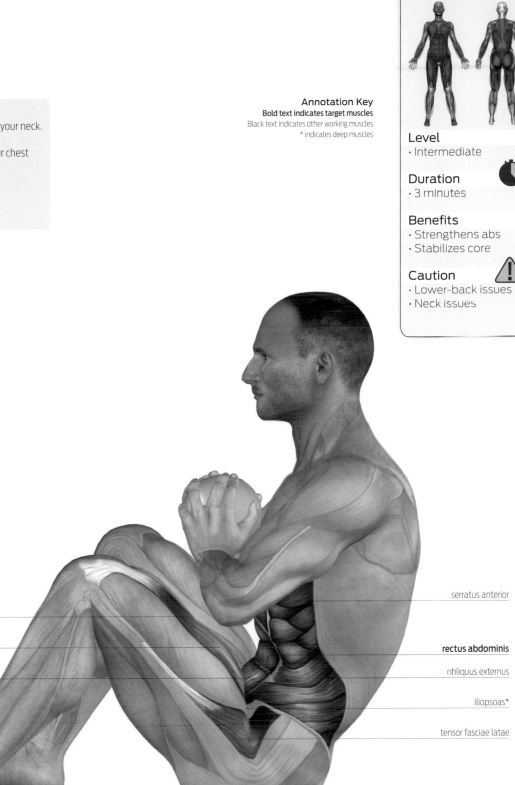

serratus anterior

rectus femoris

vastus intermedius*

rectus abdominis

transversus abdominis*

obliquus externus

iliopsoas*

tensor fasciae latae

Crunch

Like the Sit-Up, the Crunch is highly effective for isolating the rectus abdominis. Unlike the Sit-Up, however, your lower back never leaves the floor during the movement, which places less strain on the lumbar region of your spine. Lead with your abdominals, as if a string were hoisting you up by your belly button.

1 Lie on your back with your legs bent, elbows flared, and palms next to your ears.

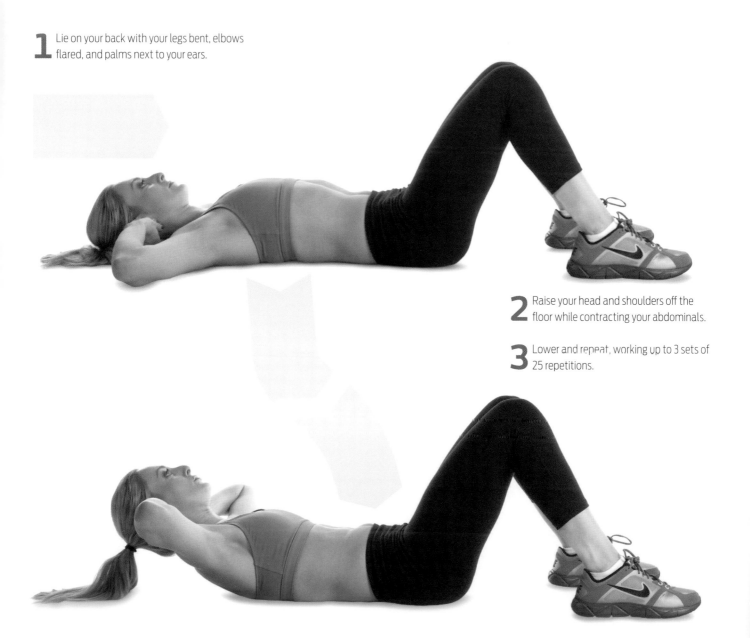

2 Raise your head and shoulders off the floor while contracting your abdominals.

3 Lower and repeat, working up to 3 sets of 25 repetitions.

Level
· Beginner

Duration
· 3 minutes

Benefits
· Strengthens abs
· Stabilizes core

Caution
· Lower-back issues
· Neck issues

Front View

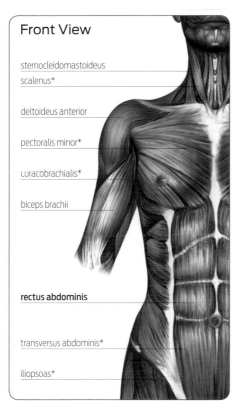

sternocleidomastoideus

scalenus*

deltoideus anterior

pectoralis minor*

coracobrachialis*

biceps brachii

rectus abdominis

transversus abdominis*

iliopsoas*

Correct form
· Keep both feet planted on the floor.
· Use your abs to drive the movement.

Avoid
· Overusing your neck.

Back View

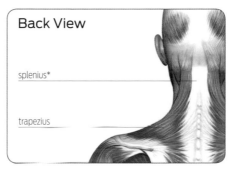

splenius*

trapezius

Annotation Key
Bold text indicates target muscles
Black text indicates other working muscles
* indicates deep muscles

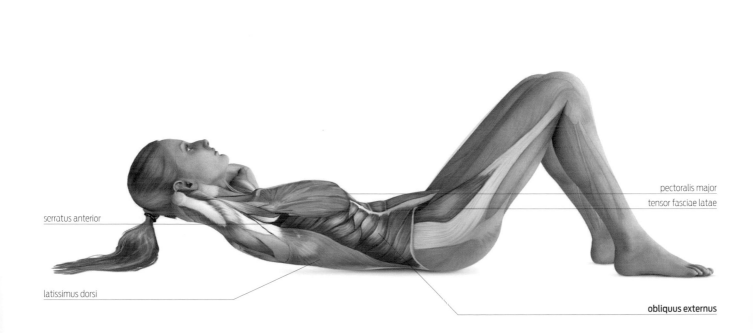

serratus anterior

latissimus dorsi

pectoralis major

tensor fasciae latae

obliquus externus

Bicycle Crunch

Bicycle Crunch is particularly effective for strengthening and toning your upper abdominals as well as your oblique muscles. Although you may be tempted to "cycle" quickly, perform each crunch smoothly and with control for best results.

1 Lie on your back with fingers at your ears, your elbows flared outward and your legs bent to form a 90-degree angle.

2 Begin to lift your shoulders and upper torso off the floor as you raise your right elbow diagonally. At the same time, bring your left knee toward your elbow and extend your right leg diagonally forward—until your right elbow and left knee meet.

Modifications

Easier: Bend both knees and place both feet on the floor, keeping them anchored there throughout the exercise. Leading with your abdominals, raise your entire torso off the floor as you bring your left elbow to your right knee. Lower and repeat, alternating sides.

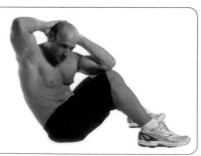

Correct form
· Raise your elbow and opposite knee equally, so that they meet in the middle.

Avoid
· Raising your lower back off the floor.
· Rushing through the movement.

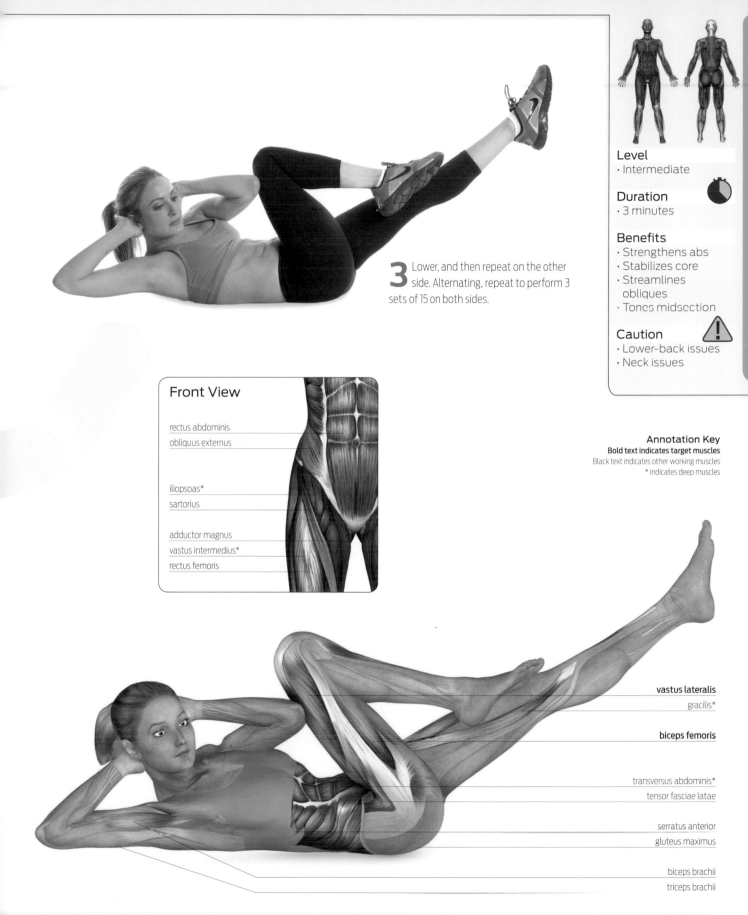

3 Lower, and then repeat on the other side. Alternating, repeat to perform 3 sets of 15 on both sides.

Level
· Intermediate

Duration
· 3 minutes

Benefits
· Strengthens abs
· Stabilizes core
· Streamlines obliques
· Tones midsection

Caution
· Lower-back issues
· Neck issues

Annotation Key
Bold text indicates target muscles
Black text indicates other working muscles
* indicates deep muscles

Front View

rectus abdominis
obliquus externus

iliopsoas*
sartorius

adductor magnus
vastus intermedius*
rectus femoris

vastus lateralis
gracilis*

biceps femoris

transversus abdominis*
tensor fasciae latae

serratus anterior
gluteus maximus

biceps brachii
triceps brachii

Diagonal Crunch with Medicine Ball

Diagonal Crunch with Medicine Ball strengthens your abdominal, oblique, and intercostal muscles. You will notice the sides of your core getting tighter and stronger through regularly practicing this challenging move.

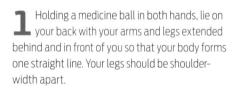

1 Holding a medicine ball in both hands, lie on your back with your arms and legs extended behind and in front of you so that your body forms one straight line. Your legs should be shoulder-width apart.

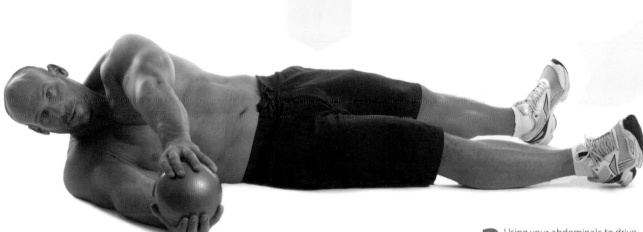

2 Using your abdominals to drive the movement, move your arms and torso to one side.

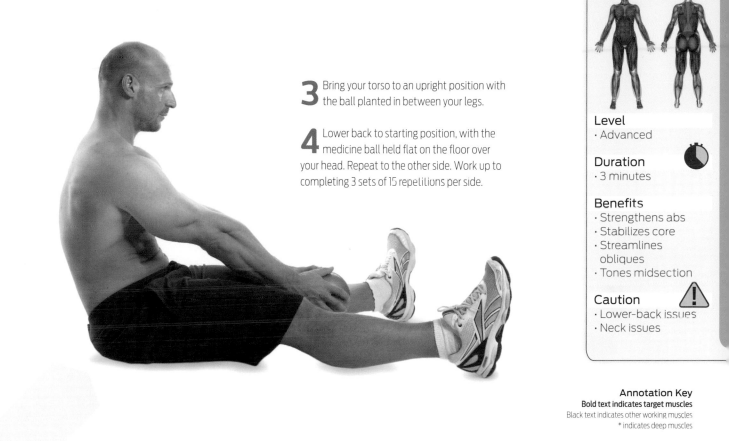

3 Bring your torso to an upright position with the ball planted in between your legs.

4 Lower back to starting position, with the medicine ball held flat on the floor over your head. Repeat to the other side. Work up to completing 3 sets of 15 repetitions per side.

Level
· Advanced

Duration
· 3 minutes

Benefits
· Strengthens abs
· Stabilizes core
· Streamlines obliques
· Tones midsection

Caution
· Lower-back issues
· Neck issues

Annotation Key
Bold text indicates target muscles
Black text indicates other working muscles
* indicates deep muscles

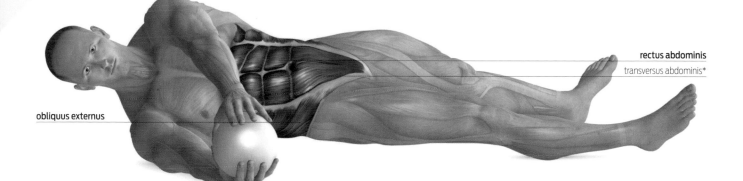

rectus abdominis
transversus abdominis*

obliquus externus

Front View

intercostales interni*
intercostales externi

obliquus internus*

Correct form
· Keep your legs and feet stable.
· Move smoothly and with control.
· Use your abdominal muscles to drive the movement.

Avoid
· Lifting your legs or feet off the floor.
· Jerking your upper body.

Fitness Ball Side Crunch

Fitness Ball Side Crunch is an advanced core-strengthening exercise. It is especially beneficial to your oblique and intercostal muscles.

1 Lie on your left side on top of a fitness ball, with your left hip and the left side of your torso supported by the ball. Bend both knees. Raise your left heel off the floor. Bring your right leg over your left, and rest your right foot in front of your left thigh. Place your fingertips on your ears with your elbows flared outward.

2 Using your abdominals to drive the movement, raise your torso until it is nearly upright.

3 Lower and repeat, building up to 15. Repeat on the other side. Aim for 3 sets of 15 per side.

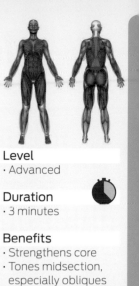

Correct form
· Aim to keep the fitness ball as stable as possible by maintaining your body position.
· Keep your arms in place.
· Keep your core strongly engaged.
· If desired, rest your back foot against a wall for help with balancing.

Avoid
· Rushing through the exercise.
· Using your legs to drive the movement.
· Allowing the ball to wobble.

Annotation Key
Bold text indicates target muscles
Black text indicates other working muscles
* indicates deep muscles

Level
· Advanced

Duration
· 3 minutes

Benefits
· Strengthens core
· Tones midsection, especially obliques

Caution
· Lower-back issues

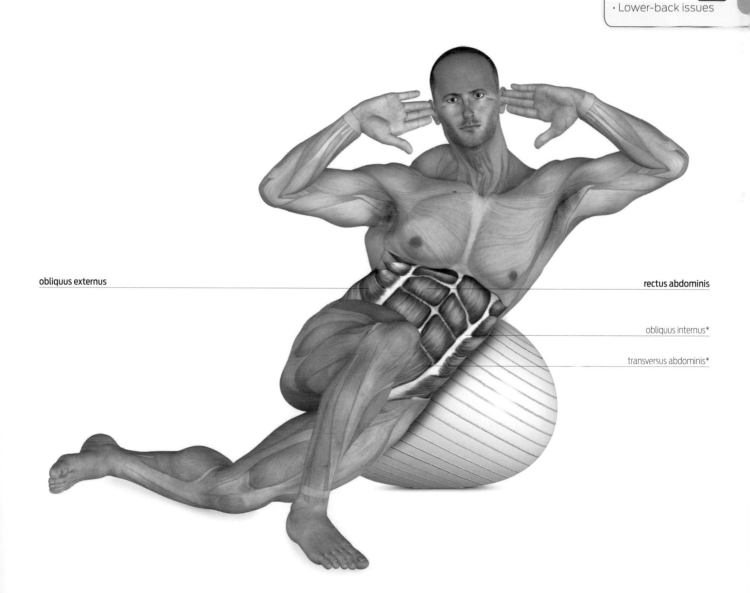

obliquus externus

rectus abdominis

obliquus internus*

transversus abdominis*

V-Up

The challenging V-Up targets both your upper and lower rectus abdominis, as it moves through its entire range of motion. Performing V-Ups is also an efficient way to strengthen your lower-back muscles and tighten your quads.

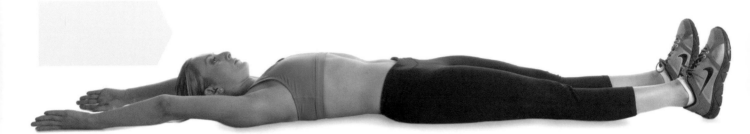

1 Lie on your back with your legs straight and your arms extended behind your head.

2 Simultaneously raise your arms and legs so that your fingertips are nearly touching your feet, while maintaining a flat back.

3 Lower and repeat, working up to 3 sets of 20 repetitions.

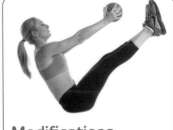

Modifications

Harder: Grasp a medicine ball in your hands, keeping it in place throughout the exercise.

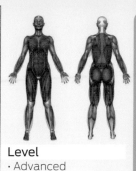

Front View

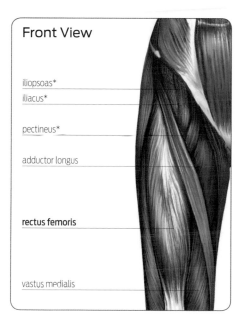

iliopsoas*

iliacus*

pectineus*

adductor longus

rectus femoris

vastus medialis

Correct form
· Keep your arms and legs straight.

Avoid
· Using a jerking motion as your raise or lower your arms and legs.

Annotation Key
Bold text indicates target muscles
Black text indicates other working muscles
* indicates deep muscles

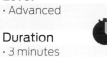

Level
· Advanced

Duration
· 3 minutes

Benefits
· Strengthens core
· Increases spinal mobility

Caution
· Lower-back issues
· Neck issues

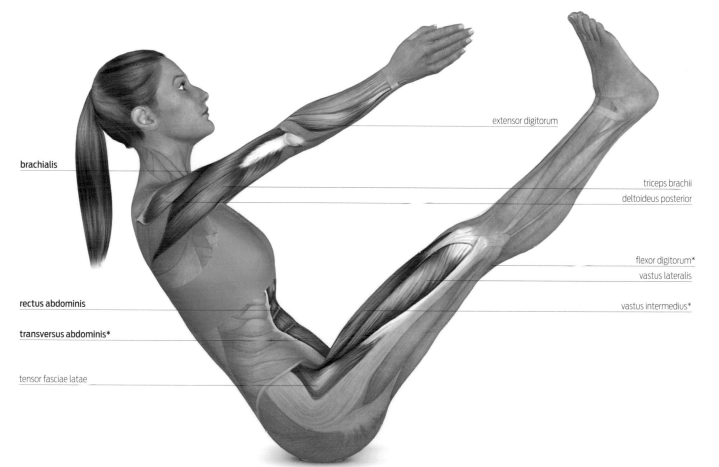

brachialis

extensor digitorum

triceps brachii

deltoideus posterior

flexor digitorum*

vastus lateralis

rectus abdominis

vastus intermedius*

transversus abdominis*

tensor fasciae latae

Fitness Ball Crunch

Fitness Ball Crunch adds a new dimension to the basic crunch exercise. By positioning yourself on top of the ball, you challenge your abs to work harder: as they work to drive the crunching movement, they also must stay engaged as you balance on top of the ball, trying not to let it wobble.

1 Lie on your back, with your feet planted wider than shoulder-distance apart, your back supported on the ball, your hands at your ears, and your elbows flared outward.

2 Simultaneously raise your arms and legs so that your arms are nearly touching your feet, while maintaining a flat back.

3 Lower and repeat, working up to 3 sets of 20.

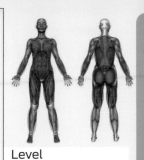

Annotation Key
Bold text indicates target muscles
Black text indicates other working muscles
* indicates deep muscles

Correct form
· Keep your legs anchored into the floor.
· Keep your lower back supported.
· Keep your body as stable as possible on
  top of the ball.

Avoid
· Allowing the ball to wobble.

Level
· Intermediate

Duration
· 3 minutes

Benefits
· Strengthens abs
· Stabilizes core

Caution
· Lower-back issues
· Neck issues

rectus abdominis

obliquus internus*

transversus abdominis*

obliquus externus

Reverse Crunch

Reverse Crunch is highly effective for isolating the lowest portion of the rectus abdominis, where most abdominal fat tends to be stored. Less is more with this exercise: your movements should be small but focused.

1 Lie on your back with your arms at your sides and your legs bent at a 90-degree angle with your feet off the floor.

2 Lift your buttocks a few inches off the mat as you bring your knees toward your chest.

3 Lower in a controlled manner. Repeat, working up to 3 sets of 20.

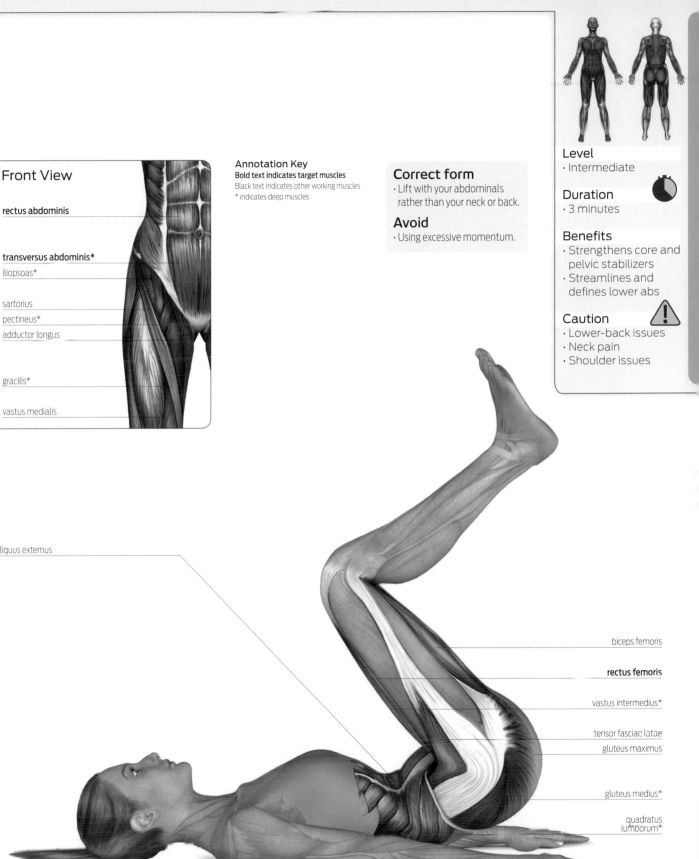

Front View

rectus abdominis

transversus abdominis*
iliopsoas*

sartorius
pectineus*
adductor longus

gracilis*

vastus medialis

Annotation Key
Bold text indicates target muscles
Black text indicates other working muscles
* indicates deep muscles

Correct form
· Lift with your abdominals rather than your neck or back.

Avoid
· Using excessive momentum.

Level
· Intermediate

Duration
· 3 minutes

Benefits
· Strengthens core and pelvic stabilizers
· Streamlines and defines lower abs

Caution
· Lower-back issues
· Neck pain
· Shoulder issues

obliquus externus

biceps femoris

rectus femoris

vastus intermedius*

tensor fasciae latae
gluteus maximus

gluteus medius*

quadratus lumborum*

Big Circles with Medicine Ball

Big Circles with Medicine Ball are highly effective for working the front of your core. Here the muscles stay engaged as they move through their range of motion.

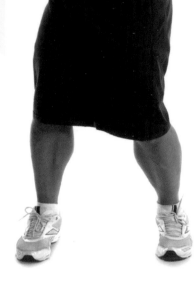

1 Stand with your feet planted shoulder-distance or slightly wider apart and a medicine ball grasped in both hands. Lift your arms overhead.

2 Continuing the circular movement, bring your arms out to the side, turning your head to follow the ball's movement with your gaze.

3 Keeping your arms extended, continue the circular movement to bring your arms down in front of you. Again, follow the ball's movement with your gaze.

4 Bring your arms to the opposite side.

5 Bring your arms overhead to starting position. Complete 30 circles, then repeat in the opposite direction for another 30.

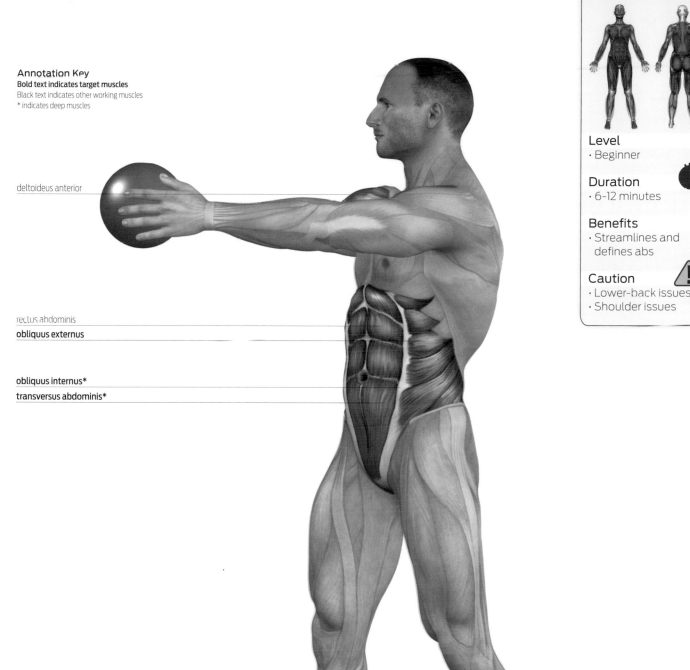

Annotation Key
Bold text indicates target muscles
Black text indicates other working muscles
* indicates deep muscles

deltoideus anterior

rectus abdominis
obliquus externus

obliquus internus*
transversus abdominis*

Level
· Beginner

Duration
· 6–12 minutes

Benefits
· Streamlines and
  defines abs

Caution
· Lower-back issues
· Shoulder issues

Correct form
· Keep your arms extended.
· Keep your torso straight.
· Keep the movement controlled.
· Keep your frontal core muscles
  actively engaged.

Avoid
· Bending your arms.
· Rushing through the movement.
· Lifting either foot off the floor.

Medicine Ball Slam

When performing Medicine Ball Slam with proper form, you will really feel the muscles of your shoulders working hard. Although this exercise is dynamic, do not get carried away and neglect your core muscles; they should stay strongly engaged throughout.

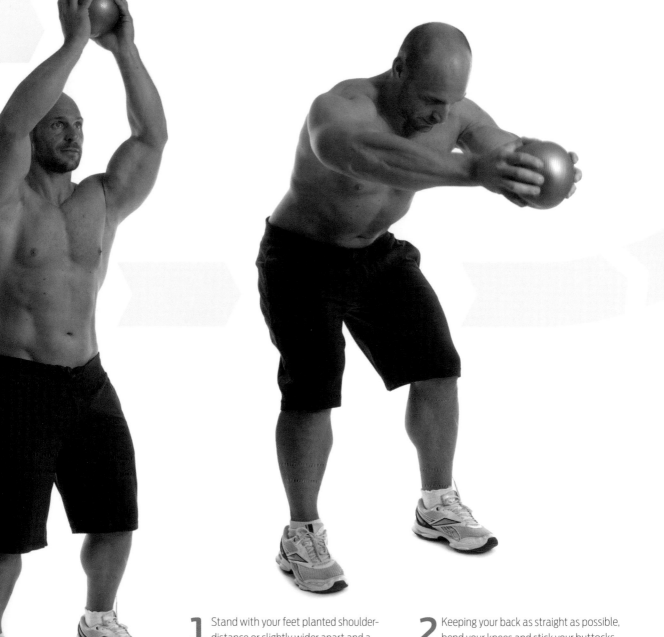

1 Stand with your feet planted shoulder-distance or slightly wider apart and a medicine ball grasped in both hands. Lift your arms overhead.

2 Keeping your back as straight as possible, bend your knees and stick your buttocks slightly outward as you bring the medicine ball down to shoulder height.

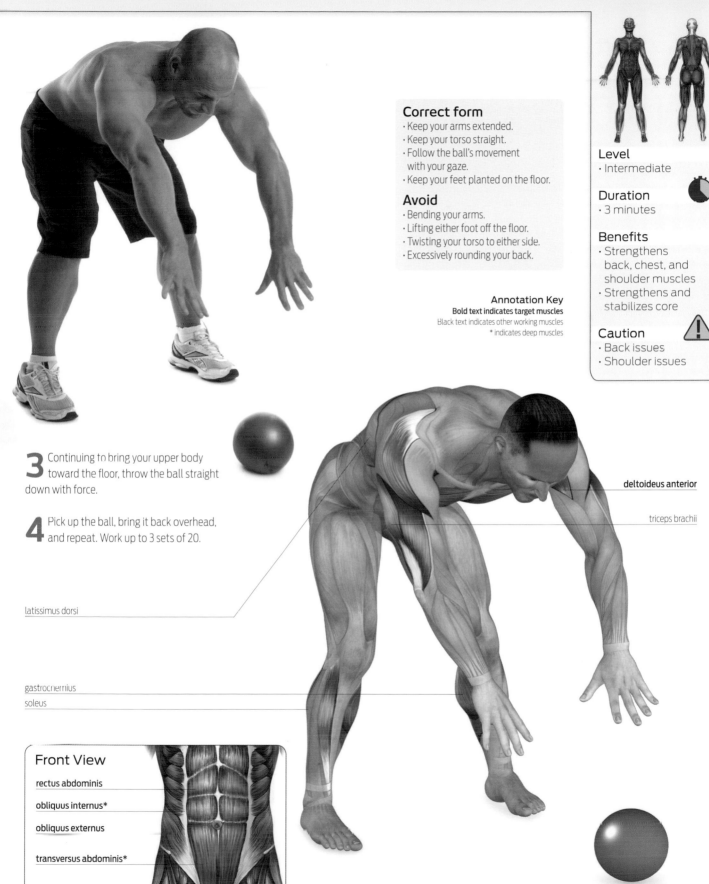

Correct form
· Keep your arms extended.
· Keep your torso straight.
· Follow the ball's movement with your gaze.
· Keep your feet planted on the floor.

Avoid
· Bending your arms.
· Lifting either foot off the floor.
· Twisting your torso to either side.
· Excessively rounding your back.

Annotation Key
Bold text indicates target muscles
Black text indicates other working muscles
* indicates deep muscles

Level
· Intermediate

Duration
· 3 minutes

Benefits
· Strengthens back, chest, and shoulder muscles
· Strengthens and stabilizes core

Caution
· Back issues
· Shoulder issues

3 Continuing to bring your upper body toward the floor, throw the ball straight down with force.

4 Pick up the ball, bring it back overhead, and repeat. Work up to 3 sets of 20.

deltoideus anterior

triceps brachii

latissimus dorsi

gastrocnemius

soleus

Front View
rectus abdominis

obliquus internus*

obliquus externus

transversus abdominis*

Kneeling Crunch with Band

Kneeling Crunch with Band utilizes a resistance band to help engage and strengthen your core muscles. Form is crucial; to reap the greatest benefit, use your abs to drive the movement while keeping the rest of your body stable and aligned. To protect your knees, be sure to use a mat.

1 Loop a resistance band around a nearby stable object, and grasp the handles in both hands. Kneel on your mat, with your heels lifted. Bend your elbows and place the handles next to your ears.

2 Engaging your abdominals, bend forward from the hips until your torso is fully contracted.

3 Rise back to starting position. Repeat, building up to 3 sets of 25.

Correct form
· Keep your hands beside your ears.
· Keep your torso straight.
· Keep your abdominals strongly engaged.

Avoid
· Excessively rounding your back.
· Twisting your torso to either side.

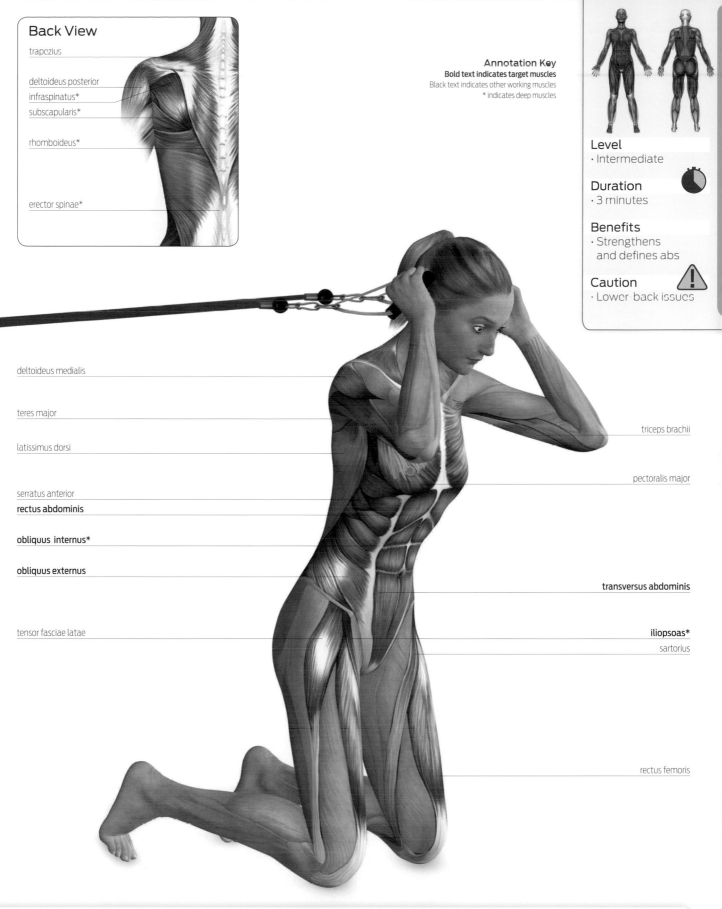

Back View

trapezius

deltoideus posterior
infraspinatus*
subscapularis*

rhomboideus*

erector spinae*

Annotation Key
Bold text indicates target muscles
Black text indicates other working muscles
* indicates deep muscles

Level
· Intermediate

Duration
· 3 minutes

Benefits
· Strengthens
  and defines abs

Caution
· Lower back issues

deltoideus medialis

teres major

latissimus dorsi

serratus anterior
rectus abdominis

obliquus internus*

obliquus externus

tensor fasciae latae

triceps brachii

pectoralis major

transversus abdominis

iliopsoas*
sartorius

rectus femoris

One-Armed Band Pull

One-Armed Band Pull makes use of the resistance band to target the front of your core. The pull movement also benefits your back, particularly the latissimus dorsi.

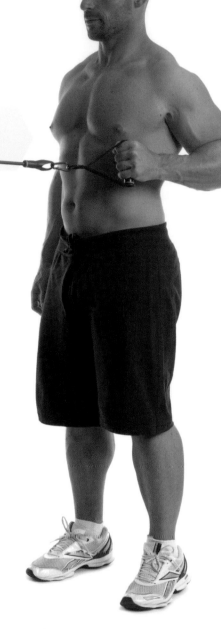

1 Attach one end of a resistance band to a stable object, and grasp the other handle in one hand. Stand straight, with your feet planted shoulder-width apart, and extend the arm that is holding the band in front of you.

Correct form
· Keep your torso straight.
· Anchor your feet to the floor.

Avoid
· Twisting your torso.
· Rushing through the movement.

2 Bend your elbow as you bring the band toward your body in a rowing motion. Continue until the band is just below your chest.

3 Extend your arm back to starting position, and then repeat to perform 15 repetitions. Transfer the band to the other arm, and repeat, working up to 3 set of 15 per side.

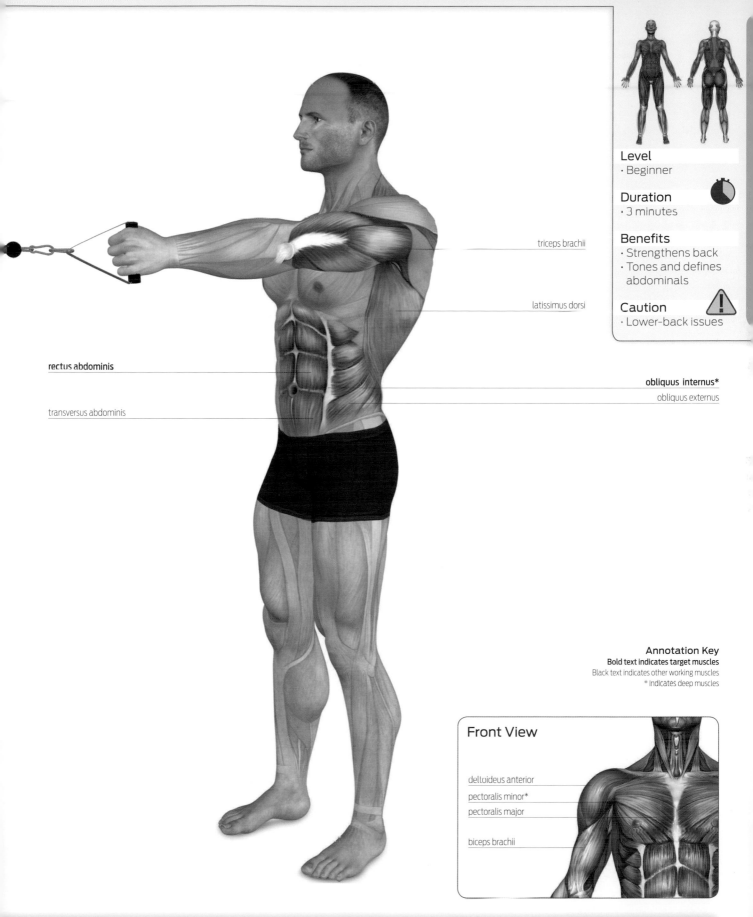

Level
· Beginner

Duration
· 3 minutes

Benefits
· Strengthens back
· Tones and defines
  abdominals

Caution
· Lower-back issues

triceps brachii

latissimus dorsi

rectus abdominis

transversus abdominis

obliquus internus*
obliquus externus

Annotation Key
Bold text indicates target muscles
Black text indicates other working muscles
* Indicates deep muscles

Front View

delloideus anterior

pectoralis minor*

pectoralis major

biceps brachii

Penguin Crunch

Penguin Crunch, also called Penguin Heel Reach, targets your oblique muscles. Because it incorporates lateral movement of the abdominals, it is a great exercise to prepare you for any sport that requires rotational movement, such as swimming or diving.

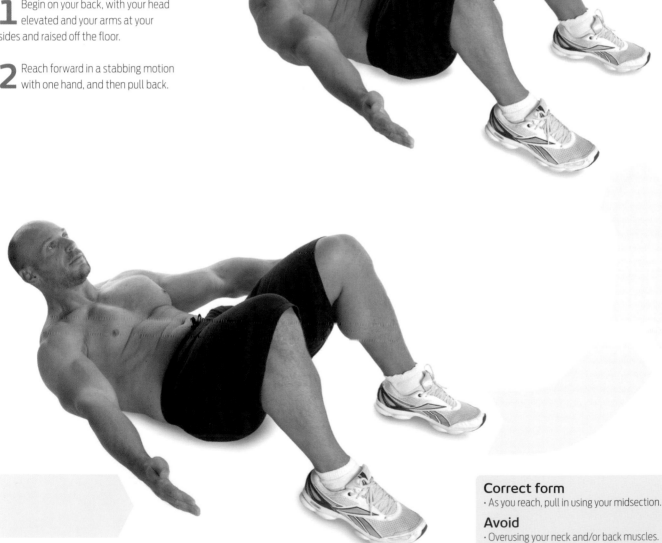

1 Begin on your back, with your head elevated and your arms at your sides and raised off the floor.

2 Reach forward in a stabbing motion with one hand, and then pull back.

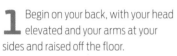

Correct form
· As you reach, pull in using your midsection.

Avoid
· Overusing your neck and/or back muscles.

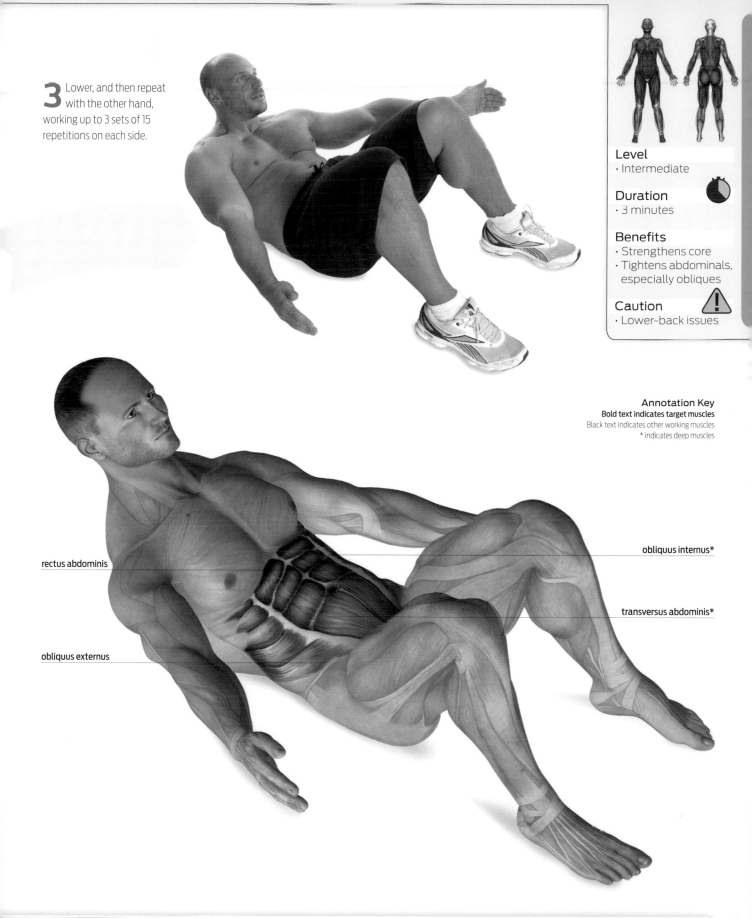

3 Lower, and then repeat with the other hand, working up to 3 sets of 15 repetitions on each side.

Level
· Intermediate

Duration
· 3 minutes

Benefits
· Strengthens core
· Tightens abdominals, especially obliques

Caution
· Lower-back issues

Annotation Key
Bold text indicates target muscles
Black text indicates other working muscles
* indicates deep muscles

rectus abdominis

obliquus externus

obliquus internus*

transversus abdominis*

Wood Chop with Band

Wood Chop with Band is an effective exercise for strengthening your oblique muscles. Using the band adds an element of resistance to the movement, enhancing your results.

1 Attach one end of the band to a stable object. Stand straight while holding the other end of the band in both hands, your arms fully extended. Rotate your torso to one side, bringing the ball with you.

2 Rotate to the other side, raising your arms as you turn. Feel your abdominals contract.

3 Lower your arms as you bring your torso back to center.

4 Repeat through the same range of motion on the other side, working up to 3 sets of 20 per side.

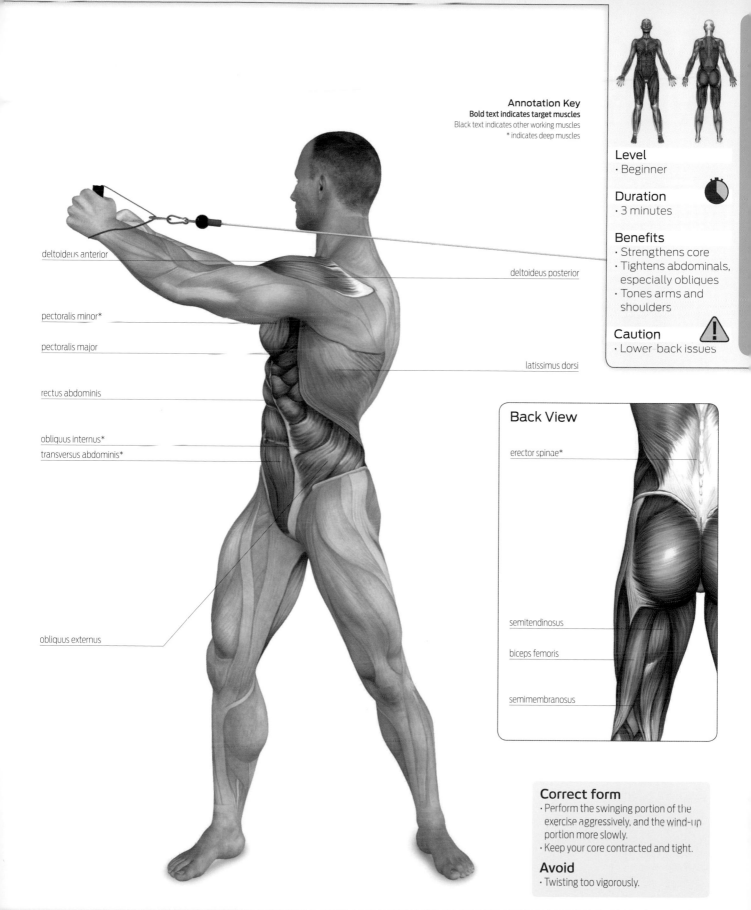

Annotation Key
Bold text indicates target muscles
Black text indicates other working muscles
* indicates deep muscles

Level
· Beginner

Duration
· 3 minutes

Benefits
· Strengthens core
· Tightens abdominals, especially obliques
· Tones arms and shoulders

Caution
· Lower-back issues

deltoideus anterior

deltoideus posterior

pectoralis minor*

pectoralis major

latissimus dorsi

rectus abdominis

obliquus internus*

transversus abdominis*

obliquus externus

Back View

erector spinae*

semitendinosus

biceps femoris

semimembranosus

Correct form
· Perform the swinging portion of the exercise aggressively, and the wind-up portion more slowly.
· Keep your core contracted and tight.

Avoid
· Twisting too vigorously.

Wood Chop with Fitness Ball

Wood Chop with Fitness Ball is another take on a gym classic. Perform this version of the Wood Chop to strengthen your abdominals, especially the oblique muscles. This exercise also works your arm and shoulder muscles.

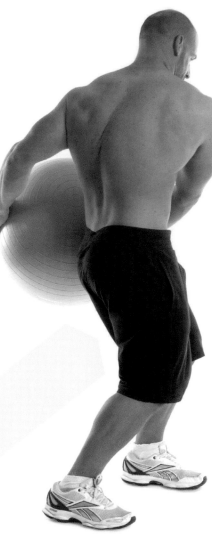

1 Stand while holding a fitness ball, your arms fully extended. Rotate your torso to one side, bringing the ball with you.

2 Lower the ball across your body, and then follow through by rotating to the other side and raising the ball as you turn, as if swinging a baseball bat, while feeling your abdominals contract.

3 Lower the ball as you return your core to the center.

4 Repeat through the same range of motion on the other side, working up to 3 sets of 20 per side.

Correct form
· Perform the swinging portion of the exercise aggressively, and the wind-up portion more slowly.
· Keep your core contracted and tight.

Avoid
· Twisting too vigorously.

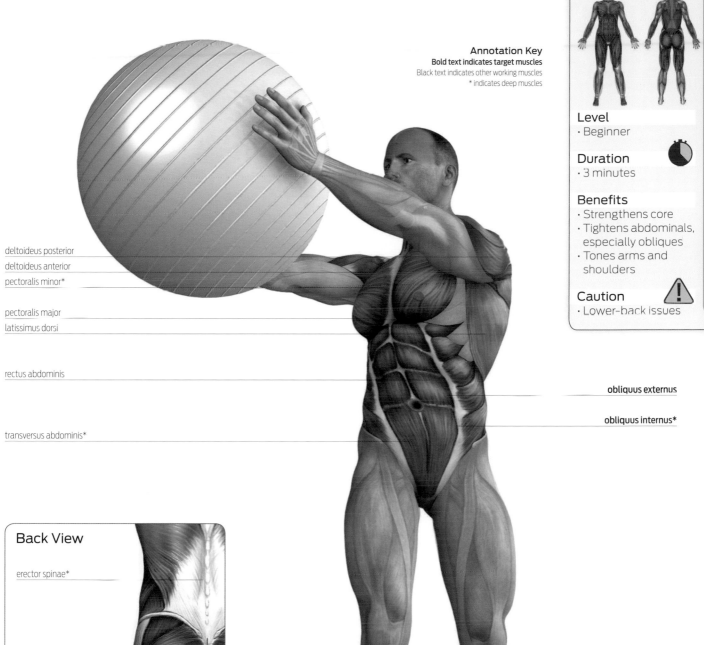

Annotation Key
Bold text indicates target muscles
Black text indicates other working muscles
* indicates deep muscles

Level
· Beginner

Duration
· 3 minutes

Benefits
· Strengthens core
· Tightens abdominals, especially obliques
· Tones arms and shoulders

Caution
· Lower-back issues

deltoideus posterior
deltoideus anterior
pectoralis minor*

pectoralis major
latissimus dorsi

rectus abdominis

transversus abdominis*

obliquus externus

obliquus internus*

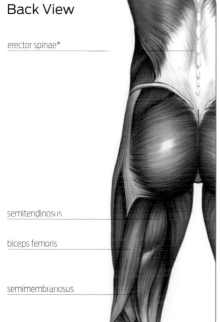

Back View

erector spinae*

semitendinosus

biceps femoris

semimembranosus

Medicine Ball Standing Russian Twist

Medicine Ball Standing Russian Twist is an effective exercise for strengthening the major muscles of the your core. Challenge yourself to keep the rest of your body stable and aligned as you keep your core as active and engaged as possible.

1 Stand with your legs slightly wider than shoulder-distance apart. Keep your knees soft, bending them very slightly. Hold a medicine ball in front of you with arms extended.

2 Rotate your arms and torso to one side, back to center, and then to the other side.

3 Return to center and repeat, working up to 3 sets of 20 rotations.

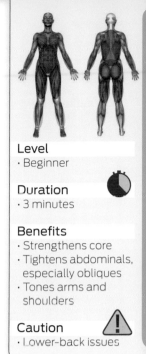

Level
· Beginner

Duration
· 3 minutes

Benefits
· Strengthens core
· Tightens abdominals, especially obliques
· Tones arms and shoulders

Caution
· Lower-back issues

Annotation Key
Bold text indicates target muscles
Black text indicates other working muscles
* indicates deep muscles

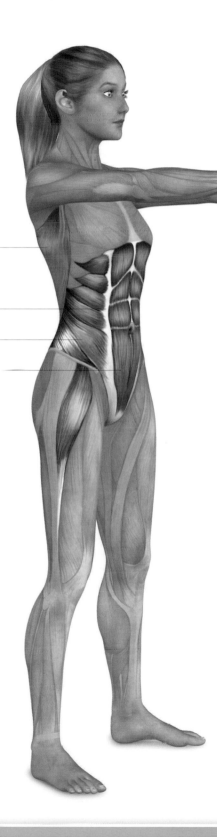

latissimus dorsi

obliquus internus*

obliquus externus

transversus abdominis

Correct form
· Twist in a smooth, controlled motion.
· Keep your arms extended.
· Keep both feet anchored to the floor.
· Follow the movement of the ball with your gaze.

Avoid
· Letting go of the ball.
· Locking your arms or legs.
· Hunching your shoulders or slumping forward.

Fitness Ball Seated Russian Twist

Fitness Ball Seated Russian Twist is effective for strengthening the major muscles of your core, including your obliques, lower-back extensors, abdominals, and deep core stabilizers.

1 Sit with your legs apart while holding a fitness ball at arm's length. Lean back slightly to activate your core.

2 Rotate from side to side, keeping your back as flat as possible.

Correct form
· Twist smoothly and with control.

Avoid
· Rounding your back.
· Rushing through the movement.

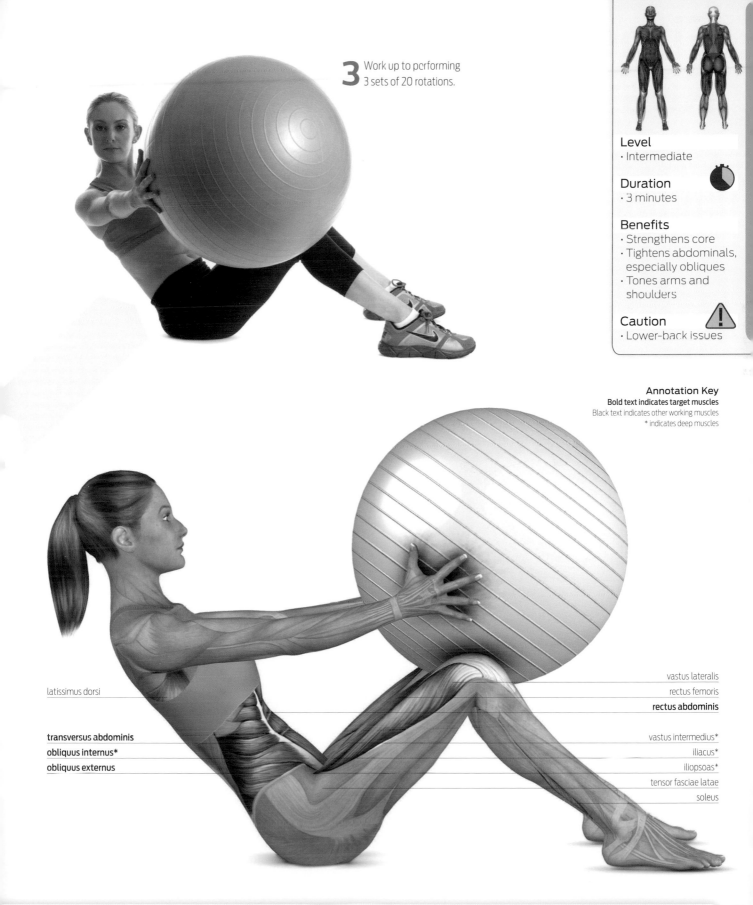

3 Work up to performing 3 sets of 20 rotations.

Level
· Intermediate

Duration
· 3 minutes

Benefits
· Strengthens core
· Tightens abdominals, especially obliques
· Tones arms and shoulders

Caution
· Lower-back issues

Annotation Key
Bold text indicates target muscles
Black text indicates other working muscles
* indicates deep muscles

latissimus dorsi

transversus abdominis
obliquus internus*
obliquus externus

vastus lateralis
rectus femoris
rectus abdominis

vastus intermedius*
iliacus*
iliopsoas*
tensor fasciae latae
soleus

Fitness Ball Russian Twist

Fitness Ball Russian Twist offers a fun, unique way to strengthen your core—and whittle your waistline. It targets all of your abdominals, but because it incorporates rotation, it places an emphasis on the obliques.

1 Sit on your fitness ball, with feet planted shoulder-width apart. Roll forward until your neck is supported on the ball. Extend your arms to full lockout directly above your chest.

2 Turn one hip out to the side while also turning your torso and your arms.

3 Return to the center.

Correct form
· Move slowly and with control.

Avoid
· Allowing your upper back to hang off the fitness ball, unsupported.

4 Repeat to the other side, working up to 3 sets of 15 repetitions per side.

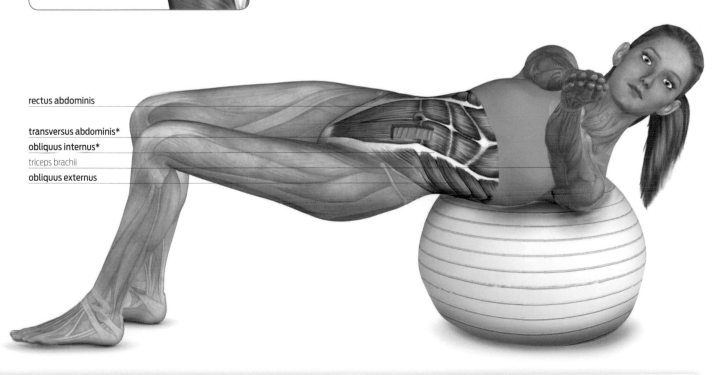

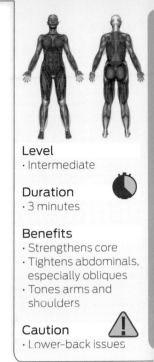

Level
· Intermediate

Duration
· 3 minutes

Benefits
· Strengthens core
· Tightens abdominals, especially obliques
· Tones arms and shoulders

Caution
· Lower-back issues

Annotation Key
Bold text indicates target muscles
Black text indicates other working muscles
* indicates deep muscles

Back View

trapezius

deltoideus medialis

deltoideus posterior

latissimus dorsi

Front View

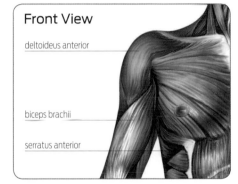

deltoideus anterior

biceps brachii

serratus anterior

rectus abdominis

transversus abdominis*

obliquus internus*

triceps brachii

obliquus externus

Fitness Ball Alternating Leg Tuck

Fitness Ball Alternating Leg Tuck is a powerful strengthener for your core. It benefits all of your powerhouse muscles, particularly targeting the lower abdominal area.

1 Sit upright on a fitness ball, with your feet planted in front of you, slightly wider than hip-distance apart, and your hands on the ball at your sides.

2 Raise one leg upward, bringing it toward your chest.

3 Lower the leg. Repeat on the other side, building up to 3 sets of 20 repetitions per leg.

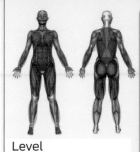

Correct form
· Aim to touch your knee to your chest.
· Keep your torso and back straight.
· Maintain the bend in your knee as you
  raise your leg.
· Gaze forward.

Avoid
· Arching your back or curving it forward.

Annotation Key
Bold text indicates target muscles
Black text indicates other working muscles
* indicates deep muscles

Level
· Intermediate

Duration
· 4 minutes

Benefits
· Strengthens core
· Streamlines and
  defines abs

Caution
· Lower-back issues

obliquus internus*

rectus abdominis

obliquus externus

transversus abdominis

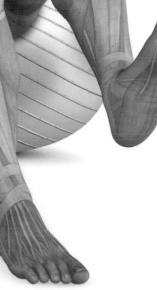

Leg Raise

Leg Raise targets the transversus abdominis, that tough-to-reach lower abdominal area. This core-strengthener is easy to perform effectively, even for most beginners. Carry out this exercise regularly to see a reduction in abdominal fat.

Correct form
· Keep your upper body braced.
· Lift your legs back to starting position just as slowly as you lower them.

Avoid
· Using momentum, or your lower back, to drive the movement.

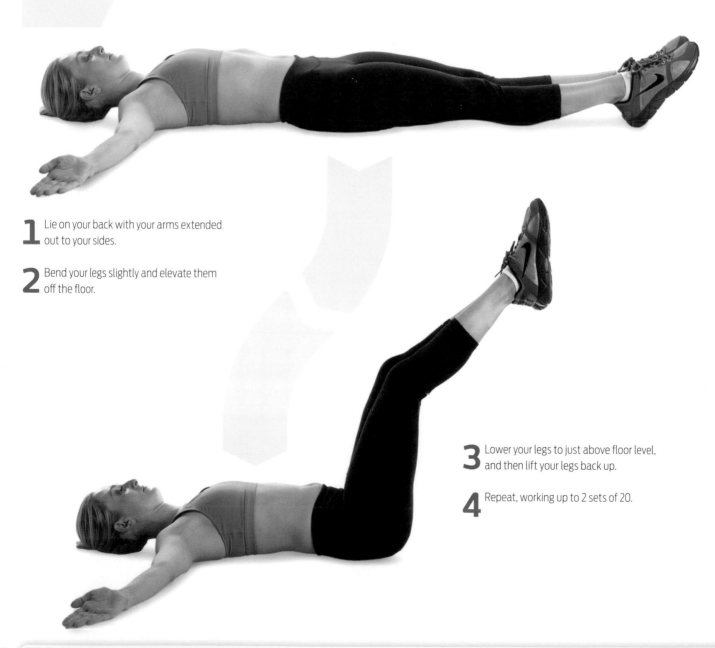

1 Lie on your back with your arms extended out to your sides.

2 Bend your legs slightly and elevate them off the floor.

3 Lower your legs to just above floor level, and then lift your legs back up.

4 Repeat, working up to 2 sets of 20.

Front View

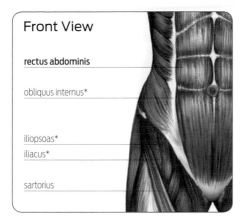

rectus abdominis

obliquus internus*

iliopsoas*
iliacus*

sartorius

Annotation Key
Bold text indicates target muscles
Black text indicates other working muscles
* indicates deep muscles

Modifications

Easier: Instead of raising both legs, raise one leg at a time.

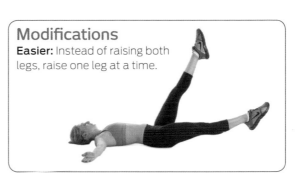

Level
· Beginner

Duration
· 2 minutes

Benefits
· Strengthens core
· Streamlines and defines abs

Caution
· Lower-back issues

vastus lateralis

rectus femoris

vastus intermedius*

transversus abdominis*

obliquus externus

Side Leg Raise

Side Leg Raise is especially beneficial for your obliques and hip adductors. Concentrate on keeping the rest of your body still as you move your top leg a few inches up and then back down—moving with smooth control.

1 Begin on your side, with your legs stacked one on top of the other. Bend your bottom arm, brace your forearm against the floor, and place the hand of your top arm on your hip. Your torso should be raised off the floor, facing forward.

2 Raise your top leg a few inches.

3 Slowly lower the leg back to your starting position. Repeat to perform 20 raises. Switch sides and repeat, working up to 3 sets of 20 per side.

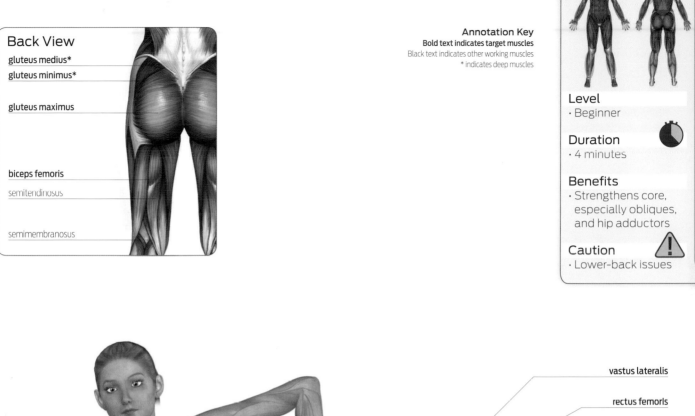

Back View

gluteus medius*

gluteus minimus*

gluteus maximus

biceps femoris

semitendinosus

semimembranosus

Annotation Key
Bold text indicates target muscles
Black text indicates other working muscles
* indicates deep muscles

Level
· Beginner

Duration
· 4 minutes

Benefits
· Strengthens core, especially obliques, and hip adductors

Caution
· Lower-back issues

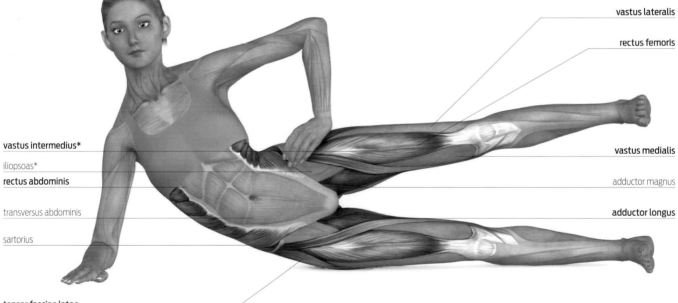

vastus intermedius*

iliopsoas*

rectus abdominis

transversus abdominis

sartorius

tensor fasciae latae

vastus lateralis

rectus femoris

vastus medialis

adductor magnus

adductor longus

Correct form
· Keep your top leg directly over your bottom leg throughout the exercise.
· Keep your torso straight.
· Keep your hips stacked.

Avoid
· Rushing through the movement.
· Tilting your top hip back or forward.

Body Saw

The core-strengthening Body Saw is harder than it looks. Challenge yourself to keep your body in a straight line as you shift back and forth like a saw. The better your form, the harder your abdominals and lower-back muscles will work.

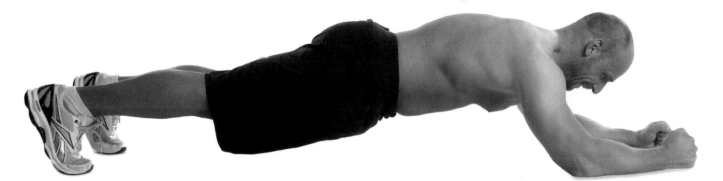

1 Begin facedown, balancing on your toes and your forearms.

2 Shift your body backward, pressing into the floor with your forearms as you reposition your feet.

3 Shift your body forward to return to starting position. Repeat, working up to 3 sets of 20.

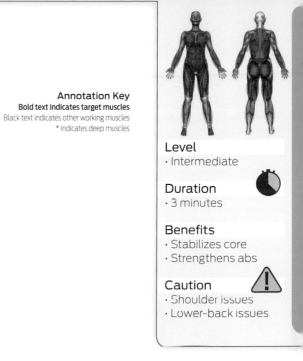

Annotation Key
Bold text indicates target muscles
Black text indicates other working muscles
* indicates deep muscles

Level
· Intermediate

Duration
· 3 minutes

Benefits
· Stabilizes core
· Strengthens abs

Caution
· Shoulder issues
· Lower-back issues

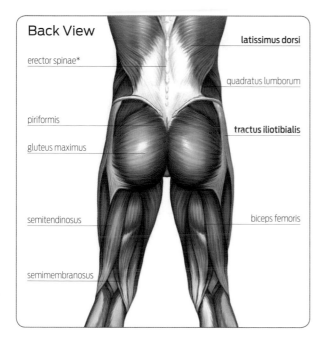

Back View

erector spinae*

latissimus dorsi

quadratus lumborum

piriformis

tractus iliotibialis

gluteus maximus

semitendinosus

biceps femoris

semimembranosus

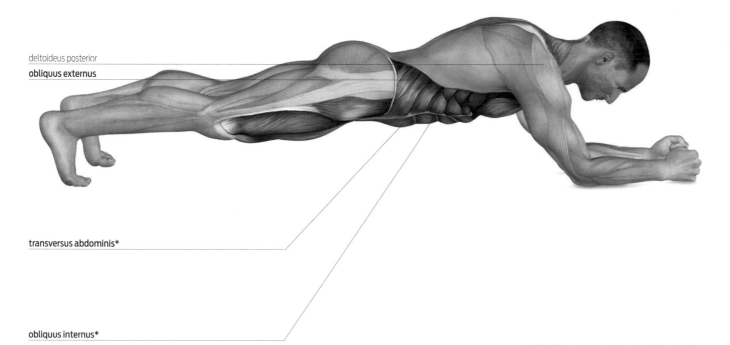

deltoideus posterior
obliquus externus

transversus abdominis*

obliquus internus*

Correct form
· Keep your body in one straight line.
· Gaze toward the floor.

Avoid
· Arching your back, or curving it forward.

Side Bend

Side Bend is a potent core-strengthening exercise that targets your oblique muscles. Lean only as far to the side as you can go while keeping your torso straight. If you find your torso twisting, this means your form needs to be corrected as your abdominals are not being challenged enough.

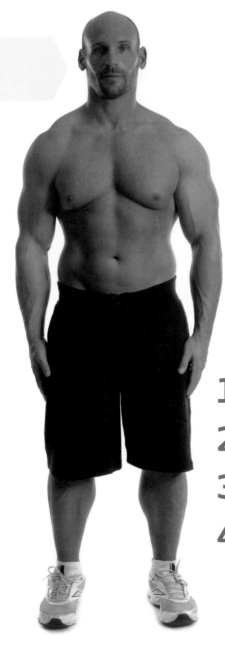

1 Stand with your feet planted shoulder-width apart and your arms at your sides.

2 Leading with your arm, lean over to one side while keeping your torso facing forward.

3 Engaging your abdominal muscles, lift your upper body back to center to stand tall.

4 Repeat on the other side. Alternating, work up to completing 3 sets of 20 per side.

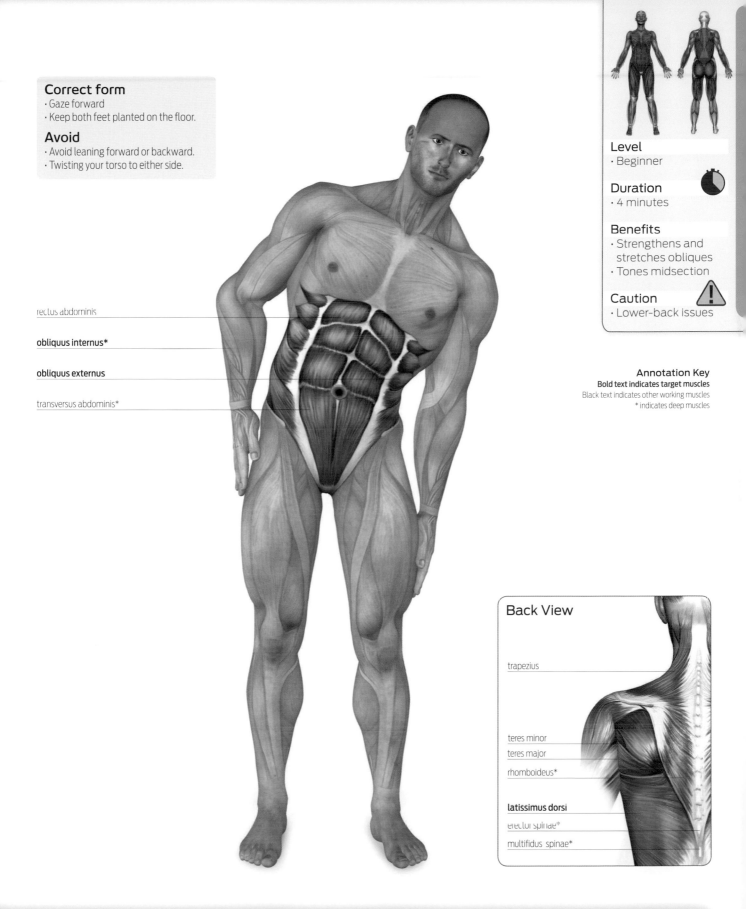

Correct form
· Gaze forward
· Keep both feet planted on the floor.

Avoid
· Avoid leaning forward or backward.
· Twisting your torso to either side.

Level
· Beginner

Duration
· 4 minutes

Benefits
· Strengthens and stretches obliques
· Tones midsection

Caution
· Lower-back issues

Annotation Key
Bold text indicates target muscles
Black text indicates other working muscles
* indicates deep muscles

rectus abdominis

obliquus internus*

obliquus externus

transversus abdominis*

Back View

trapezius

teres minor

teres major

rhomboideus*

latissimus dorsi

erector spinae*

multifidus spinae*

149

Vertical Leg Crunch

When carrying out Vertical Leg Crunch, you should feel a strong sense that your abs are not just getting stronger but becoming streamlined and defined, too. With your legs up, your abdominals do almost all the work. Keep your movement smooth as you lower yourself to the floor, so that your core stays active throughout all stages of the exercise.

1 Lie on your back, with your arms extended behind your head and your legs extended in front of you so that your body forms one straight line.

2 Bring your arms over your head so they are reaching straight upward, your hands directly above your shoulders and your arms forming a 90-degree angle with the floor. Raise your legs until they are parallel to your arms.

3 Using your abdominals to drive the movement, lift your shoulders off the floor, reaching your extended fingers towards your toes.

4 Lower and repeat, aiming to carry out 3 sets of 20.

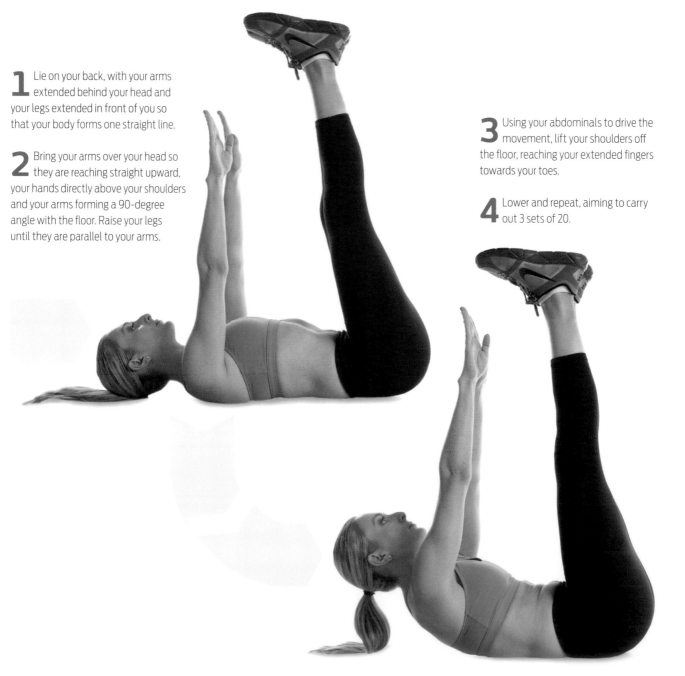

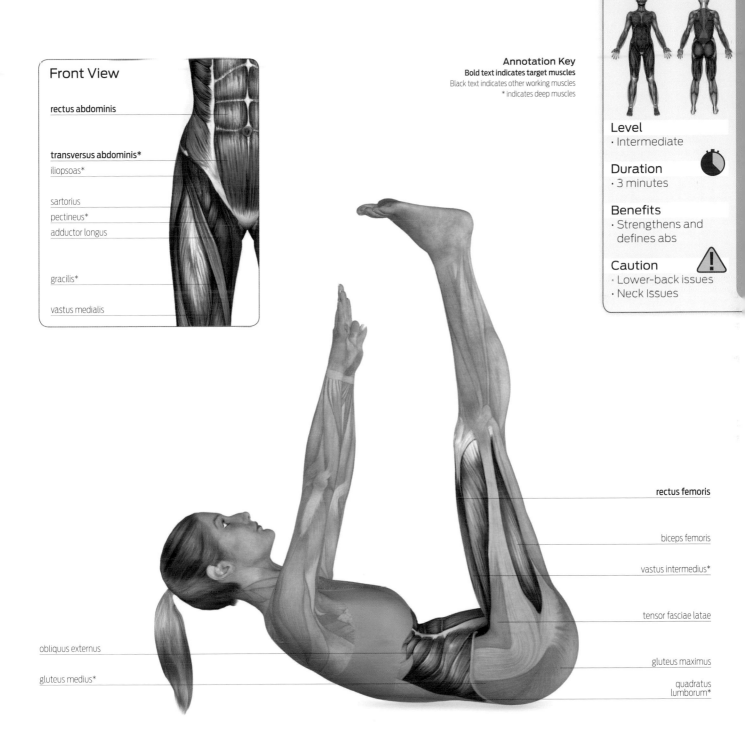

Front View

rectus abdominis

transversus abdominis*
iliopsoas*

sartorius
pectineus*
adductor longus

gracilis*

vastus medialis

Annotation Key
Bold text indicates target muscles
Black text indicates other working muscles
* indicates deep muscles

Level
· Intermediate

Duration
· 3 minutes

Benefits
· Strengthens and
  defines abs

Caution
· Lower-back issues
· Neck Issues

rectus femoris

biceps femoris

vastus intermedius*

tensor fasciae latae

gluteus maximus

quadratus
lumborum*

obliquus externus

gluteus medius*

Correct form
· Keep your arms and legs extended.
· Lower your upper back just as slowly as you raised it.
· Press your legs together as if they were a single leg.

Avoid
· Using your lower-back muscles to drive the movement.

Band Roll-Down with Twist

Thoroughly working your entire core, Band Roll-Down with Twist is a powerful strengthener. Although the movement may seem small, when performed correctly you will really feel its effects in your midsection.

1 Sit with your legs slightly bent, a resistance band looped beneath your heels. Grasp the handle with both hands and bring them to your ears.

2 Bring your elbows to your thighs as you contract your trunk, lowering your shoulders and upper back.

Correct form
· Elongate your upper body in starting position.
· Keep the handles of the resistance band next to your ears.
· Keep your legs and feet in place.

Avoid
· Rounding your back as you twist your torso to the side.

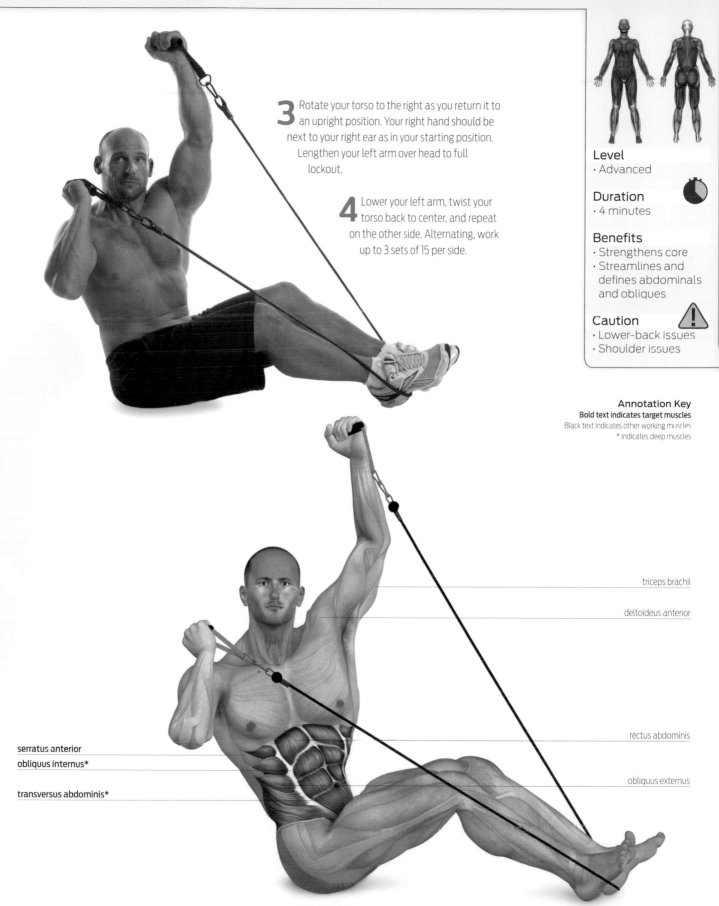

3 Rotate your torso to the right as you return it to an upright position. Your right hand should be next to your right ear as in your starting position. Lengthen your left arm over head to full lockout.

4 Lower your left arm, twist your torso back to center, and repeat on the other side. Alternating, work up to 3 sets of 15 per side.

Level
· Advanced

Duration
· 4 minutes

Benefits
· Strengthens core
· Streamlines and defines abdominals and obliques

Caution
· Lower-back issues
· Shoulder issues

Annotation Key
Bold text indicates target muscles
Black text indicates other working muscles
* indicates deep muscles

triceps brachii

deltoideus anterior

rectus abdominis

obliquus externus

serratus anterior

obliquus internus*

transversus abdominis*

Good Mornings

Good Mornings are effective moves for strengthening your lower back. Weight lifters commonly use a barbell to perform Good Mornings, but here your own body weight provides the resistance for the exercise.

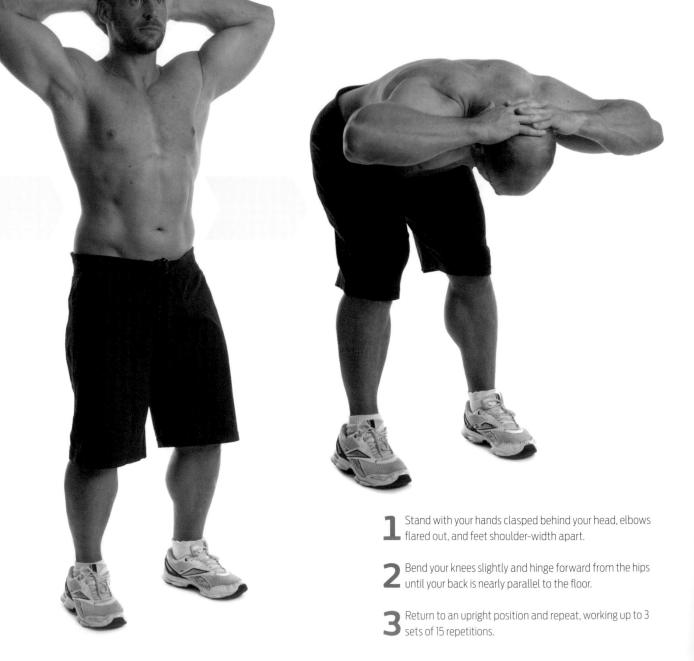

1 Stand with your hands clasped behind your head, elbows flared out, and feet shoulder-width apart.

2 Bend your knees slightly and hinge forward from the hips until your back is nearly parallel to the floor.

3 Return to an upright position and repeat, working up to 3 sets of 15 repetitions.

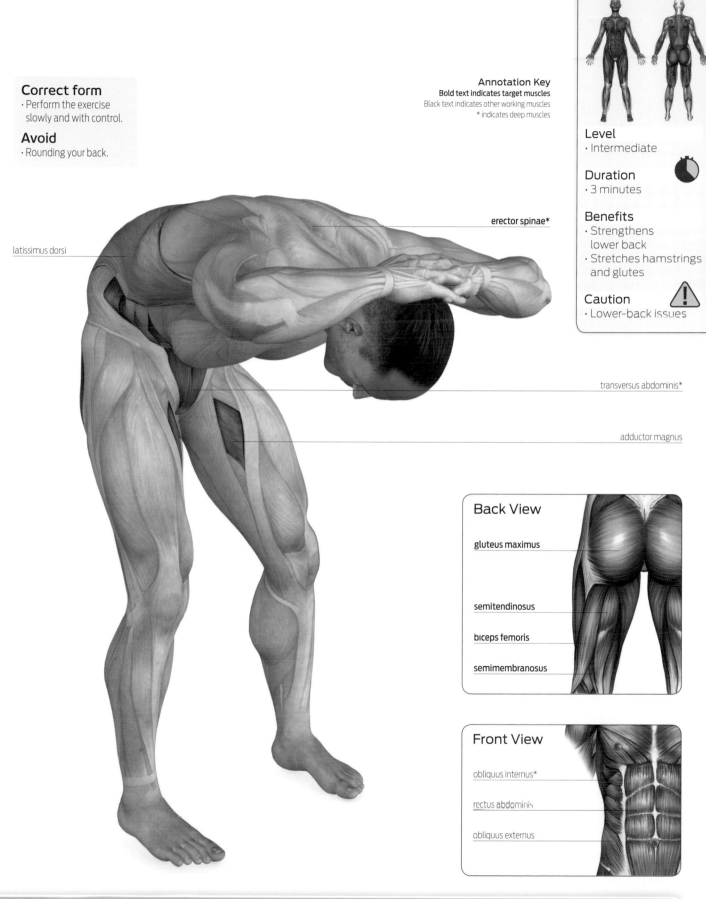

Correct form
· Perform the exercise
  slowly and with control.

Avoid
· Rounding your back.

Annotation Key
Bold text indicates target muscles
Black text indicates other working muscles
* indicates deep muscles

Level
· Intermediate

Duration
· 3 minutes

Benefits
· Strengthens
  lower back
· Stretches hamstrings
  and glutes

Caution
· Lower-back issues

erector spinae*

latissimus dorsi

transversus abdominis*

adductor magnus

Back View

gluteus maximus

semitendinosus

biceps femoris

semimembranosus

Front View

obliquus internus*

rectus abdominis

obliquus externus

Superman

Superman engages just about every muscle in your body, but it is especially effective at stretching and strengthening the hip flexors. It is also an effective exercise for your back, strengthening both the full extent of the erector spinae, as well as the multifidus spinae. Beware though—this move is harder than it looks.

1 Lie facedown on your stomach with your arms and legs extended on the floor.

2 Raise your arms and your legs simultaneously, squeezing your glutes at the top.

Correct form
· Raise your arms and legs as high as possible.

Avoid
· Overstressing your neck.

3 Lower, and then repeat, working up to 3 sets of 15.

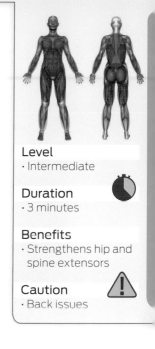

Level
· Intermediate

Duration
· 3 minutes

Benefits
· Strengthens hip and
  spine extensors

Caution
· Back issues

Back View

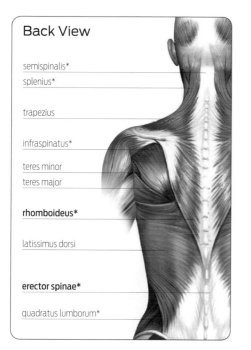

semispinalis*
splenius*
trapezius
infraspinatus*
teres minor
teres major
rhomboideus*
latissimus dorsi
erector spinae*
quadratus lumborum*

Front View

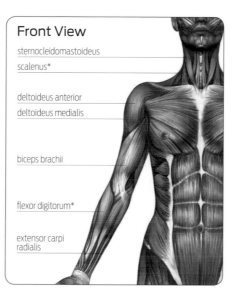

sternocleidomastoideus
scalenus*
deltoideus anterior
deltoideus medialis
biceps brachii
flexor digitorum*
extensor carpi
radialis

Annotation Key
Bold text indicates target muscles
Black text indicates other working muscles
* indicates deep muscles

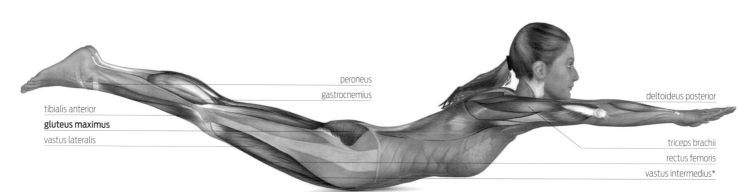

peroneus
gastrocnemius
tibialis anterior
gluteus maximus
vastus lateralis
deltoideus posterior
triceps brachii
rectus femoris
vastus intermedius*

Back View

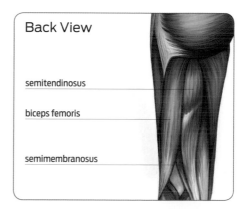

semitendinosus
biceps femoris
semimembranosus

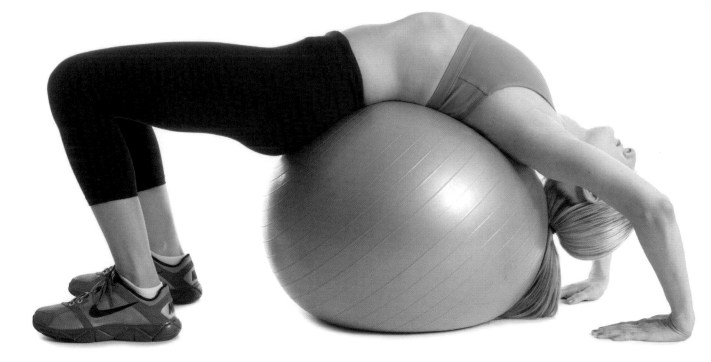

Contents

Cool-downs

At the end of a long workout session, your body deserves a great cool-down. The cool-down is your time to reflect on your workout, in the process stretching those muscles that have been strengthened, lengthened, tightened, and toned. After pushing yourself to perform numerous repetitions, to work harder, lift heavier, and balance longer, take the time to let your muscles recover. This is where, for instance, the Back Arch Stretch and Fitness Ball Abdominal Stretch, not to mention the ultra-rejuvenating Child's Pose, come in. More than mere relaxation, these stretches help to lock in the progress you've made throughout your workout.

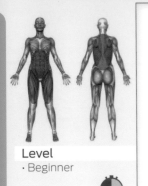

Back Arch Stretch

Back Arch Stretch is an excellent back cool-down exercise. At the end of a long core-training workout, it offers a great stretch for the muscles of your upper and lower back.

Level
· Beginner

Duration
· 1 minute

Benefits
· Stretches back

Caution
· Wrist pain

Correct form
· Keep your abdominals tucked.

Avoid
· Stressing your lower-back muscles by using them to drive the movement.

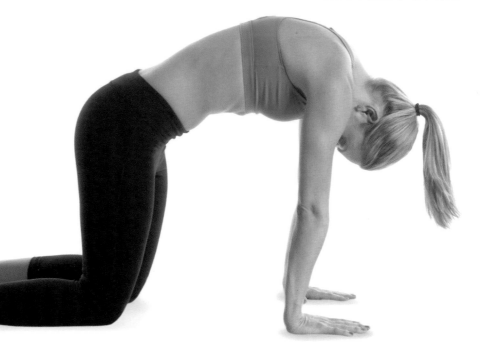

1 Kneel on all fours, with your palms planted hip-distance apart and your knees directly below your hips.

2 Suck in your stomach, imagining it touching the back of your diaphragm.

3 Raise your back as high as you can. Hold this position for 30 seconds.

4 Release, and then repeat for an additional 30 seconds.

Back View

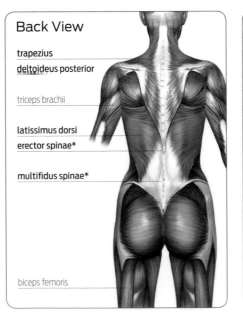

trapezius
deltoideus posterior

triceps brachii

latissimus dorsi
erector spinae*

multifidus spinae*

biceps femoris

Front View

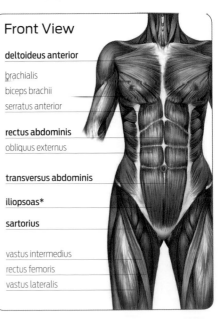

deltoideus anterior

brachialis
biceps brachii
serratus anterior

rectus abdominis
obliquus externus

transversus abdominis

iliopsoas*

sartorius

vastus intermedius
rectus femoris
vastus lateralis

Annotation Key
Bold text indicates target muscles
Black text indicates other working muscles
* indicates deep muscles

Child's Pose

Child's Pose will effectively stretch your entire back. You can come into this pose at the end of a workout—or at any point in your core-training regimen where you need to rest and reinvigorate your body and mind.

Correct form
· Keep your torso straight.

Avoid
· Hyperextending your lower back.
· Twisting your torso.

Level
· Beginner

Duration
· 1 minute

Benefits
· Stretches back

Caution
· Knee injury

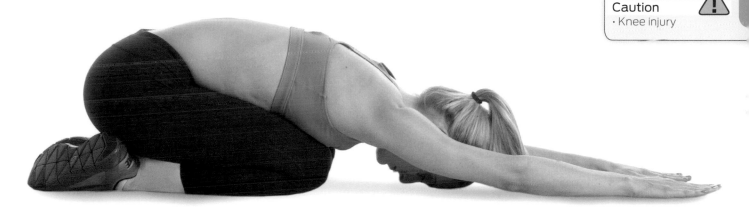

1 Begin facedown with your legs bent, your thighs near your chest and your arms outstretched in front of you.

2 Lean your weight back onto your hips, and elongate your arms as far you can reach. Hold for 30 seconds.

3 Release, and then repeat for an additional 30 seconds.

Annotation Key
Bold text indicates target muscles
Black text indicates other working muscles
* indicates deep muscles

Back View
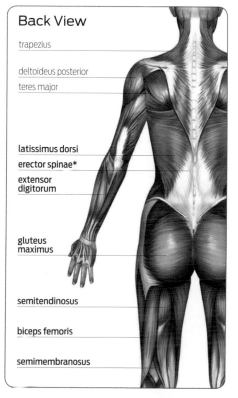

trapezius
deltoideus posterior
teres major
latissimus dorsi
erector spinae*
extensor digitorum
gluteus maximus
semitendinosus
biceps femoris
semimembranosus

Front View
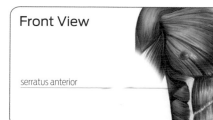

serratus anterior

Front View
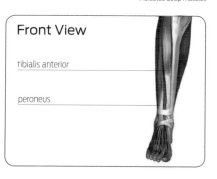

tibialis anterior
peroneus

Fitness Ball Abdominal Stretch

Fitness Ball Abdominal Stretch makes use of the ball to optimize its impact on your abs. In particular, this stretch benefits your rectus abdominis.

1 Begin on your back on top of a fitness ball, with your feet planted shoulder-width apart and your arms bent, hands beside your head.

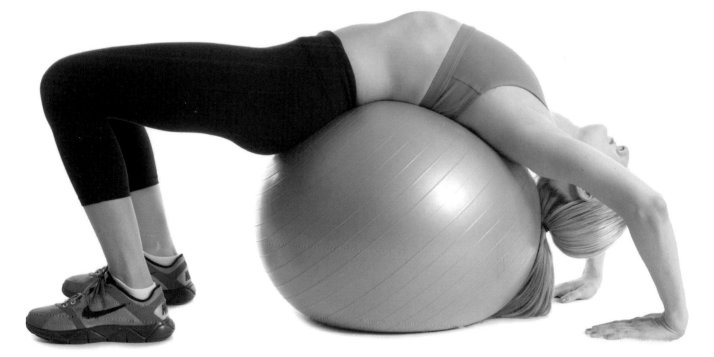

Correct form
· Ensure that your entire back remains supported by the ball.
· Anchor your feet to the floor.
· Maintain your body position as you reach backward.

Avoid
· Raising your pelvis excessively high.
· Allowing the ball to wobble.

2 Reach your arms backward until your palms are on the floor.

3 Lower your hips and stretch your pelvis toward the ceiling. Hold for 30 seconds.

4 Release, and then repeat for an additional 30 seconds.

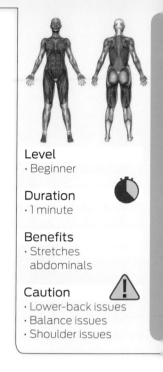

Back View

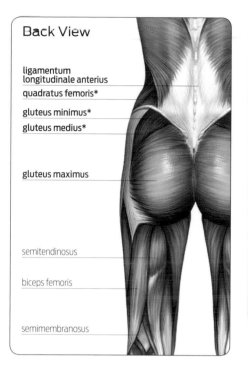

- ligamentum longitudinale anterius
- **quadratus femoris***
- **gluteus minimus***
- **gluteus medius***
- **gluteus maximus**
- semitendinosus
- biceps femoris
- semimembranosus

Front View

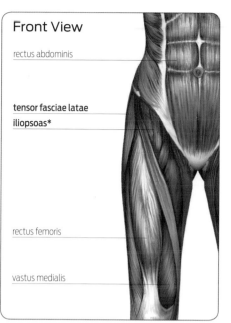

- rectus abdominis
- tensor fasciae latae
- **iliopsoas***
- rectus femoris
- vastus medialis

Level
- Beginner

Duration
- 1 minute

Benefits
- Stretches abdominals

Caution
- Lower-back issues
- Balance issues
- Shoulder issues

Annotation Key
Bold text indicates target muscles
Black text indicates other working muscles
* indicates deep muscles

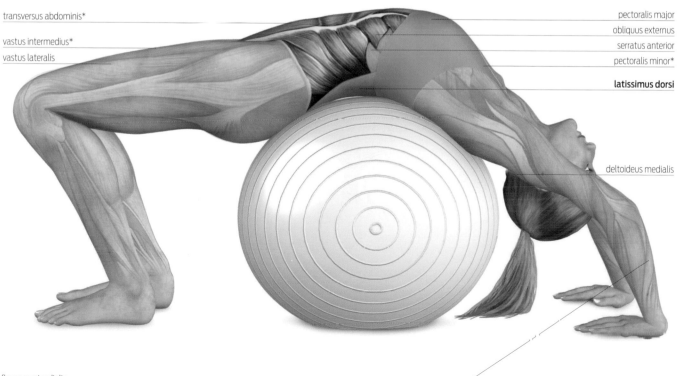

- transversus abdominis*
- vastus intermedius*
- vastus lateralis
- flexor carpi radialis
- pectoralis major
- obliquus externus
- serratus anterior
- pectoralis minor*
- **latissimus dorsi**
- deltoideus medialis

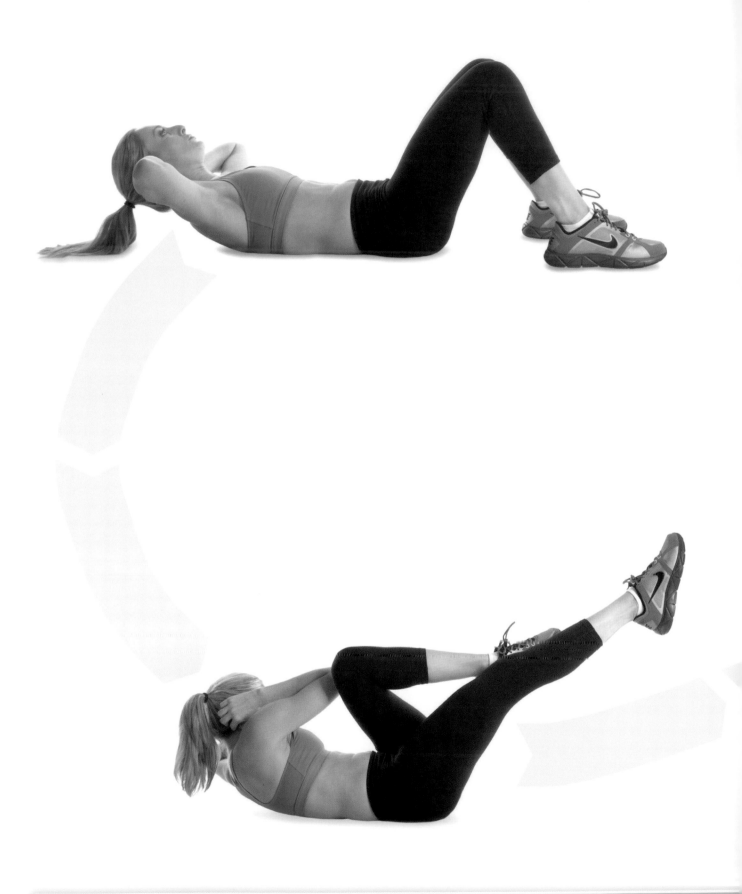

Workouts

Contents

You have now accumulated a wealth of information about core training. You've warmed up and cooled down, you've stabilized and strengthened—and, along the way, you've picked up an inkling of which exercises will work for you. The following workouts will help you to make core training a way of life. Addressing a range of different needs—from beginner to advanced, upper abs to lower abs, and much more—there is likely to be a workout or two that works for you. Once you get comfortable with these workouts, try making them even more challenging by adding more repetitions, additional exercises, or longer holds. With the knowledge you've gained you can tailor your workout to fit you to a T. When it comes to stabilizing and strengthening your powerhouse, the most effective results come from challenging yourself more and more, every single day.

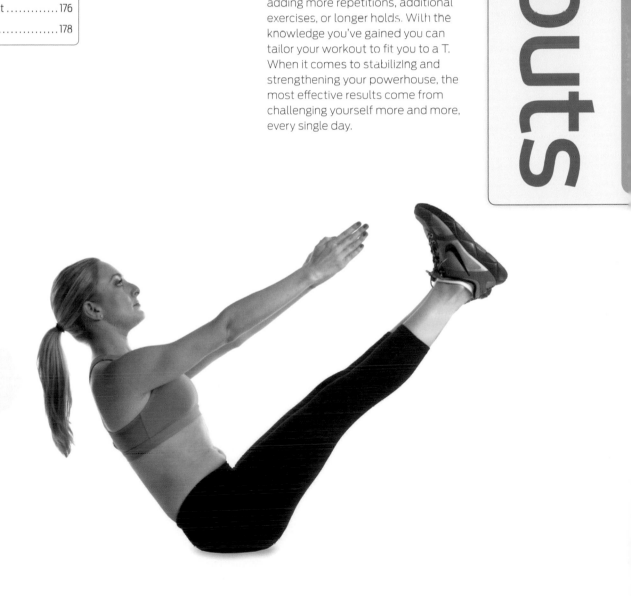

Beginner's Workout

The Beginner's Workout is a great introduction to core training, and with simple adjustments to the number of sets and repetitions it's suitable for exercisers of all levels.

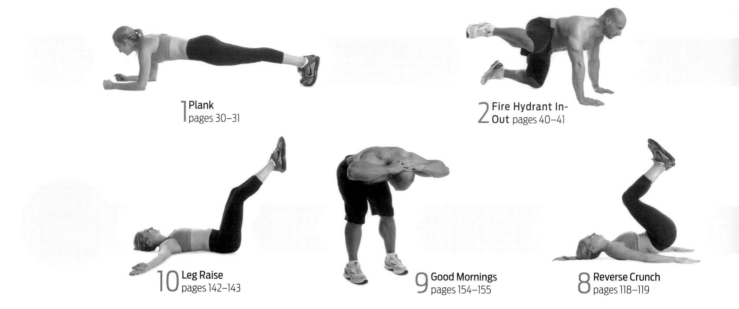

1 Plank
pages 30–31

2 Fire Hydrant In-Out pages 40–41

10 Leg Raise
pages 142–143

9 Good Mornings
pages 154–155

8 Reverse Crunch
pages 118–119

Over-Fifty Workout

Core training knows no age limits, and this workout is particularly suited to mature exercisers just embarking on a fitness regime—or anyone looking for a balanced sequence of low-impact moves.

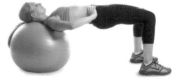

1 Fitness Ball
Hyperextension pages 54–55

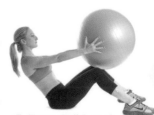

2 Fitness Ball Bridge
pages 90–91

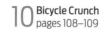

10 Bicycle Crunch
pages 108–109

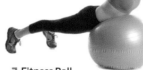

9 Fitness Ball Rollout
pages 52–53

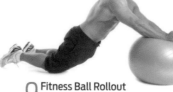

8 Fitness Ball Seated
Russian Twist pages 136–137

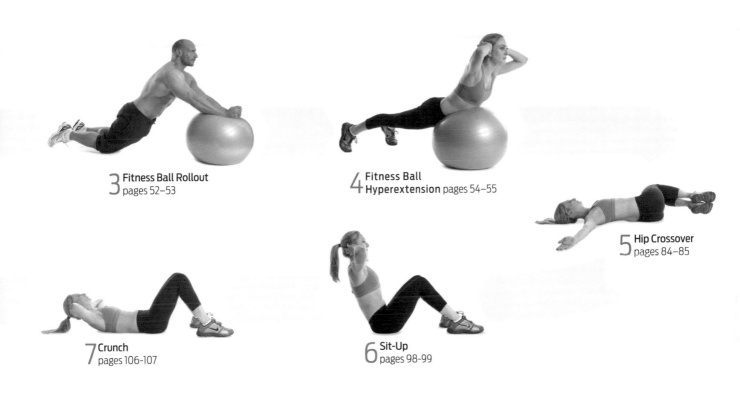

3 **Fitness Ball Rollout**
pages 52–53

4 **Fitness Ball Hyperextension** pages 54–55

5 **Hip Crossover**
pages 84–85

7 **Crunch**
pages 106-107

6 **Sit-Up**
pages 98-99

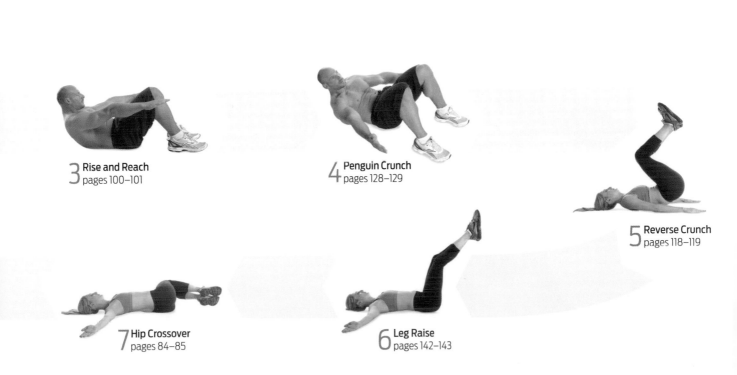

3 **Rise and Reach**
pages 100–101

4 **Penguin Crunch**
pages 128–129

5 **Reverse Crunch**
pages 118–119

7 **Hip Crossover**
pages 84–85

6 **Leg Raise**
pages 142–143

Upper-Abdominal Workout

This workout strengthens and defines the upper abs, helping you to achieve the "six-pack" look.

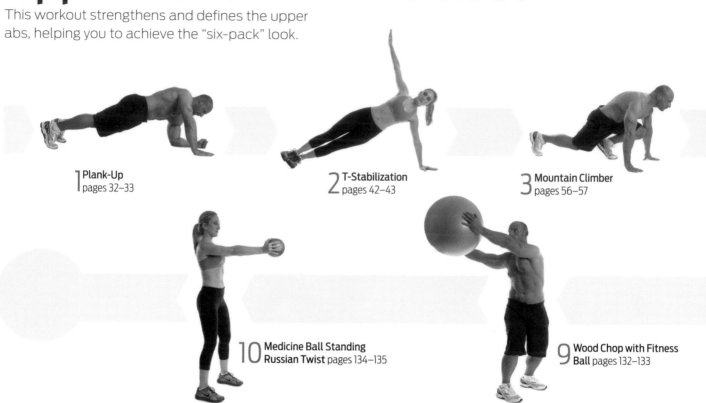

1 **Plank-Up** pages 32–33

2 **T-Stabilization** pages 42–43

3 **Mountain Climber** pages 56–57

10 **Medicine Ball Standing Russian Twist** pages 134–135

9 **Wood Chop with Fitness Ball** pages 132–133

Lower-Abdominal Workout

Targeting the hard-to-reach transversus abdominis, this workout will strengthen and tone your lower abdominal muscles.

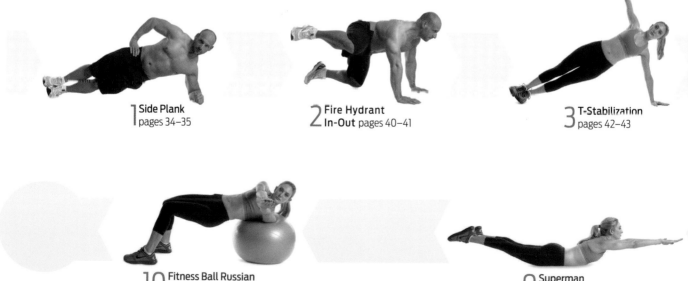

1 **Side Plank** pages 34–35

2 **Fire Hydrant In-Out** pages 40–41

3 **T-Stabilization** pages 42–43

10 **Fitness Ball Russian Twist** pages 138–139

9 **Superman** pages 156–157

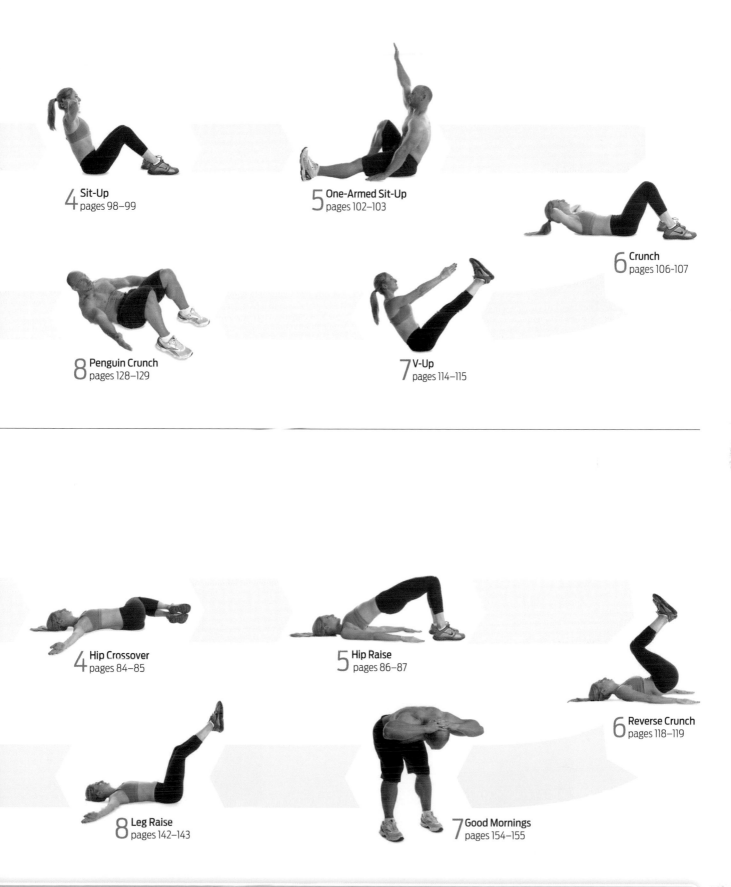

4 **Sit-Up**
pages 98–99

5 **One-Armed Sit-Up**
pages 102–103

6 **Crunch**
pages 106-107

8 **Penguin Crunch**
pages 128–129

7 **V-Up**
pages 114–115

4 **Hip Crossover**
pages 84–85

5 **Hip Raise**
pages 86–87

6 **Reverse Crunch**
pages 118–119

8 **Leg Raise**
pages 142–143

7 **Good Mornings**
pages 154–155

Global Workout

Featuring a balanced mix of core stabilizing and strengthening exercises, this workout offers the best of both worlds.

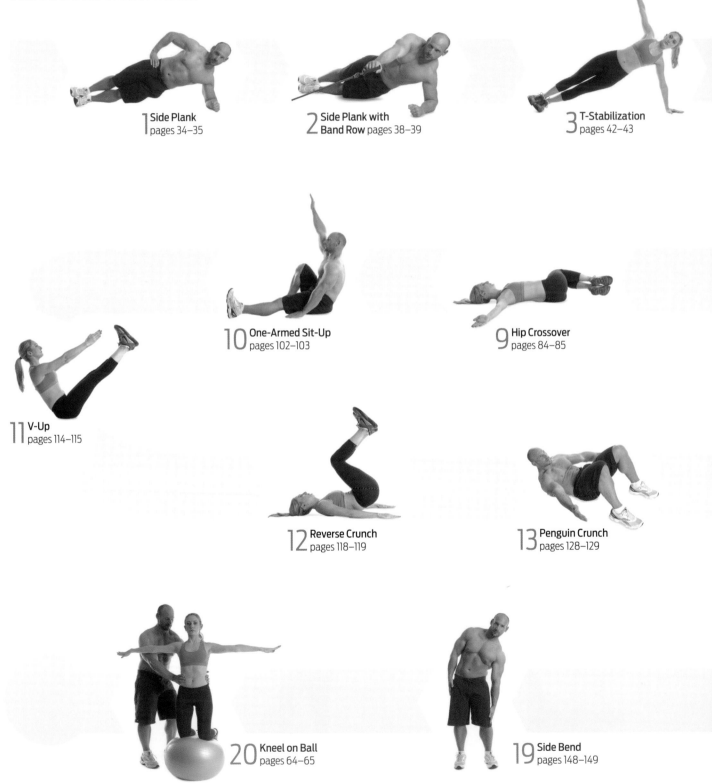

1 Side Plank
pages 34–35

2 Side Plank with Band Row pages 38–39

3 T-Stabilization
pages 42–43

10 One-Armed Sit-Up
pages 102–103

9 Hip Crossover
pages 84–85

11 V-Up
pages 114–115

12 Reverse Crunch
pages 118–119

13 Penguin Crunch
pages 128–129

20 Kneel on Ball
pages 64–65

19 Side Bend
pages 148–149

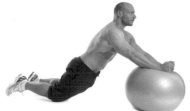

4 Fitness Ball Rollout
pages 52–53

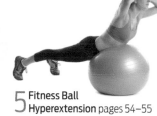

5 Fitness Ball
Hyperextension pages 54–55

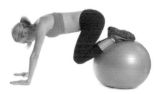

6 Fitness Ball
Band Fly pages 76–77

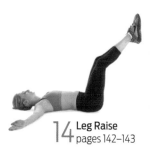

8 Standing One-Legged
Row pages 94–95

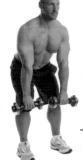

7 Stiff-Legged Deadlift
pages 92–93

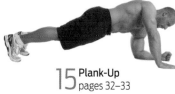

14 Leg Raise
pages 142–143

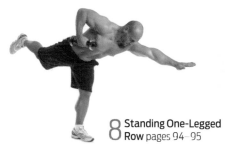

15 Plank-Up
pages 32–33

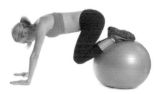

16 Fitness Ball Jackknife
pages 48–49

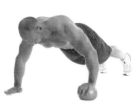

18 Medicine Ball Walkover
pages 74–75

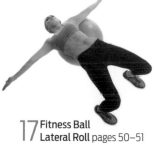

17 Fitness Ball
Lateral Roll pages 50–51

Sports Workout

This challenging workout gears up your core for the rotational performance that many sports demand.

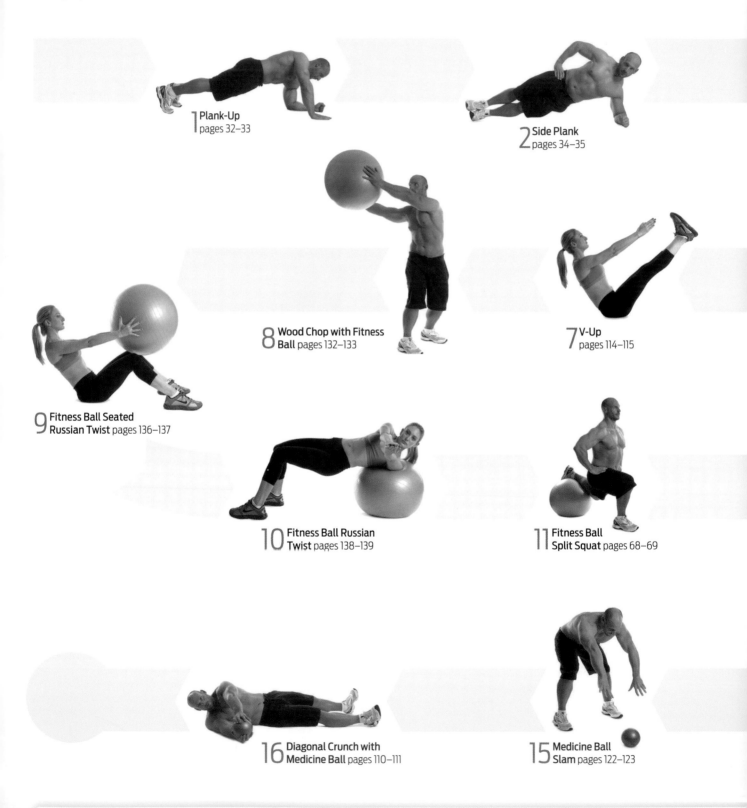

1 Plank-Up
pages 32–33

2 Side Plank
pages 34–35

8 Wood Chop with Fitness Ball pages 132–133

7 V-Up
pages 114–115

9 Fitness Ball Seated Russian Twist pages 136–137

10 Fitness Ball Russian Twist pages 138–139

11 Fitness Ball Split Squat pages 68–69

16 Diagonal Crunch with Medicine Ball pages 110–111

15 Medicine Ball Slam pages 122–123

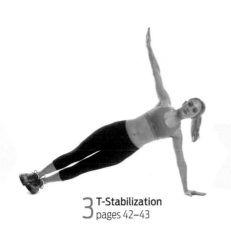

3 **T-Stabilization** pages 42–43

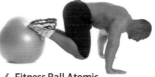

4 **Fitness Ball Atomic Push-Up** pages 44–45

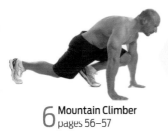

6 **Mountain Climber** pages 56–57

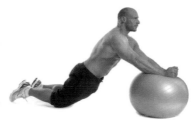

5 **Fitness Ball Rollout** pages 52–53

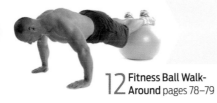

12 **Fitness Ball Walk-Around** pages 78–79

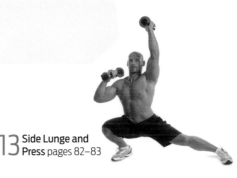

13 **Side Lunge and Press** pages 82–83

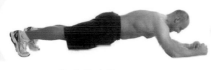

14 **Body Saw** pages 146–147

Warrior Workout

A demanding workout that challenges the insatiable diehard to maximize core stability, strength, athleticism, and abdominal visibility.

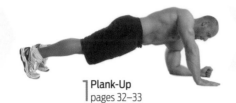

1 Plank-Up
pages 32–33

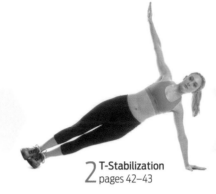

2 T-Stabilization
pages 42–43

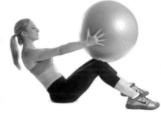

9 Fitness Ball Seated
Russian Twist pages 136–137

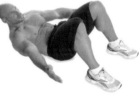

8 Penguin Crunch
pages 128–129

10 Leg Raises
pages 142–143

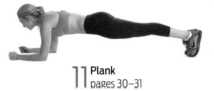

11 Plank
pages 30–31

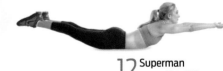

12 Superman
pages 156–157

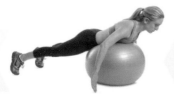

19 Fitness Ball Prone Row to
External Rotation pages 70–71

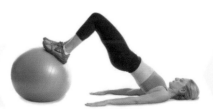

18 Fitness Ball Hip Raise
pages 88–89

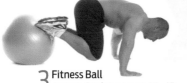

3 **Fitness Ball**
Atomic Pushup pages 44–45

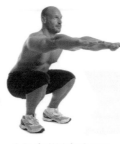

4 **Body-Weight Squat**
pages 58–59

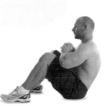

5 **Medicine Ball Sit-Up**
pages 104–105

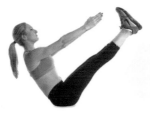

7 **V-Up**
pages 114–115

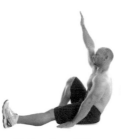

6 **One-Armed Sit-Up** pages 102–103

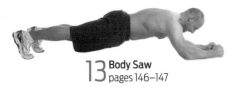

13 **Body Saw**
pages 146–147

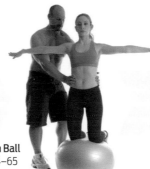

14 **Kneel on Ball**
pages 64–65

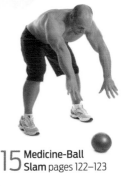

15 **Medicine-Ball Slam** pages 122–123

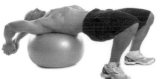

17 **Medicine Ball Pullover**
on Fitness Ball pages 80–81

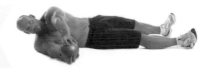

16 **Diagonal Crunch with**
Medicine Ball pages 110–111

Beach-Bod Bikini Workout

The perfect blend of core exercises—read ripped and defined abs for the beach season, while preparing women to show off a slim waist and trim tummy.

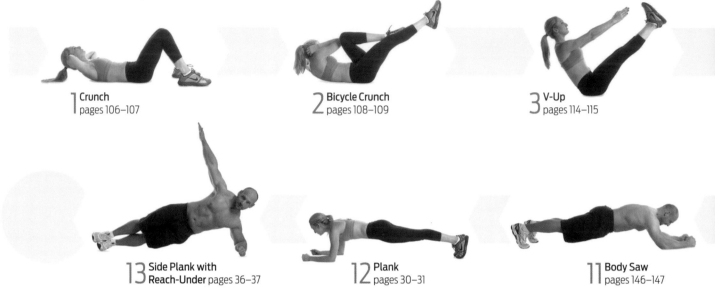

1 **Crunch**
pages 106–107

2 **Bicycle Crunch**
pages 108–109

3 **V-Up**
pages 114–115

13 **Side Plank with Reach-Under** pages 36–37

12 **Plank**
pages 30–31

11 **Body Saw**
pages 146–147

Balance and Postural Workout

Perform this workout regularly to strengthen both the major and minor muscles that assist your posture and balance.

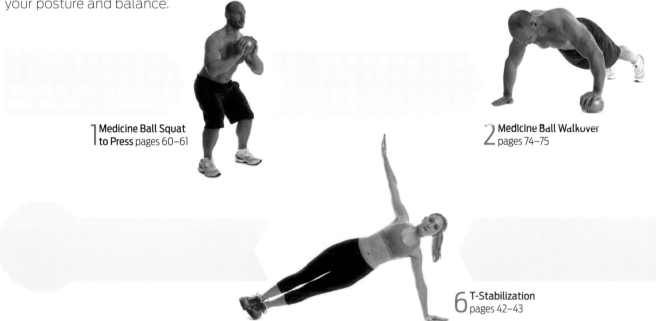

1 **Medicine Ball Squat to Press** pages 60–61

2 **Medicine Ball Walkover** pages 74–75

6 **T-Stabilization**
pages 42–43

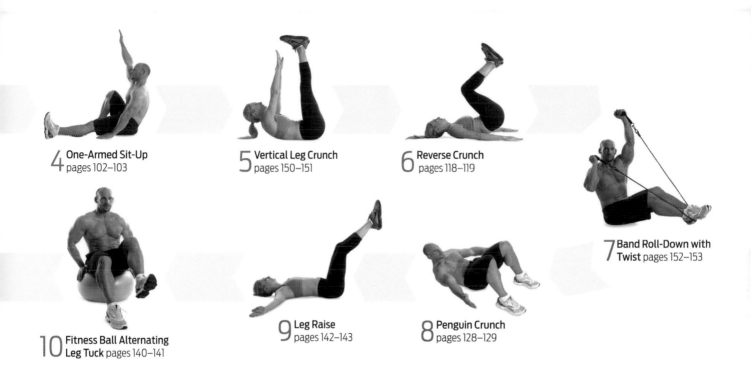

4 **One-Armed Sit-Up**
pages 102–103

5 **Vertical Leg Crunch**
pages 150–151

6 **Reverse Crunch**
pages 118–119

7 **Band Roll-Down with Twist** pages 152–153

10 **Fitness Ball Alternating Leg Tuck** pages 140–141

9 **Leg Raise**
pages 142–143

8 **Penguin Crunch**
pages 128–129

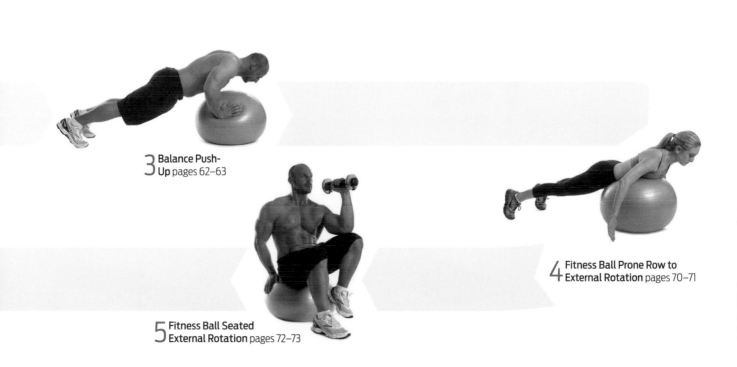

3 **Balance Push-Up** pages 62–63

5 **Fitness Ball Seated External Rotation** pages 72–73

4 **Fitness Ball Prone Row to External Rotation** pages 70–71

Power Workout

This strenuous workout will build core strength, allowing you to power through whatever physical challenge come your way.

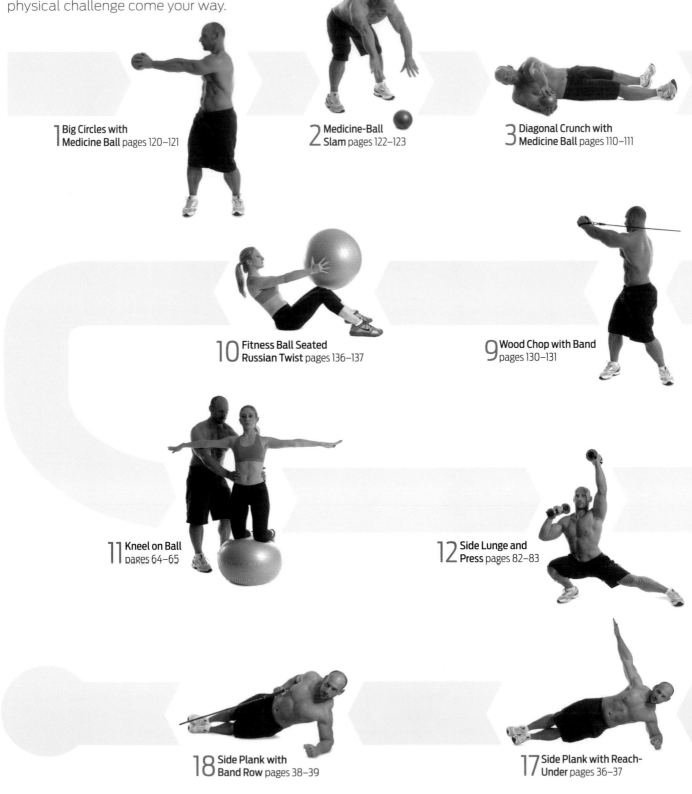

1 Big Circles with Medicine Ball pages 120–121

2 Medicine-Ball Slam pages 122–123

3 Diagonal Crunch with Medicine Ball pages 110–111

10 Fitness Ball Seated Russian Twist pages 136–137

9 Wood Chop with Band pages 130–131

11 Kneel on Ball pages 64–65

12 Side Lunge and Press pages 82–83

18 Side Plank with Band Row pages 38–39

17 Side Plank with Reach-Under pages 36–37

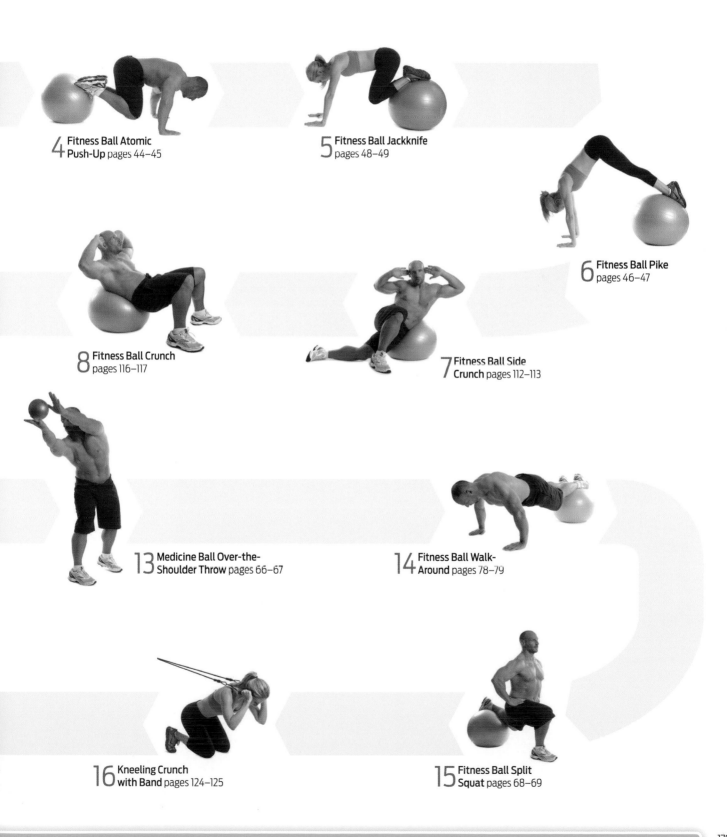

4 Fitness Ball Atomic Push-Up pages 44–45

5 Fitness Ball Jackknife pages 48–49

6 Fitness Ball Pike pages 46–47

8 Fitness Ball Crunch pages 116–117

7 Fitness Ball Side Crunch pages 112–113

13 Medicine Ball Over-the-Shoulder Throw pages 66–67

14 Fitness Ball Walk-Around pages 78–79

16 Kneeling Crunch with Band pages 124–125

15 Fitness Ball Split Squat pages 68–69

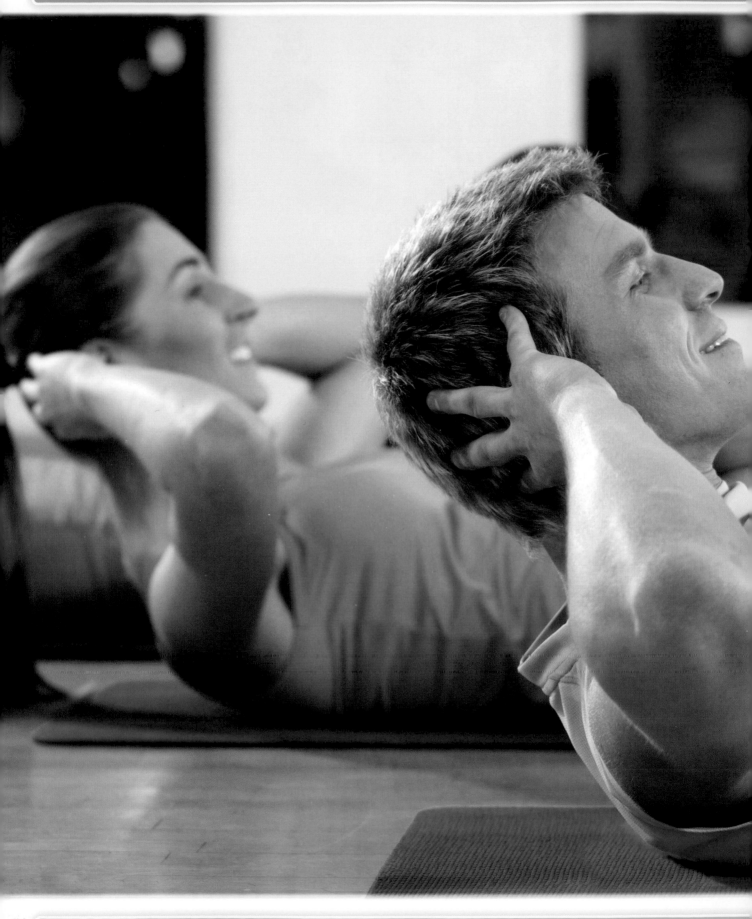

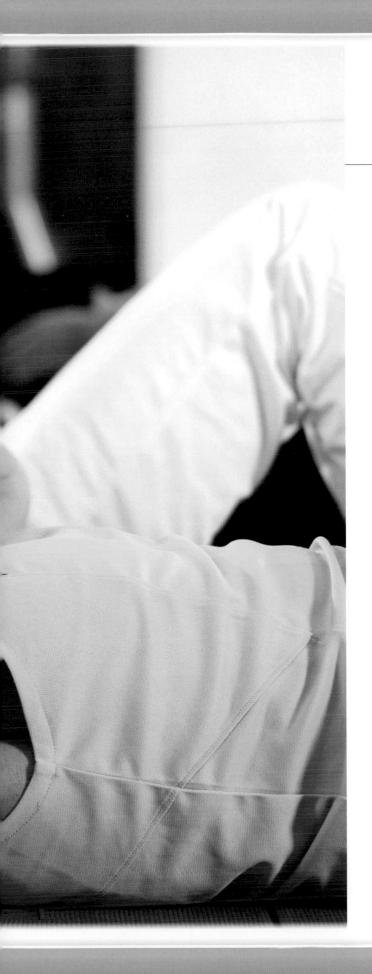

Conclusion

Congratulations! You've now learned how to perform a wide range of dynamic, challenging, and multifaceted exercises. Equipped with the tools in this book, you have all you need to both stabilize and strengthen those all-important core muscles, which you rely on every single day.

So what comes next?

It's now time to make core training a regular part of your life. You can join a health club, but if you have a corner of the living room, some workout clothes, and perhaps a mat, then your home gym is complete. And through exploring this book, you have learned all about what your core muscles do and how to work them most effectively. The rest is up to you.

Don't be limited by the workouts shown here. After grasping the basics of core training, and exploring an array of exercises, try creating your own fitness routines based on your needs. However you choose to incorporate core training into your daily life, don't forget: in setting aside time to work your core, you're moving further down the path to a fitter, leaner, better-functioning, stronger physique.

Glossary

GENERAL TERMINOLOGY

abduction: Movement away from the body.

adduction: Movement toward the body.

anterior: Located in the front.

cardiovascular exercise: Any exercise that increases the heart rate, making oxygen and nutrient-rich blood available to working muscles.

cervical spine: The upper area of the spine immediately below the skull.

cooldown: An exercise performed at the end of the workout session that works to cool and relax the body after more vigorous exertion.

core stabilizer: An exercise that calls for resisting motion at the lumbar spine though activation of the abdominal muscles and deep stabilizers; improves core strength and endurance.

core strengthener: An exercise that allows for motion in the lumbar spine, while working the abdominal muscles and deep stabilizers; improves movement such as running or walking.

core: Refers to the deep muscle layers that lie close to the spine and provide structural support for the entire body. The core is divisible into two groups: major core and minor core muscles. Major muscles reside on the trunk and include the belly area and the mid and lower back. This area encompasses the pelvic floor muscles (levator ani, pubococcygeus, iliococcygeus, pubo-rectalis, and coccygeus), the abdominals (rectus abdominis, transversus abdominis, obliquus externus, and obliquus internus), the spinal extensors (multifidus spinae, erector spinae, splenius, longissimus thoracis, and semispinalis), and the diaphragm. The minor core includes the latissimus dorsi, gluteus maximus, and trapezius (upper, middle, and lower). Minor core muscles assist the major muscles when the body engages in activities or movements that require added stability.

crunch: A common abdominal exercise that calls for curling the shoulders toward the pelvis while lying supine with hands behind head and knees bent.

deadlift: An exercise movement that calls for lifting a weight, such as a barbell, off the ground from a stabilized bent-over position.

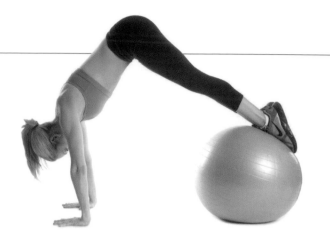

dumbbell: A basic piece of resistance equipment that consists of a short bar on which plates are secured. A person can use a dumbbell in one hand or both hands during an exercise.

exercise mat: A firm mat, usually made of foam rubber, that is at least one-half inch (1.27 cm) thick. The roll-up variety typically measures about 72 to 86 inches (180–220 cm), with widths varying from 20 or so inches to close to 40 inches (50–100 cm).

extension: The act of straightening.

extensor muscle: A muscle serving to extend a body part away from the center of the body.

external rotation: The act of moving a body part away from the center of the body.

fitness ball: A large, inflatable ball sometimes used for support during a core-training workout. It brings the core muscles into play, using them for balance and stability. Also called a Swiss ball.

flexion: The bending of a joint.

flexor muscle: A muscle that decreases the angle between two bones, as bending the arm at the elbow or raising the thigh toward the stomach.

fly: An exercise movement in which the hand and arm move through an arc while the elbow is kept at a constant angle. Fly exercises work the muscles of the upper body.

hand weights: Small weights that can be incorporated into Pilates exercises to enhance strengthening and toning benefits.

hyperextension: An exercise that works the lower back as well as the mid and upper back, specifically the erector spinae, which usually involves raising the torso and/or lower body from the floor while keeping the pelvis firmly anchored.

iliotibial band (ITB): A thick band of fibrous tissue that runs down the outside of the leg, beginning at the hip and extending to the outer side of the tibia just below the knee joint. The band functions in concert with several of the thigh muscles to provide stability to the outside of the knee joint.

internal rotation: The act of moving a body part toward the center of the body.

isometric exercise: A form of exercise involving the static contraction of a muscle without any visible movement in the angle of the joint.

lateral: Located on, or extending toward, the outside.

lumbar spine: The lower part of the spine.

medial: Located on, or extending toward, the middle.

medicine ball: A small weighted ball used in weight training and toning.

neutral position: A position in which the natural curve of the spine is maintained, typically adopted when lying on one's back with one or both feet on the mat.

neutral: Describes the position of the legs, pelvis, hips, or other part of the body that is neither arched nor curved forward.

plate: A cast-iron weight placed on a dumbbell. The weight of plates generally start at a 1¼ pounds (.56 kg) and range upward to 50 pounds (22 kg) and higher.

posterior: Located behind.

press: An exercise movement that calls for moving a weight or other resistance away from the body.

range of motion: The distance and direction a joint can move between the flexed position and the extended position.

resistance band: Any rubber tubing or flat band device that provides a resistive force used for strength training. Also called a "fitness band," "stretching band," and "stretch tube."

rotator muscle: One of a group of muscles that assists the rotation of a joint, such as the hip or the shoulder.

scapula: The protrusion of bone on the mid to upper back, also known as the "shoulder blade."

split squat: An assisted one-legged squat where the nonlifting leg is rested on the floor a few steps behind the lifting leg, as if it were a static lunge.

squat: An exercise movement that calls for moving the hips back and bending the knees and hips to lower the torso and an accompanying weight, and then returning to the upright position. A squat primarily targets the muscles of the thighs, hips, buttocks, and hamstrings.

synergistic exercise: Combinations of exercises or diet and exercise strategically used to produce optimal results in the least amount of time.

thoracic spine: The middle part of the spine.

warm-up: Any form of light exercise of short duration that prepares the body for more intense exercise.

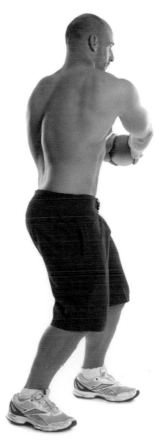

LATIN TERMINOLOGY

The following glossary list explains the Latin terminology used to describe the body's musculature. In some instances, certain words are derived from Greek, which is therein indicated.

Chest

coracobrachialis: Greek *korakoeidés*, "ravenlike," and *brachium*, "arm"

pectoralis (major and minor): *pectus*, "breast"

Abdomen

obliquus externus: *obliquus*, "slanting," and *externus*, "outward"

obliquus internus: *obliquus*, "slanting," and *internus*, "within"

rectus abdominis: *rego*, "straight, upright," and *abdomen*, "belly"

serratus anterior: *serra*, "saw," and *ante*, "before"

transversus abdominis: *transversus*, "athwart," and *abdomen*, "belly"

Neck

scalenus: Greek *skalénós*, "unequal"

semispinalis: *semi*, "half," and *spinae*, "spine"

splenius: Greek *spléníon*, "plaster, patch"

sternocleidomastoideus: Greek *stérnon*, "chest," Greek *kleís*, "key," and Greek *mastoeidés*, "breastlike"

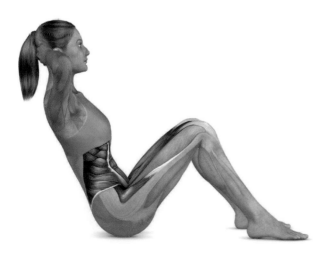

Back

erector spinae: *erectus*, "straight," and *spina*, "thorn"

latissimus dorsi: *latus*, "wide," and *dorsum*, "back"

multifidus spinae: *multifid*, "to cut into divisions," and *spinae*, "spine"

quadratus lumborum: *quadratus*, "square, rectangular," and *lumbus*, "loin"

rhomboideus: Greek *rhembesthai*, "to spin"

trapezius: Greek *trapezion*, "small table"

Shoulders

deltoideus (anterior, medial, and posterior): Greek *deltoeidés*, "delta-shaped"

infraspinatus: *infra*, "under," and *spina*, "thorn"

levator scapulae: *levare*, "to raise," and *scapulae*, "shoulder [blades]"

subscapularis: *sub*, "below," and *scapulae*, "shoulder [blades]"

supraspinatus: *supra*, "above," and *spina*, "thorn"

teres (major and minor): *teres*, "rounded"

Upper arm

biceps brachii: *biceps*, "two-headed," and *brachium*, "arm"

brachialis: *brachium*, "arm"

triceps brachii: *triceps*, "three-headed," and *brachium*, "arm"

Lower arm

anconeus: Greek *anconad*, "elbow"

brachioradialis: *brachium*, "arm," and *radius*, "spoke"

extensor carpi radialis: *extendere*, "to extend," Greek *karpós*, "wrist," and *radius*, "spoke"

extensor digitorum: *extendere*, "to extend," and *digitus*, "finger, toe"

flexor carpi pollicis longus: *flectere*, "to bend," Greek *karpós*, "wrist," *pollicis*, "thumb," and *longus*, "long"

flexor carpi radialis: *flectere*, "to bend," Greek *karpós*, "wrist," and *radius*, "spoke"

flexor carpi ulnaris: *flectere*, "to bend," Greek *karpós*, "wrist," and *ulnaris*, "forearm"

flexor digitorum: *flectere*, "to bend," and *digitus*, "finger, toe"

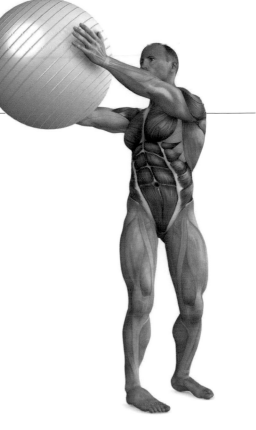

palmaris longus: *palmaris*, "palm," and *longus*, "long"

pronator teres: *pronate*, "to rotate," and *teres*, "rounded"

Hips

gemellus (inferior and superior): *geminus*, "twin"

gluteus maximus: Greek *gloutós*, "rump," and *maximus*, "largest"

gluteus medius: Greek *gloutós*, "rump," and *medialis*, "middle"

gluteus minimus: Greek *gloutós*, "rump," and *minimus*, "smallest"

iliopsoas: *ilium*, "groin," and Greek *psoa*, "groin muscle"

iliacus: *ilium*, "groin"

obturator externus: *obturare*, "to block," and *externus*, "outward"

obturator internus: *obturare*, "to block," and *internus*, "within"

pectineus: *pectin*, "comb"

piriformis: *pirum*, "pear," and *forma*, "shape"

quadratus femoris: *quadratus*, "square, rectangular," and *femur*, "thigh"

Upper leg

adductor longus: *adducere*, "to contract," and *longus*, "long"

adductor magnus: *adducere*, "to contract," and *magnus*, "major"

biceps femoris: *biceps*, "two-headed," and *femur*, "thigh"

gracilis: *gracilis*, "slim, slender"

rectus femoris: *rego*, "straight, upright," and *femur*, "thigh"

sartorius: *sarcio*, "to patch" or "to repair"

semimembranosus: *semi*, "half," and *membrum*, "limb"

semitendinosus: *semi*, "half," and *tendo*, "tendon"

tensor fasciae latae: *tenere*, "to stretch," *fasciae*, "band," and *latae*, "laid down"

vastus intermedius: *vastus*, "immense, huge," and *intermedius*, "between"

vastus lateralis: *vastus*, "immense, huge," and *lateralis*, "side"

vastus medialis: *vastus*, "immense, huge," and *medialis*, "middle"

Lower leg

adductor digiti minimi: *adducere*, "to contract," *digitus*, "finger, toe," and *minimum*, "smallest"

adductor hallucis: *adducere*, "to contract," and *hallex*, "big toe"

extensor digitorum: *extendere*, "to extend," and *digitus*, "finger, toe"

extensor hallucis: *extendere*, "to extend," and *hallex*, "big toe"

flexor digitorum: *flectere*, "to bend," and *digitus*, "finger, toe"

flexor hallucis: *flectere*, "to bend," and *hallex*, "big toe"

gastrocnemius: Greek *gastroknémía*, "calf [of the leg]"

peroneus: *peronei*, "of the fibula"

plantaris: *planta*, "the sole"

soleus: *solea*, "sandal"

tibialis anterior: *tibia*, "reed pipe," and *ante*, "before"

tibialis posterior: *tibia*, "reed pipe," and *posterus*, "coming after"

Icon Index

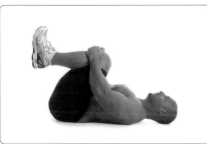

Supine Lower-Back Stretch
page 24

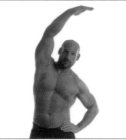

Side Stretch
page 25

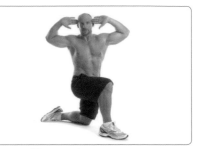

Half-Kneeling Rotation
page 26

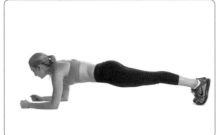

Plank
page 30

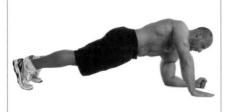

Plank-Up
page 32

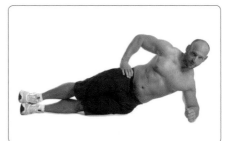

Side Plank
page 34

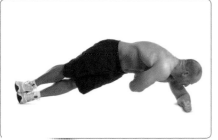

Side Plank with Reach-Under
page 36

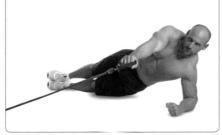

Side Plank with Band Row
page 38

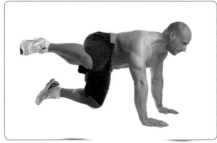

Fire-Hydrant In-Out
page 40

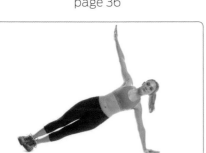

T-Stabilization
page 42

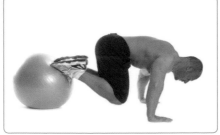

Fitness Ball Atomic Push-Up
page 44

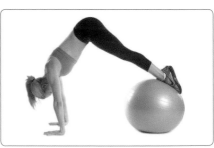
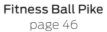

Fitness Ball Pike
page 46

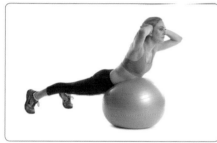

Fitness Ball Jackknife
page 48

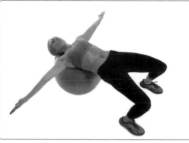

Fitness Ball Lateral Roll
page 50

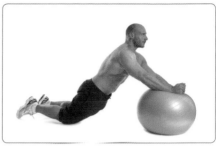

Fitness Ball Rollout
page 52

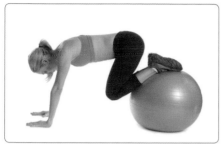

Fitness Ball Hyperextension
page 54

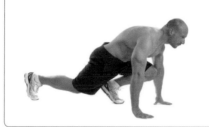

Mountain Climber
page 56

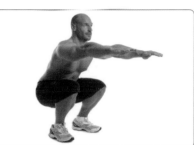

Body-Weight Squat
page 58

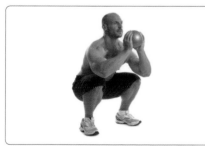

Medicine Ball Squat to Press
page 60

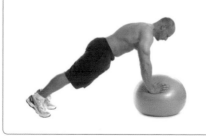

Balance Push-Up
page 62

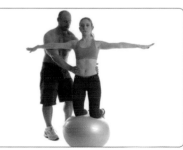

Kneel on Ball
page 64

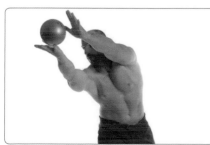

Med. Ball Over-the-Shoulder Throw
page 66

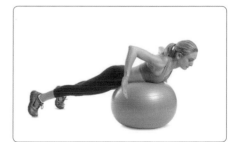

Fitness Ball Split Squat
page 68

Fitness Ball Prone Row Ext. Rotation
page 70

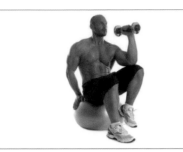

Fitness Ball Seated Ext. Rotation
page 72

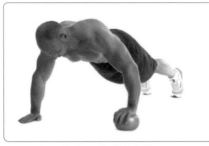

Medicine Ball Walkover
page 74

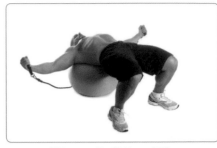

Fitness Ball Band Fly
page 76

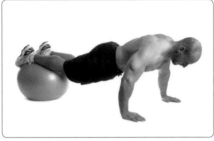

Fitness Ball Walk-Around
page 78

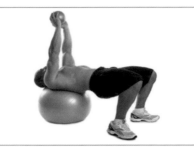

Med. Ball Pullover on Fitness Ball
page 80

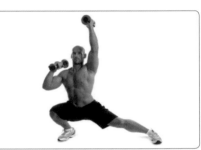

Side Lunge and Press
page 82

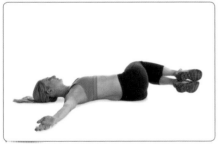

Hip Crossover
page 84

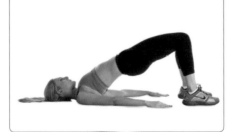

Hip Raise
page 86

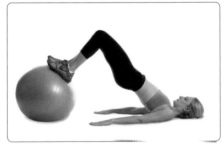

Fitness Ball Hip Raise
page 88

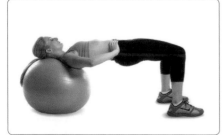

Fitness Ball Bridge
page 90

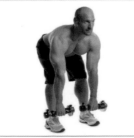

Stiff-Legged Deadlift
page 92

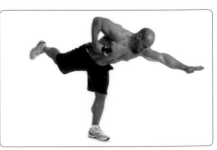

Standing One-Legged Row
page 94

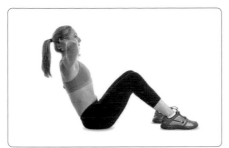

Sit-Up
page 98

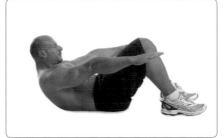

Rise and Reach
page 100

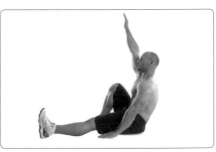

One-Armed Sit-Up
page 102

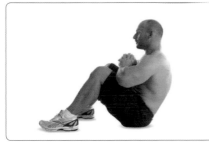

Medicine Ball Sit-Up
page 104

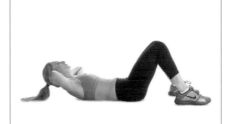

Crunch
page 106

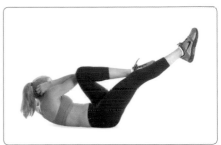

Bicycle Crunch
page 108

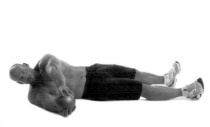

Diagonal Crunch with Med. Ball
page 110

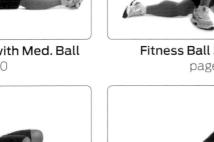

Fitness Ball Side Crunch
page 112

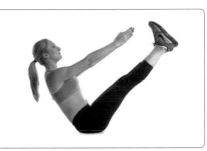

V-Up
page 114

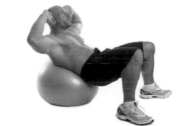

Fitness Ball Crunch
page 116

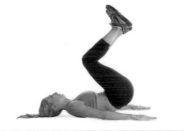

Reverse Crunch
page 118

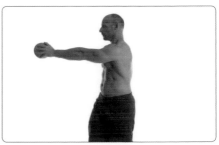

Big Circles with Medicine Ball
page 120

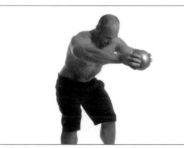

Medicine Ball Slam
page 122

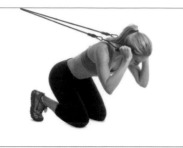

Kneeling Crunch with Band
page 124

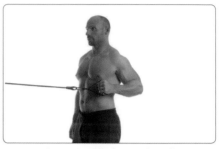

One-Armed Band Pull
page 126

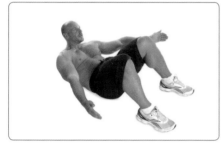

Penguin Crunch
page 128

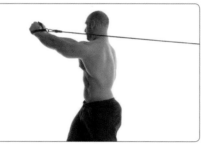

Wood Chop with Band
page 130

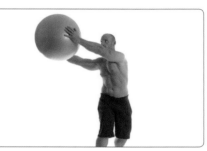

Wood Chop with Fitness Ball
page 132

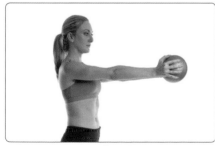

Med. Ball Standing Russian Twist
page 134

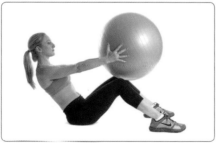

Fitness Ball Seated Russian Twist
page 136

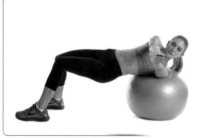

Fitness Ball Russian Twist
page 138

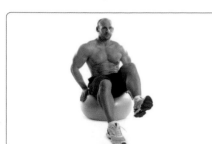

Fitness Ball Alternating Leg Tuck
page 140

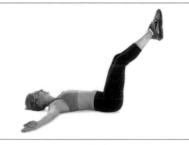

Leg Raise
page 142

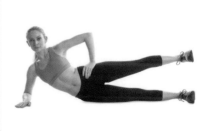
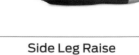

Side Leg Raise
page 144

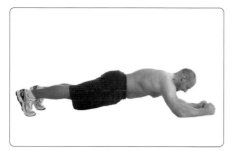

Body Saw
page 146

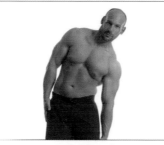

Side Bend
page 148

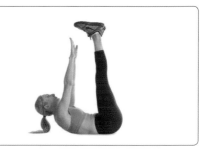

Vertical Leg Crunch
page 150

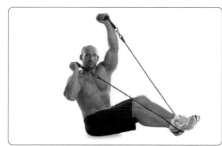

Band Roll-Down with Twist
page 152

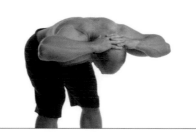

Good Mornings
page 154

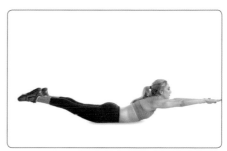

Superman
page 156

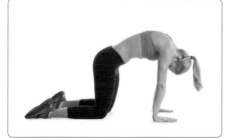

Back Arch Stretch
page 160

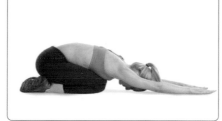

Child's Pose
page 161

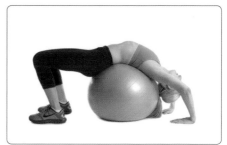

Fitness Ball Abdominal Stretch
page 162

About the author

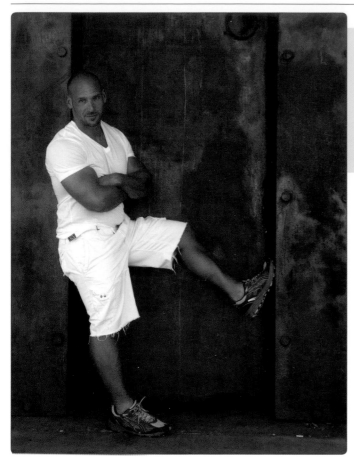

Hollis Lance Liebman has been a fitness magazine editor and national bodybuilding champion. He is a published physique photographer and has served as a bodybuilding and fitness competition judge. Currently a Los Angeles resident, Hollis has worked with some of Hollywood's elite, earning rave reviews. Visit his Web site, www.holliswashere.com, for fitness tips and complete training programs.

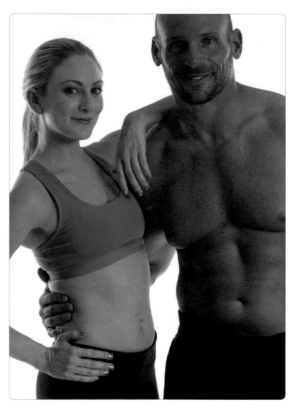

Credits

All photographs by Jonathan Conklin Photography, Inc. (jonathanconklin.net), except for the following:

Page 8 Paul Cotney/Shutterstock.com; page 11 AVAVA/Shutterstock.com; page 13 Lana K/Shutterstock.com; page 14 top Africa Studio/Shutterstock.com; page 14 bottom StockLite/Shutterstock.com; page 16 Beth Van Trees/Shutterstock.com; page 17 bottom left Valeriy Lebedev/Shutterstock.com; page 17 top left Olga Miltsova/Shutterstock.com; page 17 middle Viktor1/Shutterstock.com; page 17 bottom PHB.cz (Richard Semik)/Shutterstock.com; page 18 top left Africa Studio/Shutterstock.com; page 18 bottom left Nattika/Shutterstock.com; page 18 bottom middle joingate/Shutterstock.com; page 18 bottom right Aleksandr Stennikov/Shutterstock.com; page 19 top Liliia Rudchenko/Shutterstock.com; page 19 middle Juice Team/Shutterstock.com; page 19 bottom Valentyn Volkov/Shutterstock.com; pages 180–181 Kzenon/Shutterstock.com; page 192 left Sonia Keshishian.

All anatomical illustrations by Hector Aiza/3D Labz Animation India (www.3dlabz.com), except small insets and full-body anatomy on pages 20–21 by Linda Bucklin/Shutterstock.com, and page 9 sam100/Shutterstock.com.

Core-training model Cori D. Cohen is a registered dietitian and healthy lifestyle coach based in New York City. She provides private nutrition counseling to a diverse clientele, in addition to working with residents at a nursing and rehabilitation center. Ms. Cohen has degrees from the University of Delaware, Fashion Institute of Technology, CUNY Queens College, and LIU C. W. Post. She is currently featured as a columnist for the *Queens Courier*, where she provides readers with valuable nutrition advice.